Practical Issues in Geriatrics

Series Editor
Stefania Maggi, Aging Branch
CNR-Neuroscience Institute
Padua, Italy

This practically oriented series presents state of the art knowledge on the principal diseases encountered in older persons and addresses all aspects of management, including current multidisciplinary diagnostic and therapeutic approaches. It is intended as an educational tool that will enhance the everyday clinical practice of both young geriatricians and residents and also assist other specialists who deal with aged patients. Each volume is designed to provide comprehensive information on the topic that it covers, and whenever appropriate the text is complemented by additional material of high educational and practical value, including informative video-clips, standardized diagnostic flow charts and descriptive clinical cases. Practical Issues in Geriatrics will be of value to the scientific and professional community worldwide, improving understanding of the many clinical and social issues in Geriatrics and assisting in the delivery of optimal clinical care.

Indexed in Scopus

Alberto Pilotto · Walter Maetzler

Editors

Gerontechnology. A Clinical Perspective

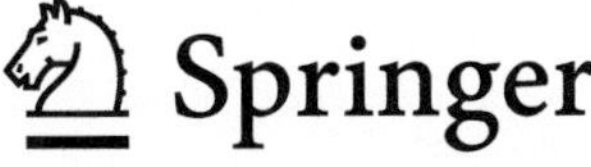 Springer

Editors
Alberto Pilotto
Department of Geriatric Care
Orthogeriatrics and Rehabilitation
Galliera Hospital
Genova, Italy

Department of Interdisciplinary Medicine
"Aldo Moro" University of Bari
Bari, Italy

Walter Maetzler
Neurology
Kiel University and University Hospital
Schleswig-Holstein
Kiel, Germany

ISSN 2509-6060   ISSN 2509-6079 (electronic)
Practical Issues in Geriatrics
ISBN 978-3-031-32248-8   ISBN 978-3-031-32246-4   (eBook)
https://doi.org/10.1007/978-3-031-32246-4

This Springer imprint is published by the registered company Springer Nature Switzerland AG
The registered company address is: Gewerbestrasse 11, 6330 Cham, Switzerland

Preface

In many parts of the world, average life expectancy is rising consistently, and at the same time technology is developing at a dramatic pace. This means completely new options for the diagnosis, treatment, and follow-up of diseases and disabilities of the older people and also new options to improve the quality of life by promoting an active and healthy aging lifestyle at population level.

The main objective of this book is to disseminate information and knowledge in the field of gerontechnology, a topic that on the one hand is considered a specific field of interest for technology experts (e.g., computer scientists, engineers, bioengineers, biostatisticians), but on the other hand often still has a relatively low diffusion of expertise among clinicians and other health professionals who are involved in the care of the older people.

Indeed, nowadays, telecare and telemedicine, domotics and robotics, artificial intelligence and decisional algorithms are all terms that have entered the common vocabulary, and for which interest has also grown in the public area, as well as in research and funding agencies. We note that outstanding results are emerging in science, which suggest that older people in particular will benefit from these technological developments. It is important to implement these successes into daily clinical practice as early as possible and to inform the population about potential new diagnostic and treatment options through these technological advances.

The book presents the technical developments that are currently beginning to influence the clinical and care management of diseases and disabilities of the older people, with the final aim to positively influence quality of life. These include *Information and Communication Technologies (ICT)*, such as electronic medical-health records and online healthcare services, *Assistive Technologies (AT)*, such as behavior and motility monitoring sensorial tools, smart homes, and telemedicine tools, and *Human–Computer Interaction Technologies (HCI)*, such as robots for supporting mobility or cognition, humanoid robots, exoskeletons, and rehabilitation robots.

The presentation of these topics has been divided into three thematic blocks: (1) Technologies in a world of aging people; (2) Specific clinical applications of the technologies in the older people; (3) Older people and technologies including the issues of education and training of older people, their caregivers and healthcare professionals on the technology challenges and possibilities as well as of the experts in technology such as engineers, informatics, and techno-designers on the basic concepts of the aging process and its effects on sensorial, behavioral, and lifestyle modifications that may occur in old age. The last two chapters venture a look into the future of geriatric medicine: they discuss the role of artificial intelligence in helping clinicians and patients to take clinical decisions, and the use of bio-technologies to understand the mechanisms of active and healthy aging, frailty, and resilience.

As the development of the topic has picked up speed again, especially in the last few years, we hope to provide the reader with a state-of-the-art overview of the most relevant recent developments across all major areas of the above pillars. We also hope that by presenting these technical developments in a condensed way, we can trigger new ideas and considerations that will further benefit the aging population in terms of their health status and quality of life.

Bari, Italy   Alberto Pilotto
Kiel, Germany   Walter Maetzler

Contents

Part III Older People and Technologies

List of Contributors

Armagan Albayrak Faculty of Industrial Design Engineering, Delft University of Technology, Delft, The Netherlands

Marina Barbagelata Department of Geriatric Care, Orthogeriatrics and Rehabilitation, Galliera Hospital, Genoa, Italy

Giacinto Barresi Rehab Technologies Lab, Istituto Italiano di Tecnologia, Genoa, Italy

Clemens Becker Unit Digitale Geriatrie, Universitätsklinikum Heidelberg, Heidelberg, Germany

Antonio Bianco Department of Public Health, Federico II University of Naples, Napoli, Italy

Kayla Bohlke Department of Bioengineering, Swanson School of Engineering, University of Pittsburgh, Pittsburgh, PA, USA

Alessio Del Bue Pattern Analysis and Computer Vision (PAVIS), Istituto Italiano di Tecnologia, Genoa, Italy

Matteo Bustreo Pattern Analysis and Computer Vision (PAVIS), Istituto Italiano di Tecnologia, Genoa, Italy

Tischa J. M. van der Cammen Faculty of Industrial Design Engineering, Delft University of Technology, Delft, The Netherlands

Honorary Research Fellow, Erasmus University Medical Center, Rotterdam, The Netherlands

Alberto Cella Department of Primary Care, Local Health Agency, Savona, Italy

Carlo Custodero Department of Interdisciplinary Medicine, "Aldo Moro" University of Bari, Bari, Italy

Department of Interdisciplinary Medicine, University of Bari "Aldo Moro", Italy

Kirsten Emmert Department of Neurology, University Medical Centre Schleswig-Holstein, Campus Kiel and Kiel University, Kiel, Germany

Luigi Ferrucci Longitudinal Studies Section, Translational Gerontology Branch, National Institute on Aging, Baltimore, MD, USA

Guido Iaccarino Department of Public Health, Federico II University of Naples, Napoli, Italy

Maddalena Illario Department of Public Health, Federico II University of Naples, Napoli, Italy

Jennifer Kudelka Neurology Department, University Hospital Schleswig-Holstein, Kiel, Germany

Vincenzo De Luca Department of Public Health, Federico II University of Naples, Napoli, Italy

Walter Maetzler Neurology Department, University Hospital Schleswig-Holstein, Kiel, Germany

Department of Neurology, Christian-Albrechts-University of Kiel, Kiel, Germany

Department of Neurology, University Medical Centre Schleswig-Holstein, Campus Kiel and Kiel University, Kiel, Germany

Arduino Alexander Mangoni Department of Clinical Pharmacology, Division of Critical and Cardiac Care, Flinders Medical Centre and Flinders University Adelaide, Adelaide, Australia

Francesco Mattace-Raso Department of Internal Medicine, Erasmus MC, University Medical Center Rotterdam, Rotterdam, The Netherlands

Lorenzo Mercurio Department of Public Health, Federico II University of Naples, Napoli, Italy

Lorenzo De Michieli Rehab Technologies Lab, Istituto Italiano di Tecnologia, Genoa, Italy

Alessandro Padovani Department of Clinical and Experimental Sciences, Neurology Unit, University of Brescia, Brescia, Italy

Alexey Petrushin Rehab Technologies Lab, Istituto Italiano di Tecnologia, Genoa, Italy

Alberto Pilotto Department of Geriatric Care, Orthogeriatrics and Rehabilitation, Galliera Hospital, Genoa, Italy

Department of Interdisciplinary Medicine, "Aldo Moro" University of Bari, Bari, Italy

Andrea Pilotto Department of Clinical and Experimental Sciences, Neurology Unit, University of Brescia, Brescia, Italy

Ervin Sejdcic The Edward S. Rogers Department of Electrical and Computer Engineering, Faculty of Applied Science and Engineering, University of Toronto, Toronto, ON, Canada

The North York General Hospital, Toronto, ON, Canada

Anisha Suri Department of Electrical and Computer Engineering, Swanson School of Engineering, University of Pittsburgh, Pittsburgh, PA, USA

Slawomir Tobis Department of Occupational Therapy, Poznan University of Medical Sciences, Poznan, Poland

Giovanni Tramontano Department of Public Health, Federico II University of Naples, Napoli, Italy

Erica Volta Department of Geriatric Care, Orthogeriatrics and Rehabilitation, Galliera Hospital, Genoa, Italy

Gubing Wang Department of Medical and Clinical Psychology, School of Social and Behavioural Sciences, Tilburg University, Tilburg, Netherlands

Richard Woodman Flinders Health and Medical Research Institute, Flinders University, Adelaide, Australia

Cinzia Zatti Department of Clinical and Experimental Sciences, Neurology Unit, University of Brescia, Brescia, Italy

Part I

Technology in a World of Aging People

Gerontechnology: Definitions and Classification

1

Alberto Pilotto, Erica Volta, Marina Barbagelata, and Carlo Custodero

1.1 Introduction

With the growing elderly population, worldwide estimated to more than double by 2050, the increased demand of healthcare for older people, also based on technology solutions, is rapidly spreading. This demographic transition brings a further challenge, namely that countries and societies all around the world must face the crescent prevalence of disabilities, chronic diseases, and frailty, i.e., all clinical conditions, driven by age-related bio-psycho-social changes, associated with a high risk for health adverse outcomes [1]. Since these conditions are multidimensional in nature, with clinical, physical, psycho-cognitive, and socio-economic factors

A. Pilotto (✉)
Department of Geriatric Care, Orthogeriatrics and Rehabilitation, Galliera Hospital, Genoa, Italy

Department of Interdisciplinary Medicine, "Aldo Moro" University of Bari, Bari, Italy
e-mail: alberto.pilotto@galliera.it

E. Volta · M. Barbagelata
Department of Geriatric Care, Orthogeriatrics and Rehabilitation, Galliera Hospital, Genoa, Italy

C. Custodero
Department of Interdisciplinary Medicine, "Aldo Moro" University of Bari, Bari, Italy

© The Author(s), under exclusive license to Springer Nature Switzerland AG 2023
A. Pilotto, W. Maetzler (eds.), *Gerontechnology. A Clinical Perspective*, Practical Issues in Geriatrics, https://doi.org/10.1007/978-3-031-32246-4_1

playing a part in their development and evolution [2], their assessment and management require a multidimensional approach based on the Comprehensive Geriatric Assessment (CGA) [3], which is the *"gold standard"* in geriatric clinical practice [2, 3].

In this scenario, the development and implementation of information and communication technologies (ICT), assistive technologies, and human-computer interaction technologies are important opportunities to provide new ways to improve the quality of life as well as new solutions to monitor health parameters and follow-up clinical disorders in older people (Fig. 1.1). Indeed, developing e-health technologies has been highlighted as a possible solution to the limited capacity of the public healthcare systems as well as the structural weakening of the private- and family-based care systems for the older citizens [4].

Nowadays, telecare and telemedicine, domotics and robotics, artificial intelligence, and decisional algorithms are all terms that have entered the common vocabulary (Table 1.1), and for which interest has also grown in public information, as well as in national and international research and implementation funding programs. However, there exists a potential gap between media information, the results of scientific research, and the application of health technologies in clinical practice.

In this chapter, we present an overview of the different definitions and classifications of technologies applied and potentially useful for older people, with a specific focus on healthcare and from a geriatric clinical point of view [5] (Table 1.2).

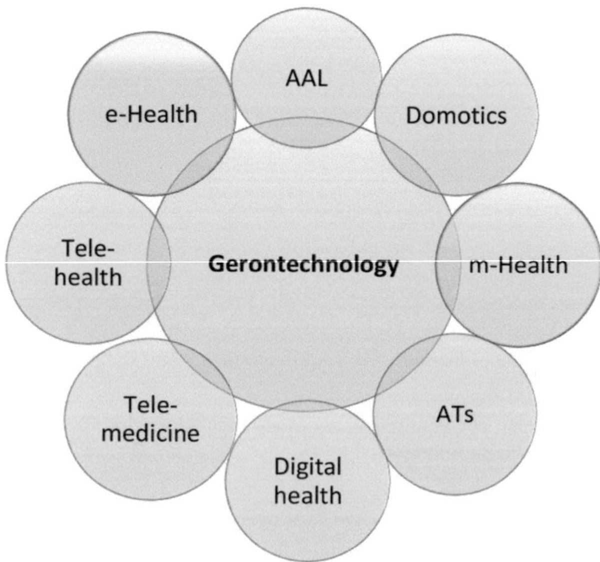

Fig. 1.1 Gerontechnology is at the core of the interdisciplinary field linking existing and developing technologies designed, applied, and implemented to satisfy the aspirations and needs of the older people to improve their healthcare, safety, and quality of life. *AAL* Ambient Assisted Living; *ATs* Assistive Technologies; *m-Health* mobile Health

Table 1.1 Gerontechnology: definitions

Terminology	Definitions
Ambient assisted living (AAL)	Products and services aimed to constitute intelligent environments to improve the quality of life of older people and help them live an active aging.
Artificial intelligence (AI)	The field of computer science that studies whether and how intelligent computer systems, able to simulate the capacity and behavior of human thought, can be realized. Examples of cognitive components considered by the AI include: Interaction with the environment, learning and adaptation, reasoning, planning, and decision-making. The main applications of AI also include machine learning and deep learning techniques.
Assistive technology	Any device or system that allows individuals to perform tasks they would otherwise be unable to do or increases the ease and safety of activities.
Big data	A broad term used to refer to the huge volume of digital information. It is not only generated by traditional information exchange and software, but also by sensors of various types embedded in a variety of environments: hospitals, metro stations, markets, and virtually every electrical device. Big data exceeds the capacity of traditional data management technologies: this presents a challenge not only for the storage of large volumes of data but also for new capabilities to analyze this huge volume of data.
Digital heath	A broad umbrella term that integrate e-health and emerging areas, such as advanced computing sciences in big data, genomics, and artificial intelligence. It is about the proper use of technology for improving the health and well-being of people at individual and population levels, and to improve patient care of patients through intelligent processing of clinical and genetic data.
Digital literacy	Skills and techniques needed to use information and communication technologies.
Domotics	Domotics (from the Latin word "domus", house) is the encounter of information technology, electrical engineering, and electronics that make an environment like a home "smart". It comprises sensors and control systems, devices and automations to increase the quality of life and comfort of the domestic space (e.g., monitoring home temperature, lighting, security systems, and many other functions).
e-health	The use of information and communications technology (ICT) to support health and related area. The term characterizes not only a technical development, but also a general attitude and thinking to improve health care by using ICT.
Exergames	Games that combine virtual, visual, and graphical support with real exercise: peoples' movements are detected by the technology giving them the opportunity to interact in the context of the game or to receive feedback and advice to improve fitness and skills. It is also used in the medical setting, e.g., for the rehabilitation of patients with neurological disorders.

(continued)

Table 1.1 (continued)

Terminology	Definitions
Genomics	The study of the complete set of DNA (including all genes) of a person or other organism. It contains all the information needed for a person to develop and grow.
Geriatrics	Branch of medicine concerned with the diagnosis, treatment, and prevention of diseases in older people and the problems specific to aging.
Gerontechnology	An interdisciplinary field linking existing and developing technologies to the aspirations and needs of older people.
Information and communication technology (ICT)	Set of technological tools and resources used to transmit, store, create, share, or exchange information. ICT includes computers, the internet (websites, blogs, and emails), live broadcasting technologies (television and webcasting), recorded transmission technologies (podcasting, audio and video players, and storage devices), and telephony (fixed or mobile and video conferencing).
Internet of things (IoT)	IoT consists of web-enabled smart devices that use integrated systems, such as processors, sensors, and communication hardware, to collect, send and act on data they acquire from their environments. The devices do most of the work without human intervention, although people can interact with them – for instance, to set them up and give them instructions or access the data.
m-health	The use of Mobile wireless technologies for health. It includes for instance wearables, such as smartwatches, and mobile apps.
Machine learning	Branch of the computer science and artificial intelligence (AI) devoted to the use of big amount of data and algorithms to imitate the way humans learn, gradually improving its accuracy, learning from the experience.
Robotics	Branch of technology that deals with the design, construction, operation, and application of robots, as well as computer systems for their control, sensory feedback, and information processing. In recent years, the field of robotics has begun to overlap with machine learning and artificial intelligence.
Smart-homes	Residences that use internet-connected devices to enable the remote monitoring and management of appliances and systems, such as lighting and heating. It is linked to the concept of domotics.
Tele-health	The use of telecommunications and virtual technology to deliver healthcare outside of traditional healthcare facilities.
Tele-medicine	The delivery of healthcare services where patients and providers are separated by distance.
Virtual reality	An artificial environment which is experienced through sensory stimuli (such as sights, sounds, and tactile) provided by both hardware (e.g., an headset) and software, and in which users can freely move and interact to perform predetermined tasks and attain goals—e.g., learning.

Table 1.2 Clinical classification of Technology in Geriatrics

Digital Health, e-Health, Information and Communication Technologies (ICT)	Assistive Technologies (AT)	Human-Computer Interaction Technologies (HCIT)
Internet systems, telephone-based support groups, webcams, and videoconferencing	Behavior monitoring tools (i.e., sensors and warning systems that alert caregivers)	Assistive robotics (i.e., robots for supporting people with mobility or cognitive limitations)
Online services and electronic medical-health records	Smart homes tools (i.e., sensors and systems to predict abnormal and potentially dangerous ambient conditions)	Humanoid robots, service robots, and companion-type robots
	Telehealth or telemedicine tools (including remote data exchange between patients and caregivers or healthcare professionals)	Exoskeletons and rehabilitation robots (i.e., to perform physical and mental activities with the aim to maintain or training physical and mental activities and rehabilitation)
	Video systems that allow patients to interact with other people	

1.2 Digital Health, e-Health, Information and Communication Technologies (ICT)

In 2019, WHO defined *Digital Health* as "a broad umbrella term encompassing e-health, information and communication technologies (ICTs) as well as developing areas such as the use of advanced computer sciences, including the topics of 'big data', genomics, and artificial intelligence" [4].

Indeed, the term "digital health" has been used in the literature since the 1990s, concerning the provision of healthcare rather than the use of technology. Also, the use of personal data and information for the care of subjects, both at population and individual levels, has been highly emphasized. A dominant concept in digital health, however, is the mobile health (mHealth), which is related to other concepts such as tele-health, e-Health, and big-data analysis and artificial intelligence (AI) in healthcare [6]. Examples of mobile health systems are mobile apps for health monitoring, contact tracing, and wearable technologies.

An interesting classification of digital health interventions has been made by the WHO in 2018 [7] presenting the different ways in which digital and mobile technologies are being used and spread to support health system needs. According to this taxonomy, ICTs and digital technology applications have been classified by four different perspectives: (1) users, (2) healthcare providers, (3) health system managers, and (4) data services. Examples of technology applications for these user groups include: for users (1) the apps that in the last 2 years were created all around the world for the COVID-19 pandemic tracking contacts and vaccination certificates [8]; for healthcare providers (2) the biometrics data collection through smartphone-based systems or electronic medical records [9]; for health system

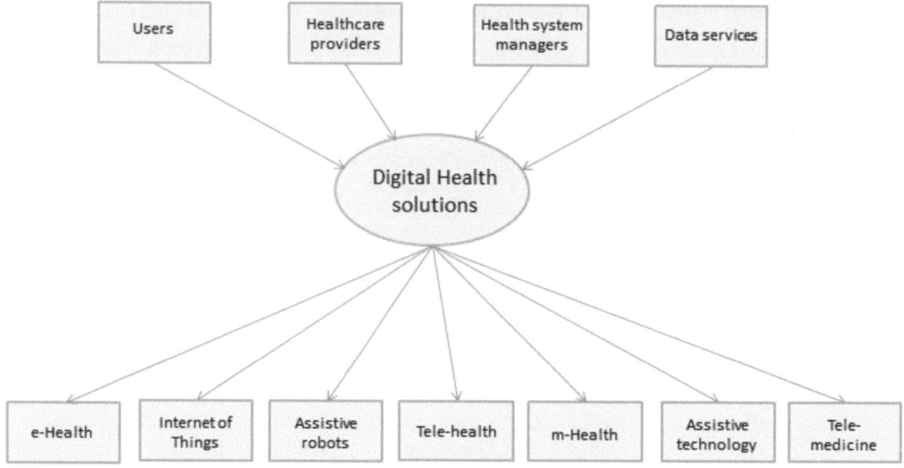

Fig. 1.2 Digital health solutions to support healthcare system needs according to four different stakeholders' perspectives: (1) users, (2) healthcare providers, (3) health system managers, (4) data services

managers (3) the implementation of sensors to monitor temperature and stability of vaccines [10]; and for data services (4) the use of predictive analytics, based on machine learning and AI algorithms [11] (Fig. 1.2).

1.3 Assistive Technologies (ATs)

Assistive technologies (ATs) can be defined as computer-based tools aimed to maintain or reach specific goals in terms of motor and cognitive functionality, quality of life, and independence. In older population, ATs represent a functional element to keep older people's independence and to increase their safety. In this umbrella term, it can be included technologies such as: (i) behavior monitoring tools, i.e., sensors and warning systems that alert caregivers whenever the care recipient changes location or behavior, (ii) smart homes tools that predict abnormal and potentially dangerous behaviors, and (iii) telehealth or telemedicine tools, including passive monitoring systems, remote data exchange between patients and caregivers or healthcare professionals, and video systems that allow patients to interact with other people staying inside or outside the home [5].

1.3.1 Tele-Health and Tele-Medicine Services

The recent COVID-19 pandemic scenario called for a reduction of the traditional medical visits and an increase in the development and implementation of *telemedicine* and *tele-health* services. Indeed, during the last years a very high number of recommendations regarding how clinical activities could change from traditional to digital-based practices, especially considering geriatric patients, have been reported. A recent review [12] suggested that while telemedicine could offer futuristic promise for essential healthcare services for older people, the extent of these services via telehealth appears to be currently limited, especially in low- and middle-income countries. Moreover, optimizing tele-health services, making them easily accessible to older people requires greater government investments and active engagement with broad participation of older people, their caregivers, physicians, and all healthcare providers, technology experts, and healthcare policymakers. Indeed, many examples of clinically useful and cost-effective applications of telemedicine and telehealth programs in clinical practice do exist including computer-assisted software and apps to facilitate diagnosis, follow-up, and management of subjects affected with geriatrics conditions including sarcopenia, mobility disorders, anorexia of aging, cognitive impairment and behavioral disorders, neurological and cardiovascular diseases [13, 14].

Another relevant topic that emerged during the COVID-19 pandemic in relation to the health of the older people is *social isolation*. It is well known that social isolation is an established risk factor for several negative health outcomes including falls, delirium, and behavioral disorders. Furthermore, it is associated with lack of clinical follow-up and poorer control of chronic conditions (such as diabetes, depression, and cardiovascular diseases) as well as a decreased adherence in prevention programs in oncology (screening and treatments) and infective diseases (vaccinations). To reduce the negative impact of social isolation among older adults, many psycho-social frameworks have been developed to provide geriatric assessment and management programs by using tele-health digital services. A home-based tele-health program may enhance older person's quality of life and it can also be used to deliver rehabilitation programs directly at home.

In this context, however, it is important to recognize, in order to reduce them, the *barriers and difficulties in implementing technological solutions* as part of routine medical care, particularly for older people: (a) limited access to *efficient internet web* may reduce the opportunity of effective telemedicine/telehealth programs especially in rural and low economic areas; (b) *high costs* of mobile (smartphone, tablets) and fixed (PC platforms) devices may increase a disparity in accessing to digital health services; (c) reduced *digital alphabetization* by older people and low level of information and training of elderly in using technology; (d) a very low grade of design adaptation of the current apps and devices to the characteristics of older people considering the age-related physiological reaction times and the psycho-physical and sensorial limitations (i.e., visual and hearing deficits).

Designing telemedicine and telehealth protocols in geriatric care should be the product of a strong interdisciplinary human-computer interaction (HCI). In fact, a deep interaction among technology professionals, healthcare professionals, older subjects, and their caregivers is required to develop greater usability and ergonomics of the currently available technologies. Moreover, a deep analysis of the designing and developing phases of technological solutions is necessary to assess whether technologies meet various requirements and needs of different end-users (e.g., healthcare professionals, patients, and caregivers) [15].

At the core of the agenda, there is indeed the promotion of internet technologies among the elderly population. Surveys all around the world reported that older adults and their caregivers are interested in acquiring ICT skills with reported positive impressions and relevant benefits linked to the use of ICT technologies by the older people improving the follow-up of chronic disorders such as hypertension and cognitive impairment, reducing social isolation and depression, and finally warranting a better quality of life and psychological well-being [16, 17]. However, a recent survey among geriatricians published by the Italian Society of Hospital and Community Geriatrics (SIGOT) [18] revealed that telemedicine and telehealth are still relatively poorly practiced mainly due to infrastructural difficulties and poor technological education for both healthcare workers and older people. All these difficulties must be addressed with attention in the next future to really exploit the efficacy of ICT application in the geriatric clinical practice.

1.3.2 ATs for "aging in place": From Exergames to Virtual Reality

The current trend in gerontology and geriatrics sciences is to encourage the concept of *"aging in place"*, where the older people remain in their own homes and communities. This is considered the best solution in terms of health, quality of life, and social connections for older people, as well as in economic terms. At the same time, aging in place also represents, as recently reported by the World Health Organization [19], a potential risk factor for injuries and negative health outcomes, since older people living alone represent a particularly vulnerable population requiring special attention.

Moreover, although it is well documented the health benefit of *physical activity* in the aging population, sedentary lifestyle is largely reported among older people. Indeed, active aging and independent living are the pillars of the policy actions of the Western countries and the development of technological solutions to help older people to be active and maintain their independency for longer times is a health policy priority.

In this context, ATs that monitor and manage the physical environment [20] and the personal characteristics of subjects including mobility and cognitive parameters [21] may have an important role in maintaining and improving the functional capabilities of older people and at the end the chances for a successful aging in place [22].

Another promising topic, developed as ICT solutions for supporting patients living with mobility difficulties and cognitive impairments and their caregivers, is represented by the ATs based on *exergames* and *virtual reality* scenarios.

In general, the term *exergames* indicates games controlled by physical activity and body movements of the player (the name exergame is derived from "exercise" + "gaming"). There is a large body of literature on exergames sustaining their application, if properly designed, as useful tools to improve seniors' engagement in physical activity, in an effective and attractive manner, by integrating different training principles and implementing motivational support. Exergames may require movement-based controller systems (e.g., haptic, or gesture-based input devices), or full-body movement interaction, demanding different motor and cognitive functions and other health parameters that are targeted by the exergame while playing. Gerontology research has provided insights into the impact of exergame-based protocols on motor and cognitive abilities of older people. A recent review provided an extensive overview of existing studies on exergames effects on older adults' physical activity [23] and thus supporting the use of exergames in geriatrics, through an increase of motivation and engagement of older people in physical activity. Further recent data suggested potential effectiveness of exergames to treat age-related chronic diseases including cognitive impairments and dementia [24]. Exergaming has also been described as an innovative and safe way to design enjoyable high-intensity training physical programs in older age. Finally, the so-called *social exergames* solutions, on the other hand, are intended to answer the needs of improving active and healthy aging in the older people by including joyful and purposeful physical activity while simultaneously stimulating social interaction to counteract isolation and loneliness.

In this area, some AT solutions are based on *videogames* and *virtual reality*. A recent review [25] reported that virtual-reality training is indeed an effective intervention to improve the functional mobility of older people compared to traditional methods. Moreover, thanks to its effect on motor activation and rehabilitation, virtual reality has promising application also in the psychogeriatric area as a beneficial tool to enhance care of the cognitive and affective disorders of older population. Indeed, in the last decades, virtual reality led to a shift from two-dimensional non-immersive perceptions to three-dimensional fully immersive experiences, allowing more sophisticated simulations of the environment. For this reason, virtual reality has been widely applied in several clinical settings including geriatrics resulting effective in screening and training of older subjects with cognitive impairment [26].

1.4 Human-Computer Interaction Technologies: Robotics and Their Assistive and Social Dimensions

Recent studies underlined that *assistive robot* can support older people during everyday tasks, contributing, at the same time, to maintain personal mobility as a supportive tool. Indeed, what robotics added to ATs is the physical interaction, when robot provides functional assistance to mobility tasks to humans with some motor difficulties [27]. Moreover, assistive robots can also support caregivers and healthcare professionals, e.g., nurses and clinicians, during their working routine, helping them with assessment and management of older patients who need repetitive tasks to improve their physical impairments [28].

In the last years, many prototypes of assistive robots have been released, to keep people independent as much as possible. The literature on assistive robotics universally stresses the importance of the designing phase of the project. Involving since the beginning the end-users in co-designing cycles of interaction allows better fit between users' needs and robot services, and thus the acceptability by the market. Co-designing with users can have different levels of participation (from drafting the initial concept together, to asking feedback on a prototype), and it has proven to enhance the usability and the acceptability of products [29].

Curiously, in the literature, there are few examples of co-designing processes that also involve caregivers and healthcare professionals. However, formal and informal caregivers are also fundamental stakeholders to be involved in the design phases as they may add relevant perspective, for their first-person involvement in the functional and healthy problems of the older subject, helping him to move in and around the house or to complete their everyday tasks. A robot might intervene to relieve caregivers' burden. Similarly, formal caregivers may have an important role, due to their expertise "on the field" on physical and cognitive problems of the older subject and his/her everyday management. Therefore, both formal and informal caregivers potentially could be the final end-users of an assistive robotic service as well as the patients [30].

Assisting the mobility of frail older people is not the only area in which assistive robots can intervene efficiently. Mental healthcare is another important area of application of assistive robotics. A recent review [31] addressed the role of social robotics in psychogeriatrics. Interestingly, the authors classified the assistive robotics used in this field as: (i) robotic pets, (ii) social robots, and (iii) telepresence robots. The first category includes all the products that have an animatronic design; social robots are those with capacity of conversation, emotion recognition, and body language projection used for robot-human interaction. Telepresence robots require a remote control, since they do not have autonomous behaviors. The final conclusions, however, indicated that robotics is still in the early stages of clinical applicability at least in psychogeriatric.

Indeed, the clinical settings where assistive and social robotics may be applied are very extended, e.g., hospitals, nursing homes, patients' and caregivers' private homes, and for different tasks.

In a future perspective, robotics can enable clinicians to treat more patients, particularly if the robots will be broadly applied in persons' houses to help observe and assist with activities of daily living, or to ensure prolongation of interventions. Additionally, robots could reduce the healthcare costs for patients. Finally, assistive and social robots may be an answer to support people who live in remote areas, where access to clinicians may be limited (e.g., rural areas), possibly reducing health disparities.

References

1. Kassebaum NJ on behalf of the Global Burden of Diseases. Ageing Collaborators. Global, regional, and national burden of diseases and injuries for adults 70 years and older: systematic analysis for the Global Burden of Disease 2019 Study. BMJ. 2019;2022:376. https://doi.org/10.1136/bmj-2021-068208.
2. Zampino M, Polidori MC, Ferrucci L, O'Neill D, Pilotto A, Gogol M, Rubenstein L. Biomarkers of aging in real life: three questions on aging and the comprehensive geriatric assessment. Geroscience. 2022;7:1–12. https://doi.org/10.1007/s11357-022-00613-4.

3. Pilotto A, Custodero C, Maggi S, Polidori MC, Veronese N, Ferrucci L. A multidimensional approach to frailty in older people. Ageing Res Rev. 2020;60:101047.
4. World Health Organization (WHO). Future of digital health: report on the WHO symposium on the future of digital health systems in the European region: Copenhagen, Denmark, 6–8 February 2019. https://apps.who.int/iris/bitstream/handle/10665/329032/9789289059992-eng.pdf. Accessed August 22, 2022.
5. Pilotto A, Boi R, Petermans J. Technology in geriatrics. Age Ageing. 2018;47:771–4.
6. Farhad F, Samadbeik M, Kazemi A. What is digital health? Review of definitions. In: Värri A, Delgado J, Gallos P, Hägglund M, Häyrinen K, Kinnunen U, et al., editors. Integrated citizen centered digital health and social care: citizens as data producers and service co-creators; 2020. p. 67–71. Online edition https://ebooks.iospress.nl/volume/integrated-citizen-centered-digital-health-and-social-care-citizens-as-data-producers-and-service-co-creators. Accessed August 22, 2022.
7. World Health Organization (WHO). Classification of digital health interventions v1. 0. Report No. WHO/RHR/18.06, 2018. https://doi.org/10.13140/RG.2.2.14531.30243. Accessed August 22, 2022.
8. Singh HJL, Couch D, Yap K. Mobile health apps that help with COVID-19 management: scoping review. J Med Internet Res Nurs. 2020;3(1):e20596. https://doi.org/10.2196/20596.
9. Hansen TK, Shahla S, Damsgaard EM, Bossen SRL, Bruun JM, Gregersen M. Mortality and readmission risk can be predicted by the record-based Multidimensional Prognostic Index: a cohort study of medical inpatients older than 75 years. Eur Geriatr Med. 2021;12(2):253–61. https://doi.org/10.1007/s41999-021-00453-z.
10. Chojnacky M. National Institute of Standards and Technology, Gaithersburg (MD). Accurate cold chain temperature monitoring using digital data logger thermometers. https://www.nist.gov/system/files/documents/2017/04/28/NIC-2012-Accurate-Cold-Chain-Temperature-Monitoring-Using-Digital-Data-Logger-Thermometers.pdf. Accessed August 20, 2022.
11. Woodman RJ, Bryant K, Sorich MJ, Pilotto A, Mangoni AA. Use of multiprognostic index domain scores, clinical data, and machine learning to improve 12-month mortality risk prediction in older hospitalized patients: prospective cohort study. J Med Internet Res. 2021;23(6):e26139. https://doi.org/10.2196/26139.
12. Patil VS, Abdulla PPJ, James JV, Ahmed JB, Rafeeque PA, Siraj MM, Mubarak KA. Telemedicine in geriatrics care during the covid-19 pandemic–a review. J Adv Med Dental Sci Res. 2021;9(11):106–9. https://doi.org/10.21276/jamdsr.
13. Merchant RA, Hui RJY, Kwek SC, et al. Rapid geriatric assessment using mobile app in primary care: prevalence of geriatric syndromes and review of its feasibility. Front Med (Lausanne). 2020;7:261.
14. Custodero C, Senesi B, Pinna A, Floris A, Vigo M, Fama M, et al. Validation and implementation of telephone-administered version of the Multidimensional Prognostic Index (TELE-MPI) for remote monitoring of community-dwelling older adults. Aging Clin Exp Res. 2021;33(12):3363–9. https://doi.org/10.1007/s40520-021-01871-6.
15. Liu N, Yin J, Wongmaanerooj M, Teo HH. The design of digital health applications for elderly users: a systematic review and future directions. PACIS–Pacific Asia Conference on Information Systems 2020 PRO 41. https://aisel.aisnet.org/pacis2020/41.
16. Pilotto A, D'Onofrio G, Benelli E, Zanesco A, Cabello A, Margeli MC, et al. On behalf of the HOPE investigators. Information and communication technology systems to improve quality of life and safety of Alzheimer's disease patients: a multicenter international survey. J Alzheimers Dis. 2011;23:131–41.
17. Sun X, Yan W, Zhou H, et al. Internet use and need for digital health technology among the elderly: a cross-sectional survey in China. BMC Public Health. 2020;20:1386. https://doi.org/10.1186/s12889-020-09448-0.
18. Cella A, Volta E, Demurtas J, Zaccaria R, Ceci M, Pilotto A, et al. The use of e-health and digital technologies in the Italian geriatric practice: a survey of the Italian Geriatric Society (SIGOT). Geriatric Care. 2021;7:10301. https://doi.org/10.4081/gc.2021.10301.

19. World Health Organization (WHO). Social isolation and loneliness among older people: advocacy brief. 2021 https://apps.who.int/iris/bitstream/handle/10665/343206/9789240030749-eng.pdf?sequence=1&isAllowed=y. Accessed August 22, 2022.
20. Patrone C, Cella C, Martini C, Pericu S, Femia R, Barla A, et al. Development of a smart post-hospitalization facility for older people by using domotics, robotics, and automated telemonitoring. Geriatric Care. 2019;5(1) https://doi.org/10.4081/gc.2019.8122.
21. Martini C, Barla A, Odone F, Verri A, Cella A, Rollandi GA, Pilotto A. Data-driven continuous assessment of frailty in older people. Front Digit Humanities. 2018;5 https://doi.org/10.3389/fdigh.2018.00006.
22. Kim KI, Gollamudi SS, Steinhubl S. Digital technology to enable aging in place. Exp Gerontol. 2017;88:25–31.
23. Kappen DL, Mirza-Babaei P, Nacke LE. Older adults' physical activity and exergames: a systematic review. Int J Human–Comp Interaction. 2019;35(2):140–67.
24. Van Santen J, Dröes RM, Holstege M, Henkemans O, Van Rijn A, De Vries R, et al. Effects of exergaming in people with dementia: results of a systematic literature review. J Alzheimer Dis. 2018;2018(63):741–60.
25. Corregidor-Sánchez AI, Segura-Fragoso A, Rodríguez-Hernández M, Jiménez-Rojas C, Polonio-López B, Criado-Álvarez JJ. Effectiveness of virtual reality technology on functional mobility of older adults: systematic review and meta-analysis. Age Ageing. 2021;50:370–9. https://doi.org/10.1093/ageing/afaa197.
26. Skurla M, Rahman A, Salcone S, Mathias L, Shah B, Forester B, Vahia I. Virtual reality and mental health in older adults: a systematic review. Int Psychogeriatr. 2022;34:143–55.
27. Fiorini L, De Mul M, Fabbricotti I, Limosani R, Vitanza A, D'Onofrio G, et al. Assistive robots to improve the independent living of older persons: results from a needs study. Disabil Rehabil Assist Technol. 2021;16(1):92–102.
28. Cella A, De Luca A, Squeri V, Parodi S, Puntoni M, Vallone F, et al. Robotic balance assessment in community-dwelling older people with different grades of impairment of physical performance. Aging Clin Exp Res. 2020;32(3):491–503. https://doi.org/10.1007/s40520-019-01395-0.
29. Winkle K, Caleb-Solly P, Turton A, et al. Mutual shaping in the design of socially assistive robots: a case study on social robots for therapy. Int J Soc Robot. 2019;12:1–20.
30. Gerłowska J, Skrobas U, Grabowska-Aleksandrowicz K, et al. Assessment of perceived attractiveness, usability, and societal impact of a multimodal robotic assistant for aging patients with memory impairments. Front Neurol. 2018;9:1–13.
31. Kulpa E, Rahman AT, Vahia IV. Approaches to assessing the impact of robotics in geriatric mental health care: a scoping review. Int Rev Psychiatr. 2021;33:1–11.

Clinical Application of Technology: Why Are they Needed, How to Implement, and What Challenges

Jennifer Kudelka and Walter Maetzler

2.1 Why Do We Need Technology?

The idea that technology could play a leading role in most areas of the healthcare system today and in the future often arouses mistrust, especially among geriatric patients. There are concerns about inaccessibility to technology, poor security of personal data, increased costs, and lack of skills to use technology [1, 2]. In order to reduce these fears, it is crucial to communicate that the implementation of technology, especially in the geriatric field, comes with enormous benefits for the patients themselves. These are presented in the following as well as in Figure 2.1.

2.1.1 What Can Technology Do for Patients?

2.1.1.1 Increase Convenience

One of the most important benefits of the use of technology in direct patient care is the increased convenience for patients [3]. By using telemedicine, it is possible to attend medical appointments from home or from any location. For working patients, this offers increased convenience, for example, by allowing them to attend a consultation appointment from their workplace. Other patients save themselves long and cost-intensive journeys, especially for specialist care, the search for a parking space, and the waiting time at the doctor's office, which is also associated with a risk of infection through contact with other patients. For example, one study showed that telemedicine visits saved patients with Parkinson's disease (PD) an average of 100 miles of travel and 3 h of time compared to in-person visits [4]. In addition, remote monitoring can potentially help reduce unplanned hospitalizations [5]. Although increased convenience is a significant factor in the compliance and

J. Kudelka (✉) · W. Maetzler
Department of Neurology, University Hospital Schleswig-Holstein, Kiel, Germany
e-mail: Jennifer.Kudelka@uksh.de

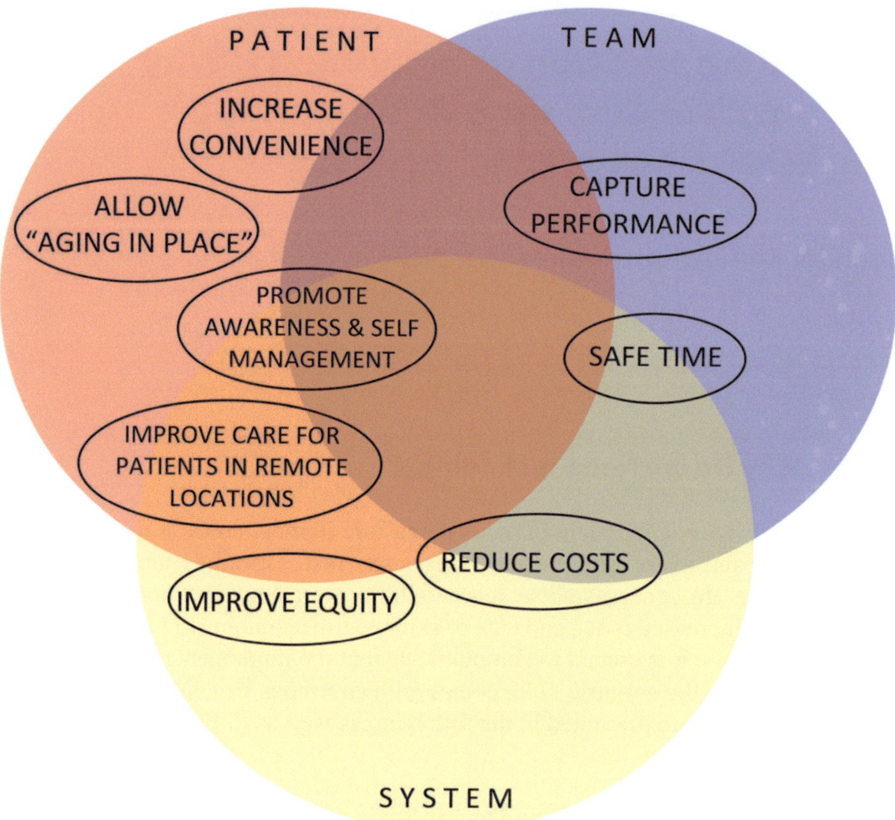

Fig. 2.1 There are many benefits related to the application of gerontechnology. Most of the benefits, however, are not only attributable to one of the three groups (patient, professional team (TEAM), healthcare system (SYSTEM)), but to several. In addition to the overlapping benefits, the figure also suggests a weighting of the benefits in favor of the patients

adherence to therapy of younger and less affected patients, geriatric patients in particular benefit most from the increased use of telemedicine. Geriatric patients, by definition, suffer from multiple chronic conditions as well as an increased age-related vulnerability. As a result of these conditions, geriatric patients are likely to have limited mobility, making it more difficult to visit a doctor. Thus, severe illness has been associated with increased effort to access healthcare services and/or poorer care from the healthcare system. Technological aids can help to soften this imbalance in the future [6].

2.1.1.2 Improve Care for Patients in Remote Locations

Technology and, in particular, information and communication technologies (ICT) and telehealth can not only help to improve the comfort of patients, for example, by preventing them from having to travel long and uncomfortable distances to see their attending physicians, but can also be of importance in the case of acute health problems. Unlike the former example, seeing the appropriate specialist in these cases is not hindered by an increased effort, but rather by an acute lack of time. One example of how telehealth can be of assistance in these cases is telestroke [7]. Since in stroke there is a defined time window in which acute treatment, such as thrombolysis therapy, can be started, there is enormous time pressure, which can be counteracted by means of technology. For example, experts in centers further away can support the physicians on site both in diagnostics (neurological examination, CT) and in the implementation and monitoring of therapy. In contrast to telestroke, which is a flagship example in the use of telehealth, telemedicine care for chronic neurological disorders has been less established, even though the prevalence of these conditions is growing significantly [6].

2.1.1.3 Allow "Aging in Place"

Technical aids should not only support patients in their direct healthcare, but also ensure that geriatric patients can remain in their familiar surroundings, resulting in greater patient satisfaction, quality of life, and reduction of healthcare costs [8]. In addition to monitoring health parameters, technology and, in particular, ICT systems can help ensure the safety of patients in their home environment: Examples include sensors that detect potential hazards such as heat, burglary, and flooding, and synchronously trigger an alarm to alert potential helpers. Furthermore, motion sensors, for example, can detect falls without fallers having to make an emergency call themselves. Although the accuracy of the systems is not yet sufficient for widespread use in clinical routine, the initial results are promising. The same applies to possible scenarios in which patients are unconscious [9]. In this respect, ICT systems not only relieve the patients themselves, but also their caregivers. A survey of caregivers of Alzheimer's patients showed that the majority of caregivers felt that implementing ICT in the patient's home would be beneficial to their personal autonomy, quality of life, and safety in everyday life and in emergency situations [10].

2.1.1.4 Promote Awareness and Self-Management

The continuous monitoring of body functions by parameters such as movement or vital signs offers, in addition to the important gain in information for physicians, the possibility of improved patients' awareness of their own disease. By looking at their data, patients can gain knowledge about their own disease and their own personalized disease progression [11], which will empower them to be more involved in treatment decisions and has the potential to facilitate shared decision-making [12].

Furthermore, artificial intelligence will be increasingly used to enable patients to receive feedback and recommendations for disease modification based on the data collected and consequently improve self-management of chronic diseases. One example that is already widely practiced is the recording of blood glucose in patients with diabetes mellitus, where continuous monitoring of blood glucose has reduced the incidence of hypoglycemia [13]. Another recent randomized controlled trial showed that digital health self-management, more specifically downloading and using an app that monitors physical activity and sends motivational messages to the user, significantly increased average daily step counts in patients with cardiovascular disease [14].

2.1.2 What Can Technology Do for Health Professionals?

2.1.2.1 Capture Performance

The continuous recording of health parameters in the home environment represents an enormous gain in information for the treating physicians, which in turn can facilitate the determination of therapy concepts. In the diagnostics currently practiced clinicians primarily rely on two variables: capacity ("How well can the patient perform?") and perception ("How do I, as a patient, perceive the limitation/health problem?"). Common clinical assessments (reflecting mainly capacity aspects, e.g., the Movement Disorder Society-revised Unified Parkinson's Disease Rating Scale (MDS-UPDRS) in PD), while of great importance for detecting symptoms and assessing disease progression, represent only a snapshot in the patient's life that is also environment- and examiner-dependent [15]. Daily life outside the hospital is almost exclusively captured by questionnaires that reflect the patient's perspective (perception measures). This is an important, but also highly subjective assessment approach. Results can sometimes be influenced by patients either not recognizing symptoms, signs or limitations, confusing them, or forgetting them. In addition, the quality of the results may be influenced by the patients' motivation to complete the questionnaires. To gain insight into the actual *performance* of patients in their daily life in addition to capacity and perception, the use of technology is crucial, e.g., body-worn sensors to record movement, vital signs, ECG or EEG. Yet, it is important to emphasize that the three pillars capacity, perception, and performance should be considered complementary and in their entirety provide a comprehensive picture of the patient's state of health [16, 17].

2.1.2.2 Save Time

The use of technology can save physicians time. Remote monitoring can help physicians prepare for appointments with patients and avoid non-essential in-clinic appointments. In addition, systems will be established in which a healthcare worker interacts with multiple patients. An example of such a model is ParkinsonTV, set up by ParkinsonNet [18] in the Netherlands with the aim to educate people with PD about their disease.

Another innovation that will revolutionize medicine is the use of artificial intelligence in the diagnostic field, for example, in radiology, pathology, or ophthalmology [5]. A promising example is the interpretation of three-dimensional optical coherence tomography (OCT) in the field of ophthalmology, where artificial intelligence has been used to diagnose sight-threatening retinal diseases. In this case, the deep learning architecture used ultimately proved to be equal or superior to the interpretation of experts [19]. Technological innovations such as these will save time for physicians, which can be used for more individualized and patient-centered care and have the potential to omit (human) errors.

2.1.3 What Can Technology Do for the HealthCare System?

2.1.3.1 Reduce Costs

The increasing aging of the world's population in the context of demographic change is associated with an enormous economic burden on the healthcare system. The example of neurological disorders, currently the third most common cause of disability and premature death worldwide, shows that further development of prevention and therapy strategies is essential not only for patients, but also for the healthcare system and the economy [20]. The use of technology such as remote monitoring and telehealth in chronic neurological disorders (e.g., PD) will help reduce costs for the healthcare system, for example, by reducing the need for in-clinic visits and decreasing hospitalization rates [21]. Moreover, many of the uses of technology already mentioned will also lower costs for the healthcare system, such as the ability to save staff in diagnostic areas where artificial intelligence can be used. These healthcare professionals can in turn be deployed in other areas of the healthcare system, where there is already a growing shortage of personnel. In addition, the use of telemedicine can save costs in the construction and maintenance of infrastructure [6].

2.1.3.2 Improve Equity

Technology, if implemented properly, can make a difference in terms of equal healthcare for all people worldwide. In the field of telemedicine, disadvantages related to place of residence can be leveled out by giving patients in remote locations access to specialists. In acute emergencies such as strokes, concepts like Telestroke [7] can also reduce the risk that the quality of treatment depends largely on where the patient suffers the stroke and how far away a suitable clinic is located.

However, telemedicine can also be used to reduce global disparities between different countries in terms of the quality of healthcare and training of healthcare workforce. Collaborations can be established between medical workforce in developing countries and specialized centers in industrialized nations, for example, by holding regular case conferences and consults [6]. A study from Nepal showed that such collaborations are technically feasible and can improve local medical treatment using expertise from afar [22].

Despite these tremendous benefits, it will be a major challenge to reap the benefits of digital medicine in a manner that is consistent with consideration of all populations. Particularly with regard to the geriatric field, it is important to focus on ensuring that all patients have access to technology and receive the necessary technical education.

2.2 How to Implement Technology

2.2.1 How to Fit Technology into Patient Lives

Despite the tremendous benefits of using technology to improve the lives and health of geriatric patients, the implementation of technology into patients' lives lags behind the rapid development of new technologies [23]. Especially geriatric patients express fear, distrust, and lack of competence regarding the use of technology [1]. Moreover, the senior technology acceptance model (STAM), developed by Chen & Chan, states that age is associated with less use of technology and user's perceived ease of use [24]. Therefore, it is of particular importance to identify the critical factors for patients' adoption of technology and to develop strategies for successful implementation.

2.2.1.1 Provide Education

Both the lack of health literacy and the lack of technical literacy among older adults make digital education of geriatric patients particularly challenging [25]. One of the challenges in the acceptance of technical aids is concerns regarding technology, for example, related to usability. Other fears are that patients would have no control over the activation or deactivation of technology or that health damages could result, for example, from suspected radiation from sensors [26]. These concerns show that education about the usefulness and functionality of technical aids and practice in using them are of great importance. A recent study showed that an intervention (2 weeks of learning) increased patients' knowledge and skills as well as eHealth literacy, and that patients' acceptance of technical aids also improved after the intervention [25].

2.2.1.2 Respect Patients' Wishes

Studies have shown that customization and maintenance of autonomy is a critical criterion for acceptance of technology by geriatric patients [27]. Therefore, it is necessary to involve them in the development of technical devices. Involvement of geriatric patients should not only be limited to trying out and evaluating technologies that have already been established (which is rather "engaging" patients), but should also include direct participation in the development and design of new technologies. Current challenges include the large age gap and resulting communication difficulties between product designers and users in the geriatric field, as well as the great diversity of geriatric users in terms of their individual background and technical understanding. Researchers agree that the inclusion of patients in the development of technologies (which is real "involvement") is urgently necessary, and further research is needed on *how* this inclusion should be carried out [28].

2.2.1.3 Include Caregivers

Research results suggest that acceptance of technology depends not only on individual factors of the users, but also on influence from family members, caregivers, and the social environment [26, 29]. In particular, spouses, children, and grandchildren can encourage geriatric patients to implement technology, such as computer devices used in telemedicine, into their daily lives. Therefore, individual family members take on specific roles: spouses often help with the daily use of the devices, children mostly support the implementation of technological devices, for example, out of concern for their parents, and grandchildren can often transfer their enthusiasm for technology to their grandparents [29]. Accordingly, the involvement of family members as well as the social environment, for example, in installing technical devices in the home environment, training them in their use, and handling the resulting data, plays a crucial role in the successful implementation of technology in geriatric care.

2.2.2 How to Choose Technology

In order to effectively and profitably implement technology into the lives of geriatric patients, a consensus must be created in the research community about the role technology should play in diagnostics and what type of technology can provide clinically relevant parameters. To achieve this, it is of major importance to establish globally valid requirements for technologies and resulting parameters so that they provide added diagnostic value in assessing the actual performance of patients in their home environment.

2.2.2.1 Define Requirements

Technologies used for remote monitoring that provide information on mobility and vital signs, for example, should be technically feasible and clinically relevant. Due to the rapidly evolving technological capabilities and the overwhelming quantity of measurable parameters, it is particularly important to filter out those that have the highest relevance to patients' health and well-being. To map the meaningfulness of sensor-based parameters, Manta et al. proposed a four-level framework consisting of *Meaningful Aspect of Health* (e.g., ability to perform ambulatory activities), *Concept of Interest* (e.g., walking capacity), *Outcome to be measured* (e.g., duration of walking bouts per day), and *Endpoint* (e.g., percent change from baseline time stepping compared to placebo) [30]. Based on this framework, it should become apparent which health problems are to be assessed and eventually improved with the aid of a digital parameter.

To define specific requirements for each outcome, we recently established four criteria that parameters used for remote monitoring in the clinical management of chronic diseases, for example, PD, should fulfill. Digital outcomes are supposed to

- Provide valid results that reflect a clinically relevant symptom
- Contribute to treatment decisions that are relevant to the patient, e.g., improvement in Health-related Quality of Life (HrQoL)
- Provide a target range by which to assess, for example, response to treatment decisions
- Be easy to use for patients and healthcare professionals [15]

These two exemplary models are intended to give an impression of how technologies can be selected to be used in the geriatric field for diagnostics, monitoring of disease progression, and therapy control.

2.2.2.2 Validate Parameters

A wide range of technologies already exist in the field of remote monitoring of diseases. However, there is a gap between the development of new technologies and the actual clinical application, which is due to the fact that there are no standardized requirements for the technical and clinical validation of digital parameters. In this context, technical validity ("criterion validity") means the comparison of new technology (e.g., body-worn sensors) with the gold standard (e.g., motor assessment under laboratory conditions) [31]. Both the accurate measurability by the devices and the functionality of the algorithms must be verified [32]. Clinical validity ("construct validity") means that a technology-based outcome captures a disease symptom as well as or better than a traditional assessment tool for measuring that same symptom. In addition, the parameter should be able to detect changes in the progression of the disease (e.g., worsening of a symptom) and should be related to relevant clinical endpoints [31].

Various publications conclude that there is a disagreement in the research community about which outcomes should be applied in clinical practice, due to a lack of consensus on how validation studies should be designed to demonstrate the clinical relevance of an outcome [9, 33, 34]. Therefore, a proposition is made for a sequence of studies that a digital outcome should complete from development to clinical use (see Table 2.1) [35].

2.2.3   How to Manage Data

With the development and implementation of technologies and algorithms that produce a variety of data in patients' daily lives, the question emerges of who owns the data, where it is stored, and who has access to it.

2.2.3.1 Build Platforms

It should be avoided that increasingly more technologies are developed that already exist in a similar format or produce outcomes that are already covered by existing technologies and algorithms. The result would be an inefficient way of doing research by putting effort into duplicating already available technologies due to a lack of data sharing [36, 37]. This poses the hazard that a patchwork of technologies will emerge that produce similar outcomes, have been validated in different ways, and are not accessible to all stakeholders. For this reason, the Movement Disorder Society (MDS) Taskforce on Technology, among others, recommends the establishment of an open-source platform where existing technology can be collected in a structured way and made available to appropriate stakeholders as needed. The benefits of this solution include improved accessibility, improved comparability of outcomes captured by different technologies, and improved feasibility of proposed validation standards [38].

Table 2.1 Requirements and "study-associated development steps" for a digital outcome parameter that is eventually used in clinical routine

Requirement	Example aim	Example study design
Establish the wearability, usability, and acceptability of the device to be used for measurement of a digital parameter	Ascertain that operation of the device is possible even with disease-related disabilities	Focus groups and qualitative interviews with participants who have used the device over sufficient time. Suggested n 10–20
Establish whether the digital parameter can be measured with accuracy in comparison with an existing gold standard	Determine whether a wearable device on the lower back can accurately measure walking speed, as defined by a stationary optical system	Cross-sectional observational study. Suggested n 20–100
Establish whether the digital parameter tests what it is intended to test by comparing measurements with other tests (clinical and/or patient-reported outcome)	Demonstrate that real-world walking speed deteriorates with increasing disease severity	Longitudinal observational studies in the target population. Suggested n 100–1000
Establish the sensitivity of the digital parameter to change, such as disease progression or treatment response	Demonstrate that step time variability measured with a device on the lower back improves with cholinergic treatment	Longitudinal observational studies or inclusion as an exploratory parameter in clinical trials
Establish the smallest change in the digital parameter that a patient and/or medical professional would consider clinically relevant	The target population and/or the treating medical team rate, e.g., on a Likert scale, whether a meaningful change (e.g., from "severe" to "moderate") of gait disability occurred during the observation period	Longitudinal observational studies or inclusion as an exploratory parameter in clinical trials

From [35], with permission

2.2.3.2 Give Patients Control

Even with evolving technology, patients today still lack adequate access to their own health data [39]. From the perspective that the introduction of new technologies "intrudes" into patients' daily lives, e.g., through remote monitoring, there is an even greater need for patients to (1) be involved in development of technology from the beginning and (2) have full access to their own data. A digital record containing information from physicians and healthcare professionals as well as the data extracted from sensors (see Fig. 2.2) should not only be accessible to patients, but should provide them with information that they can easily understand and is therefore beneficial to their health literacy and chronic disease management [40]. In addition, patients can be encouraged to provide their own data (e.g., mobility data from wearable sensors) to research institutions and benefit from it themselves [39]. Another advantage of a patient-centric dataset is that patients can decide on who they give access to which data (e.g., their caregivers or their

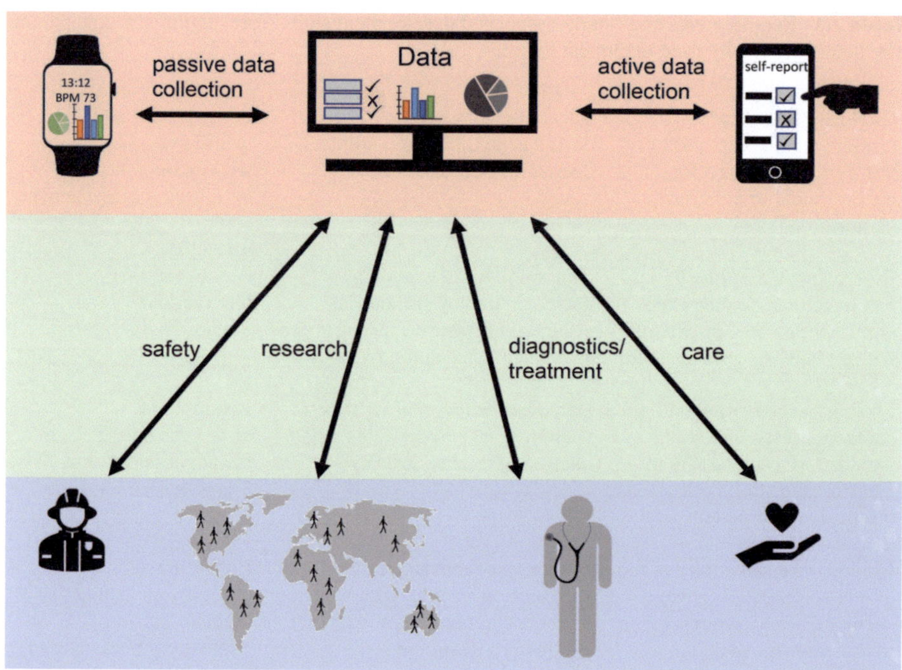

Fig. 2.2 The implementation of technology requires guidelines regarding data management. A patient-centered approach is inevitable. Collected data from the patient, such as actively collected data, e.g., via e-diaries, or passively collected data, e.g., via wearable sensors, can be made available to other stakeholders by the patient. Other stakeholders include emergency staff (e.g., access to safety data in smart homes), research institutions (e.g., access to research data), medical professionals and caregivers (e.g., access to health data). Figure adapted from Hansen et al. (2018) [40]

physicians). Such an arrangement also means a significant reduction in issues regarding data protection that could become even more pressing as new technologies are being developed.

2.3 Challenges and Opportunities

2.3.1 Ethical Aspects

Gerontechnology is an emerging field in medicine that holds immense benefits for geriatric patients. Nevertheless, it is of utmost importance to keep ethical issues in mind when implementing this field: How much should technology be able to capture about patients' lives? To what extent is technology allowed to interfere with patients' lives? How can we ensure that technology is accessible and fairly distributed to all?

2.3.1.1 Protect Rights

A recent scoping review on ethical aspects of gerontechnology identified two important issues that need to be discussed:

- The balance between the benefits of gerontechnology and the rights of patients regarding privacy, safety, and autonomy
- The risk of insecurity of older adults regarding loss of human contact, and other fears and concerns related to the use of gerontechnology [41]

Other studies confirm that these issues are criticized by geriatric patients and hinder adoption of technologies [1, 2, 26, 27].

An example to illustrate the ethical dilemma that can arise from technology implementation is GPS tracking of patients with dementia or cognitive impairment. On the one hand, GPS tracking enables early detection of danger and alerting of help, thus increasing the patient's safety. On the other hand, such "surveillance" also represents a restriction of privacy and can lead to the loss of human contact, for example, when caregivers consider technologies as a substitute for their personal care. In the case of patients with dementia, the issue becomes even more complex, as they may be cognitively incapable of weighing up the advantages and disadvantages and making an autonomous decision as to whether they want to use technology in their everyday lives. As a result, caregivers are often authorized to make these decisions for patients. Caregivers, in turn, often consider the safety of patients as more important than their autonomy [42].

This example highlights the urgent need to consider ethical aspects when implementing technologies, especially in the geriatric setting. It is important to ensure that the technologies have a noticeable benefit in the lives of patients, that patients are integrated into the development of technologies, and that strict data protection rules are applied.

2.3.2 Technical Aspects

2.3.2.1 Rethink Validation

Regarding the validation of parameters, there are already propositions (see Sect. 2.2) about the requirements, sizes, and designs of studies needed. This includes, among other aspects, the comparison with the current clinical gold standard for recording a symptom, dysfunction, sign, or disability [31]. A challenge is posed by the fact that objective measurement instruments, e.g., the remote monitoring of fluctuating symptoms, most probably outperform subjective clinical assessments in the accuracy of their measurement, for example, if the symptoms do not occur at the time of the examination by a physician [38]. Research results suggest that the relationship between technology-based measures and clinical assessments is complex and that they may not highly correlate simply because they (are supposed to) measure different constructs [36]. Even though these scenarios may require new validation approaches, it should be emphasized that new technologies offer the potential to make previously unrecognized symptoms objectively measurable, opening up entirely new options for medical management.

2.3.3 Political Aspects

2.3.3.1 Ensure Access

Equity in the digital future means that all people should use healthcare technologies equally, regardless of their location or characteristics such as age or gender. Unfortunately, recent studies show that this aim has not yet been achieved: for example, it has been revealed that especially older people, women, children, people in poor economic situations, and people in remote locations have limited access to assistive technology (AT) [43]. In addition, there are large differences between the availability of AT in various countries: Especially in low-income countries such as Botswana or Swaziland, there is a lack of technologization [44].

The Topol Review, an NHS report designed to prepare the healthcare system in the UK for technologization, identifies healthcare equality as one of the biggest challenges in the digital future. According to the report, there is both the potential to eradicate inequalities through technology, but also to fuel inequalities further [5]. Thus, technologies can be seen as both a challenge and an opportunity to make healthcare more equitable worldwide, since digital features such as telemedicine can again improve the quality of healthcare for people in low-income countries or people in remote locations (see Sect. 1.3).

2.3.3.2 Integrate into the Healthcare System

Even though ensuring that there is a globally equal access to technology looks like an ethical issue, however, it is actually a political challenge. An important instrument to achieve this goal is to reimburse costs expended on health maintenance and prevention technologies. In order to create the appropriate structures, recognition of digital outcomes by regulatory authorities such as the European Medicines Agency (EMA) or the U.S. Food and Drug Administration (FDA) is required, with defined, globally valid standards that can be adopted by technology manufacturers and health insurance companies. Thus, a cost-effectiveness analysis should demonstrate that the benefits of technologies through the positive effects on the course of disease and the HrQoL of patients exceed the initially high costs for the healthcare system in the long term [15, 31, 36].

In summary, the benefits of the use of gerontechnology for all stakeholders are evident and useful requirements and frameworks for implementation of technology have been proposed. Yet, several steps are needed to integrate technological innovations such as telemedicine or wearable devices into the actual healthcare of geriatric patients: Measures must be taken to:

- Strengthen the acceptance of the use of technologies in everyday life among geriatric patients
- Create standardization of procedures that result in the validation and official approval of digital outcomes
- Respect ethical considerations such as privacy and autonomy and ensure that *no one* is left out in our digital future of medicine—especially not geriatric patients

References

1. Nymberg VM, et al. 'Having to learn this so late in our lives…' Swedish elderly patients' beliefs, experiences, attitudes and expectations of e-health in primary health care. Scand J Prim Health Care. 2019;37:41–52.
2. Yusif S, Soar J, Hafeez-Baig A. Older people, assistive technologies, and the barriers to adoption: a systematic review. Int J Med Inform. 2016;94:112–6.
3. Chen K, Chan A. Use or non-use of Gerontechnology—a qualitative study. Int J Environ Res Public Health. 2013;10:4645–66.
4. Dorsey ER, et al. Randomized controlled clinical trial of 'virtual house calls' for Parkinson disease. JAMA Neurol. 2013;70:565–70.
5. Topol, E. The Topol review–preparing the healthcare workforce to deliver the digital future. (2019).
6. Dorsey ER, Glidden AM, Holloway MR, Birbeck GL, Schwamm LH. Teleneurology and mobile technologies: the future of neurological care. Nat Rev Neurol. 2018;14:285–97.
7. Levine SR, Gorman M. 'Telestroke': the application of telemedicine for stroke. Stroke. 1999;30:464–9.
8. Schulz R, et al. Advancing the aging and technology agenda in gerontology. Gerontologist. 2015;55:724–34.
9. Pilotto A, Boi R, Petermans J. Technology in geriatrics. Age Ageing. 2018;47:771–4.
10. Pilotto A, et al. Information and communication technology systems to improve quality of life and safety of Alzheimer's disease patients: a multicenter international survey. J Alzheimers Dis. 2011;23:131–41.
11. Van Uem JMT, et al. A viewpoint on wearable technology-enabled measurement of wellbeing and health-related quality of life in Parkinson's disease. J Parkinsons Dis. 2016;6:279–87.
12. Davis S, Roudsari A, Raworth R, Courtney KL, Mackay L. Shared decision-making using personal health record technology: a scoping review at the crossroads. J Am Med Inform Assoc. 2017;24:857–66.
13. Bolinder J, Antuna R, Geelhoed-Duijvestijn P, Kröger J, Weitgasser R. Novel glucose-sensing technology and hypoglycaemia in type 1 diabetes: a multicentre, non-masked, randomised controlled trial. Lancet. 2016;388:2254–63.
14. Park LG, et al. Mobile health intervention promoting physical activity in adults post cardiac rehabilitation: pilot randomized controlled trial. JMIR Form Res. 2021;5:e20468.
15. Maetzler W, Klucken J, Horne M. A clinical view on the development of technology-based tools in managing Parkinson's disease. Mov Disord. 2016;31:1263.
16. Maetzler W, et al. Modernizing daily function assessment in Parkinson's disease using capacity, perception, and performance measures. Mov Disord. 2021;36:76–82.
17. Warmerdam E, et al. Long-term unsupervised mobility assessment in movement disorders. Lancet Neurol. 2020;19:462–70.
18. Bloem BR, et al. ParkinsonNet: a low-cost health care innovation with a systems approach from The Netherlands. Health Aff. 2017;36:1987–96.
19. De Fauw J, et al. Clinically applicable deep learning for diagnosis and referral in retinal disease. Nat Med. 2018;24:1342–50.
20. Deuschl G, et al. The burden of neurological diseases in Europe: an analysis for the global burden of disease study 2017. Lancet Public Heal. 2020;5:e551–67.
21. Papapetropoulos S, Mitsi G, Espay AJ. Digital health revolution: is it time for affordable remote monitoring for Parkinson's disease? Front Neurol. 2015;6
22. Graham LE, et al. Telemedicine—the way ahead for medicine in the developing world. Trop Dr. 2003;33:36–8.
23. Fozard JL, Wahl HW. Age and cohort effects in gerontechnology: a reconsideration. Geron. 2012;11:10–21.
24. Chen K, Chan AHS. Gerontechnology acceptance by elderly Hong Kong Chinese: a senior technology acceptance model (STAM). Ergonomics. 2014;57:635–52.

25. Xie B. Effects of an eHealth literacy intervention for older adults. J Med Internet Res. 2011;13:e90.
26. Peek STM, et al. Factors influencing acceptance of technology for aging in place: a systematic review. Int J Med Inform. 2014;83:235–48.
27. Frennert SA, Forsberg A, Östlund B. Elderly People's perceptions of a Telehealthcare system: relative advantage, compatibility, complexity and observability. J Technol Hum Serv. 2013;31:218–37.
28. Bjering H, Curry J, Maeder A. Gerontechnology: the importance of user participation in ICT development for older adults. Stud Health Technol Inform. 2014;204:7–12.
29. Luijkx K, Peek S, Wouters E. "Grandma, you should do it—its cool" older adults and the role of family members in their acceptance of technology. Int J Environ Res Public Health. 2015;12:15470–85.
30. Manta C, Patrick-Lake B, Goldsack JC. Digital measures that Matter to patients: a framework to guide the selection and development of digital measures of health. Digit Biomarkers. 2020;4:69–77.
31. Del Din S, Kirk C, Yarnall AJ, Rochester L, Hausdorff JM. Body-worn sensors for remote monitoring of Parkinson's disease motor symptoms: vision, state of the art, and challenges ahead. J Parkinsons Dis. 2021;11:S35–47.
32. Viceconti M, et al. Toward a regulatory qualification of real-world mobility performance biomarkers in parkinson's patients using digital mobility outcomes. Sensors (Switzerland). 2020;20:1–13.
33. Fröhlich H, et al. From hype to reality: data science enabling personalized medicine. BMC Med. 2018;16:150.
34. Bateman DR, et al. Categorizing health outcomes and efficacy of mHealth apps for persons with cognitive impairment: a systematic review. J Med Internet Res. 2017;19:e301.
35. Maetzler W, Pilotto A. Digital assessment at home—mPower against Parkinson disease. Nat Rev Neurol. 2021;17:661. https://doi.org/10.1038/s41582-021-00567-9.
36. Espay AJ, et al. Technology in Parkinson's disease: challenges and opportunities. Mov Disord. 2016;31:1272–82.
37. Stephenson D, Badawy R, Mathur S, Tome M, Rochester L. Digital progression biomarkers as novel endpoints in clinical trials: a multistakeholder perspective. J Parkinsons Dis. 2021;11:S103–9.
38. Espay AJ, et al. A roadmap for implementation of patient-centered digital outcome measures in Parkinson's disease obtained using mobile health technologies. Mov Disord. 2019;34:657–63.
39. Mandl KD, Kohane IS. Time for a patient-driven health information economy? N Engl J Med. 2016;374:205–8.
40. Hansen C, Sanchez-Ferro A, Maetzler W. How mobile health technology and electronic health records will change care of patients with Parkinson's disease. J Parkinsons Dis. 2018;8:S41–5.
41. Sundgren S, Stolt M, Suhonen R. Ethical issues related to the use of gerontechnology in older people care: a scoping review. Nurs Ethics. 2020;27:88–103.
42. Landau R, Auslander GK, Werner S, Shoval N, Heinik J. Families and professional caregivers views of using advanced technology to track people with dementia. Qual Health Res. 2010;20:409–19.
43. Du Toit R, et al. A global public health perspective: facilitating access to assistive technology. Optom Vis Sci. 2018;95:883–8.
44. Matter RA, Eide AH. Access to assistive technology in two southern African countries. BMC Health Serv Res. 2018;18:792.

Technology Support to Integrated Care for the Management of Older People

3

Vincenzo De Luca, Antonio Bianco, Giovanni Tramontano, Lorenzo Mercurio, Maddalena Illario, and Guido Iaccarino

3.1 Introduction

"Integrated care" is the combined set of methods, processes, and models that seek to achieve greater efficiency and value in healthcare systems, effectively addressing fragmentation in patient services and enabling better coordinated and continuous care, particularly in older adults which present an increasing incidence of chronic diseases and complex needs. Integrated care seeks to improve the patient experience, the outcomes of care, and the effectiveness of health systems (known as the "triple aim") by linking or coordinating services and providers along the continuum of care [1]. In order for health authorities to successfully achieve this "triple aim", they should be supported in developing the organizational and technological capabilities needed to successfully implement integrated care. Integrated care reflects an organizational principle for health with the aim of improving care through better coordination of the services provided [2]. The search for methods to integrate care more effectively is a pressing political concern. The related economic burden mandates the experimentation of new forms of service provision, that are sustainable and that allow to face the new demographic challenges. The aging trends in our populations are indeed paralleled by a rise in multimorbidity and comorbidity, and

V. De Luca · L. Mercurio
Department of Public Health, Federico II University of Naples, Napoli, Italy

A. Bianco · G. Iaccarino (✉)
Interdepartmental Reserch Center on Hypertension and related conditions, Federico II University of Naples, Naples, Italy
e-mail: guiaccar@unina.it

G. Tramontano
Research and Development Unit, Federico II University Hospital, Naples, Italy

M. Illario
Department of Public Health, Federico II University of Naples, Napoli, Italy

Research and Development Unit, Federico II University Hospital, Naples, Italy a stratification of chronic diseases correlated with each other. The European societies have created many models to address integration of care, but they are divided into organizational clusters such as Health, Social Care, Housing, and others, each one organized, delivered, and recorded separately by organizations and their staff who are separately funded, managed, and regulated. As a result, patients are surrounded by uncoordinated "islands of excellence" when what is needed is coordinated care [3] (Fig. 3.1).

In order to develop effective, accessible, and resilient health systems, the European Commission declared that integration of care should take place both between different levels of healthcare (primary care, hospital care, etc.) and between health and social care, particularly with regard to elderly people or people with chronic illnesses [4].

Integrated care models have been tested in different forms in different health systems around the world [5], however, there is little evidence available. Integrated care does not lend itself easily to scientific evaluation and analysis, because it does not rely on individual interventions that can be isolated from other elements of practice. This makes the implementation of controlled studies difficult [6]. Evidence from case studies has shown that innovative care service integration approaches have led to a reduction in the number of emergency admissions as well as in the length of stay in hospital for older people [7, 8]. Analysis of good practice in the field in care integration has shown that the validity of approaches depends especially on a context-sensitive implementation strategy and a carefully tailored digital support infrastructure [9]. Home care program clearly demonstrates the importance of close integration of clinical, public health, and other services if the needs of patients with chronic conditions are to be met to a reasonable extent [10] .

Fig. 3.1 Integrated home care domains

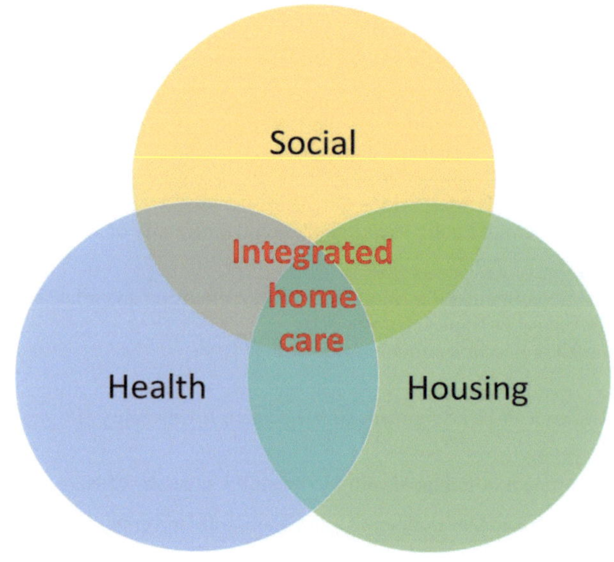

3.1.1 Technology for Integrated Care

Information and communication technologies (ICT) have often been attributed to the role of a key lever for integrated care [11]. Through its inherent functionalities, ICT generally provides the potential to facilitate information transfer, eliminate redundant paperwork, and monitor progress. Simply adding ICT to existing service delivery processes is not enough unless accompanied by a multidimensional approach that is consistent with the organizational and social context [12]. Digital solutions can contribute both to more efficient use of healthcare resources and to better targeted, more integrated, and safer healthcare [13, 14]. However, the traditional dividing lines between health and social care do not seem to have been crossed so far when it comes to implementing ICT-based services to support independent living and home care for those with chronic conditions. Most integrated services tend to be firmly situated within one or the other area of social or healthcare [15].

3.2 Health Management and Self-Monitoring

The current evolution of healthcare systems places great emphasis on patient empowerment and self-care. The chronic care model (CCM) argues that better health outcomes can be achieved with an informed and activated patient and a proactive team. It is the productive interactions between the two sides of the model that lead to better health outcomes [16]. Clinical information systems and decision support tools play a key role. The patient is supported by self-management tools activated by community resources. A proactive healthcare team that regularly communicates with self-activated patients is a desirable component of effective chronic disease management [17, 18] (Fig. 3.2).

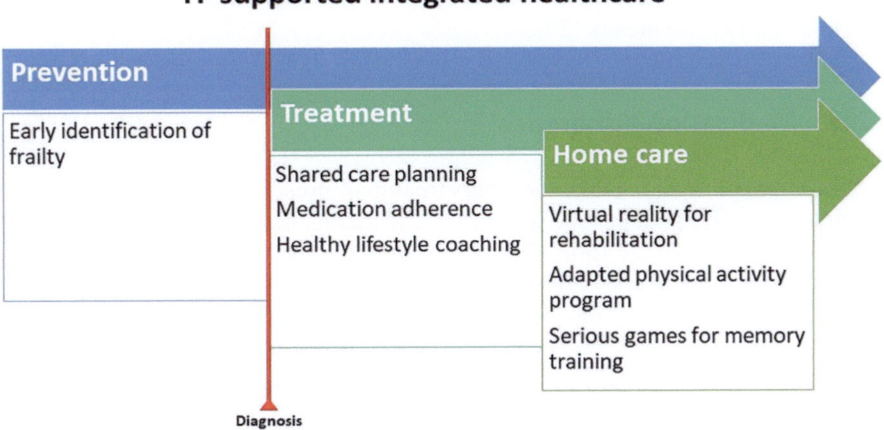

Fig. 3.2 IT-supported integrated healthcare

3.2.1 Early Identification of Frailty in the Community-Dwelling Older Adults

Early screening of frailty, based on the older adult's first contact with primary care services, community, and specialists, is pivotal to guide them to subsequent in-depth investigations with respect to the identified domains of frailty (physical, cognitive, nutritional, social). Easy to use, validated tools are available for the early identification of frailty in the over 65 population that can be used in different contexts, which can be linked to other in-depth tools for the assessment of specific dimensions [19]. ICT tools support the health professionals by linking the elements of the screening tool to further scales aimed at assessing the compromised domains, and enabling them to develop appropriate intervention strategies.

3.2.2 Shared Care Plan

The shared care plan (SCP) provides the health professionals, the patient, and other stakeholders with a common document to help manage the disease. The document provides two points of view – that of the patient and that of the professionals. The SCP represents a structured way in which patients and their doctors and other professionals can organize the management of the patient's disease. Additional actors may be involved as observers (e.g., informal caregivers, nursing assistants, and social workers) or as co-creators of the care plan (e.g., physiotherapists, nurses, or specialists). A professional acts as administrator of the care plan and allows access to other interested parties, under express consent. The SCP is an online document that can be used by the doctor during visits, or by the patient at home. The SCP allows to set and track goals, schedule events, manage alerts and notifications, medication and dosage, as well as view, generate, and export reports. The SCP is connected with medical devices that allow automatic measurement and upload of the patient's clinical parameters [20].

3.2.3 Medication Adherence

Mobile apps allow to manage the drugs treatment prescribed by professionals in a simple way. The patients access a tab of the medication, with the possibility of scheduling notices of the shots [21]. Some apps are connected with national drug nomenclatures and offer a barcode reader to access all the information of a medication. The app can be connected to the smart pillbox via Bluetooth and allows patient to program alarms with the mobile app. When it is time to take the pills, the pillbox will beep and the patient receives a notification. The smart pillbox has lights that indicate which pills to take and how many [22].

3.2.4 Healthy Lifestyle Support

Mobile apps for personalized coaching offer the opportunity for patients to be coached on physical activity, nutrition, and other lifestyles (such as smoking, drinking, drug abuse, and others) in line with personal preferences. Harmful effects (such as intolerances and unwanted food-drug interactions) can be avoided, and the patient can receive comprehensive long-term coaching. Similarly, personalized coaching solutions allow instruction in activities to prevent and avoid a sedentary lifestyle and receive useful and comprehensive long-term coaching. Lifestyles are the first level of intervention for chronic patients. Therefore, interactive coaching is more than just a list of tips as it allows to measure progress and classify a patient's behavior in order to identify possible alerts to be communicated to users. Coaching on healthy nutrition is based on the patient's meal intake data. The patient's preferences are also taken into account. The solution monitors the patient's adherence to nutritional advices. Similarly, coaching on physical activity is based on the data provided by the patient. Validated devices are used to enable the patient to record his data (Fitbit, SmartWatch, etc.). Tracking is done automatically (e.g., type of exercise, duration, distance, intensity, steps, floors, sleep, heart rate). The system continuously provides positive feedback to the patient and keeps track of goals. The system provides warnings to the patient (e.g., low daily activity or excessive sedentariness in activities of daily living).

Prescription of diet and physical activity provided by healthcare professionals are probably the most unattended medical prescriptions. ICT enables the possibility to increase this adherence, with the use of digital solutions that integrate prescription and monitoring of the activities related to these prescriptions. For instance, the dietary modules developed within the solutions DIAWATCH and DM4all for the Horizon2020 pre-commercial procurement "PROEMPOWER" [20] allowed patients to receive information regarding the daily diet and on the other hand, allowed the healthcare provider to monitor these items periodically or analyze summary reports and provide feedback to the patient during visits. Interestingly, these solutions were both considered particularly effective and usable by the patients, that reported a positive experience during the testing phase and increased ability to manage their condition.

3.2.5 Adapted Physical Activity Program

Adapted physical activity (APA) programs are personalized physical exercise programs designed for patients with chronic conditions, aimed at correcting sedentary lifestyles and subsequently preventing or mitigating frailty and disability [23]. In recent years, ICT solutions have contributed to the development of APA programs with which professionals can prescribe physical exercises and remotely monitor patient's adherence. Patients access the exercise program from home via a web-based platform interface or mobile app, which contains video tutorials of the exercises. The platform allows exchanges between patients and the physician through a dedicated communication channel. Then, data of adherence can be utilized to confirm the adoption of a healthier and more active lifestyle at the time of visit with the specialist. This platform has achieved better results when used in programs of e-rehabilitation, than standard rehabilitation programs [24].

3.2.6 Virtual Reality for Rehabilitation

A virtual reality (VR) therapy system, when combined with conventional rehabilitation, enables functional and neurological rehabilitation for older adults and persons with physical limitations [25]. The system incorporates an advanced 3D camera and a specialized computer to capture the patient's movements and allows them to interact in a virtual world. The user carries out his/her own rehabilitation program while participating in interactive games in the VR. This system has been used to address the cognitive impairment of the older patient by incorporating activities that use memory and executive function. VR helps make therapy more fun and engaging for patients and motivates them to exercise more and longer. Combining VR with natural interaction opens up new horizons and capabilities, extending the impact to intelligent monitoring and VR scenarios that have so far been limited by technological restrictions.

3.2.7 Serious Games for Memory Training

Technology-based cognitive training and rehabilitation have shown promising beneficial effects on various domains of cognition with moderate to large effect sizes [26]. Serious games are used to preserve the abilities of older adults by stimulating their brains and feelings. These games are designed to train various types of skills such as alert, selective, and focused attention, or auditory, visual, and tactile perception, or short and long-term memory. Language, imagination, and spatial-temporal orientation are considered the abilities least affected by aging, while attention, executive functions, and memory are the most relevant in relation to their sensitivity to deterioration during aging [27]. Games for older adults are designed with the need to provide simple instructions and to offer self-adjustment of the level of difficulty to avoid feelings of frustration and boredom. Additional social dynamics borrowed from games can facilitate the development of networks among patients by creating social connections and virtual communities that could be powerful clinical resources for elderly patients [28].

3.3   Housing

Ambient Assisted Living (AAL) systems improve the quality of life of patients and person with disabilities, enabling them to live healthier and more independently for longer, and supporting caregivers and medical staff in caring for them [29]. Monitoring daily activities of chronic patients and older adults, such as sleeping, walking, and bathing, are good indicators of their physical capabilities and provide important information for medical staff. Such systems are able to detect any abnormality, such as a sudden fall, and provide immediate activation. A home environment monitoring system is therefore a crucial step in future healthcare applications.

3.3.1   Home Environments Monitoring

Living environment monitoring facilitates the integration of care and the prevention of acute events that can drastically worsen the health status of older patients. It is based on the combination of components that collect information from home environment in which the older adults live (for example, smoke, water leaks, movements, etc.) and medical devices, measuring clinical parameters. An active 24/7 monitoring system provides protection to the home even when the patient is away. This is particularly important in the case of older patients who tend to lose their short-term memory, and are more likely to leave, for example, a frying pan on the cooker or an open tap in the bathroom. The monitoring module analyses the data generated by movement sensors installed in various rooms of the older adult's home and builds, over a certain period of time, a model of normal behavior for each patient living alone. Sudden and substantial changes from the normal pattern are detected and reported to the caregiver, to verify the actual occurrence of an incident before the emergency procedure is launched. The behavioral analysis and monitoring modules make use of "Nonlinear Time Series Prediction" to process the graphs generated by the motion detectors, and of neural networks to detect different patterns in the collected data. The behavioral analysis can also combine the movement pattern with other data collected by the monitoring system, such as clinical parameters, reaction times of cognitive training games, opening/closing doors or windows, etc.

3.3.2   Alert Systems

These systems may be integrated with other functionalities, also available on the smartphone, which allow monitoring the patient at home and outside, such as: the integrated panic button; the integrated fall detector based on a 3-axis motion sensor; medication reminders; the positioning and geo-referencing system. A Contact

Centre, using a web-based component, can activate and deactivate monitored persons, defining their profile, entering and modifying the rules according to which the system generates alerts for monitored patients, or subgroups of them, or even for individuals. Healthcare professionals (HCP) have access to data according to their profile and their relationship with the monitored persons. It is possible to predefine which call numbers can force hands-free communication in case of emergency. Thanks to the smartphone, the older adult may be monitored and located anywhere within the GPS and mobile phone coverage. A decision support system (DSS), operating on the basis of a set of personalized rules that depend on the specific profile of each older adults, may define under which conditions alarms or warnings should be generated, e.g., when the value of a single measurement (e.g., blood pressure or room temperature) or a combination of measurements (e.g., weight and heart rate) fall outside a predefined range or show changes in excess of a certain percentage over a predefined period of time (trends). The data collected by sensors can also be combined with information from external sources, e.g., weather forecasts. Thus, the DSS can send, for example, a message to all older adults who have already experienced an episode of hyperthermia or dehydration in the past, warning that tomorrow is expected to be a particularly hot day and therefore those people are strongly advised to stay at home during the hottest hours of the day and drink at least two liters of water. When a risk situation is detected according to the rules that have been entered into the system, the DSS is designed to activate the care pathways, customized for a given subgroup of people (e.g., people living in a specific apartment block), or even for each individual. The care pathway may vary from informing the next-door neighbor, to informing the social worker on duty or the GP that a specific intervention is needed. Messages can be sent through different means: phone call, SMS, e-mail, other text message, etc. Alarms are classified according to their severity and life or health threat character, which influence the priority and maximum delay within which the problem must be handled. DSS response protocols are based on the principle of automatic problem recognition and escalation. Thus, if the first message is not acknowledged by the receiver within a certain time (this is a configurable parameter), the next action in the escalation procedure is triggered and so on until one of the receivers confirms that it will take care of the problem. The last resort is always the transfer of the alarm to a human operator in the contact center that will take responsibility for it.

3.3.3 Domotic Services

Domotic services help the older adults to manage their home in spite of physical impairments that may progressively affect their ability to use the most common features of the home, such as windows, front door, blinds, lighting, heating, etc. All these functions can be controlled by a central, user-friendly, touchscreen-based software that runs on the fixed base unit and, at the same time, displays information about the home such as temperature and humidity. The individual wireless monitors and actuators may be easily installed in most flats and houses built in the last

50 years and using single-lock windows and doors, and provide support to older adults for their daily life. The various components can be mixed and matched according to the individual needs of each user.

The light control module allows different light sources to be controlled from a fixed or remote base unit. The door lock/unlock actuator is very similar to the radio control used to lock/unlock car doors, and works just as simply and conveniently as one of these. Access to a flat for a specific person (e.g., a cleaner or repairman) can be enabled/disabled depending on the time of day. The climate control module may help to save energy and maintain a constant room temperature. The radio-programmable wall thermostat measures the room temperature and wirelessly controls the heating via electronic radio actuators mounted on the radiators. The ventilation of a room can be controlled from a chair via the fixed base unit or be started automatically at a given time.

3.4   Social Inclusion

Social inclusion is about making all people feel included and valued in their society or community. When individuals or groups of individuals are excluded, or feel on the margins of society, there is often a direct impact on their health. Some diseases or disabilities themselves can also cause people to be excluded. Social exclusion depends on a person's or community's ability to connect with the wider society [30]. Older people are especially vulnerable to loneliness and social isolation, and this can have a serious effect on health (depression, decline in physical health, and well-being).

3.4.1   E-Inclusion Services

The inclusion services for older adults living alone are based on a videoconferencing environment which interacts with the end-users using the paradigm most familiar to the current generation of older adults, i.e., the TV set. Selecting the videoconference channel with the TV remote control, the older adult is presented with the list of correspondents he has included in his/her community and who are connected to the network. The older adult can start a videoconference by simply pressing a button on the simplified TV remote control, or can be called by one of his/her authorized correspondents. The correspondents are inserted or removed from the community at the older adult's request, avoiding making complex manipulations. The system is closed, under the control of the older adult, so that no one can intrude the privacy unless explicit invitation. In addition to the basic function of videoconferencing, the system can also provide the older adults with multimedia content such as pictures or video messages sent by family and friends, educational videos (e.g., video clips showing the functioning of the medical devices provided). The system can also be used to provide simple information services such as the local weather forecast for the next two days or special events organized by local authorities for older people [31].

3.4.2 Socially Assistive Robots

Socially Assistive Robots (SAR) designed for social interaction with humans play an important role with respect to health and psychological well-being of older adults. Robotic technologies are useful in home care for various reasons, a functional, therapeutic, and social. SARs can help the older adults with activities of daily living [32], or are more generally used for improving the psychological state and general well-being of their users [33]. SAR can be used to improve dementia patient' general sense of well-being and alleviate acute mood disorders [34]. Such robots are developed to function as an interface for older adults to digital technology, and to help increase their quality of life by providing assistance and companionship.

3.4.3 Daily Scheduler

The Daily Scheduler is a piece of software which helps the older adult to organize his/her own daily activities by showing what type of activity is scheduled for when. The Daily Scheduler is managed by the formal or informal caregiver who has responsibility for the older adult, and interacts with the diaries of the various caregivers and professionals who look after the older adult. Changes in, e.g., the time of a home visit by a nurse using an electronic diary are reflected in the schedule of the older adult. Reminders are generated to help the older adult to organize his/her routine (e.g., getting dressed to go out, take medications, etc.). The main purpose of the Daily Scheduler is to relieve the older adult from the anxiety that is typical of their age when they know that they have to do something and are afraid to forget about it.

3.4.4 Educational Items

Patients and informal caregivers, not having specific formal education, need to be provided with context-sensitive information on what to do in specific circumstances. Digital solution can support integrated home care including the possibility to send educational articles to a variety of receiving terminals such as the TV, smartphones, tablets, etc. Educational articles can be triggered by situations detected by the monitoring and alarm management services and are an integral part of integrated care pathways.

3.5 Data Sharing

3.5.1 Workflow Management

The implementation of integrated and innovative care pathways cuts the barriers between one care organization and another and activates the most appropriate resource at any given time. Considering the target population of home care services, this must be interpreted in a broad sense and self-care should include care provided

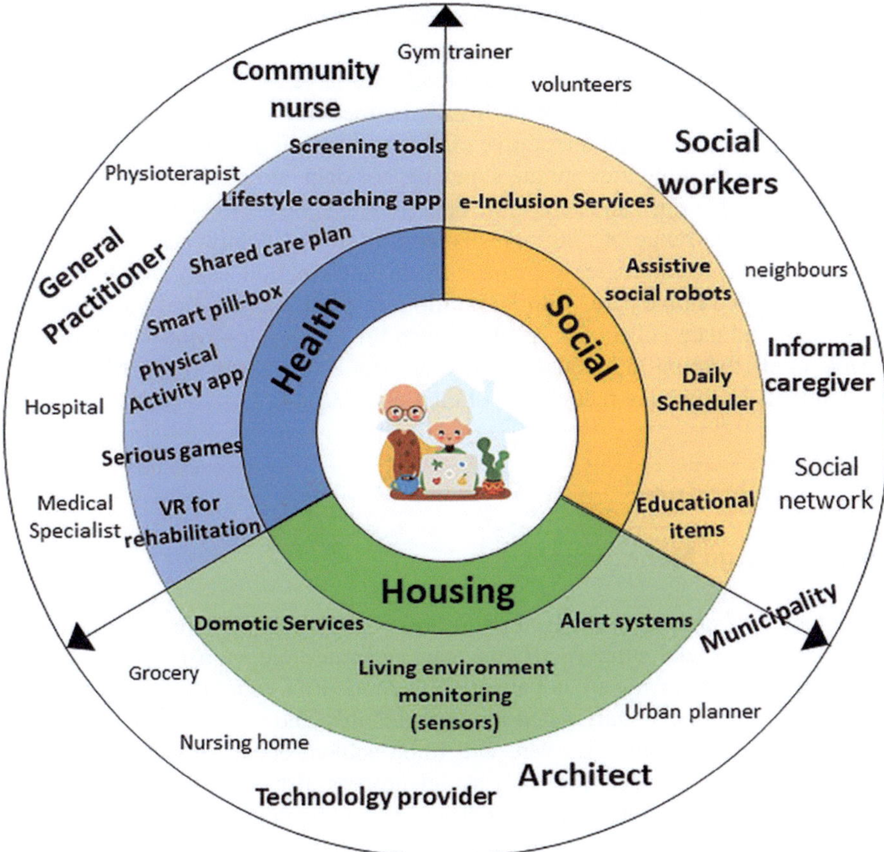

Fig. 3.3 Multi-professional framework for IT-supported home care

by community nurses, informal caregivers, social workers, gym trainers, peers organizations, charity's volunteers, etc. (Fig. 3.3).

Such integrated care pathways require the presence of a workflow management service that activates different resources when they are needed by interacting with the resource planning services of health and social care providers. Essential information about the older adults who should benefit from integrated care services is currently scattered in a large number of databases and is not even always digitized. Making this information available to social workers, health professionals, and other relevant professionals, where and when needed, represents the biggest challenge for implementing integrated home care services. The use of ICT systems to integrate services between professionals from different organizations clashes with legacy systems which are very difficult to integrate. ICT may allow for multilevel, role-based access system that takes into account the relationship between the caregiver and the care recipient, with an audit trail to ensure that authorized professionals only access personal information when they need it.

3.5.2 Interoperability and Semantic Integration

Current data resources are designed and made available as additional products and have limited access and interoperability. This does not allow full exploitation of potential results, as well as integrative efforts and long-term reusability. In the era of "Big Data", defining appropriate standards for data and metadata collections is still a challenge for open and accessible data sources. The heterogeneity of information and the wide range of ontologies is leading to the identification of Artificial Intelligence (AI) technologies to manage all this information, especially in the context of integrated home care, with its multiple devices, sensors, and tools for self-assessment and data collection. AI algorithms for the development of risk models capable of performing individual risk and staging analysis can support healthcare professionals in changing medication or care plan [35].

3.6 Governance

3.6.1 Change Management

The interaction among multi-sectoral professionals and the role played by the patient and the social support network can generate confusion in processes and resistance. Team members are not always able to identify with their profession, and this generates conflicts. Only when the team identity and the professional identity are integrated in a meaningful way will improvement occur [36]. Acceptance of technologies for integrated care is a social process, driven by inter-professional negotiations about the role and ownership of the technology and data. The strong boundaries between professions are a particularly relevant factor, especially in light of the distinct training and consideration they have for technologies [37].

3.6.2 Policy Implementation

In addition to innovative organizational model to support workflows management and collaborative service provision, regional adoption of ICT-supported integrated care requires a strategy for governance and reimbursement of ICT-supported integrated care services and continuous patient monitoring at home [38]. In Campania, Local Health Agencies and Municipalities are the "actors" of the integrated system of social-health interventions and services. The territorial districts of the Local Health Agencies are the context in which the primary care services related to the healthcare and social services are ensured, as well as the coordination with the hospitals. The Zone Plans (Piani di Zona) are the tool through which the Municipalities of the Social Territorial Cluster (Ambito Sociale Territoriale), in collaboration with the Local Health Agency, design the integrated system of interventions and social services, setting the strategic objectives, the organizational set-up, the financial and human resources to be used, the monitoring and evaluation methods. Despite the efforts for pilot experiences, the governance system of integrated care in Campania suffers from the institutional separation between social and health organizations. This siloed care provision generates fragmented services and does not allow a holistic approach for management of chronic disease in community-dwelling older adults [39].

In Catalonia, the "Integrated Attention Care Plan for health and social care (PAISS)" promotes the transformation of the model of social and healthcare to ensure integrated and people-centered care. In addition, this model guarantees that any person, at any time of life, is evaluated from a holistic perspective, promoting the maximum level of personal autonomy [40]. To this regard, a number of digital tools are already available in the region, supporting different procedures for integrated care. However, connectivity and full integration along the network of public providers is not always available. Catalonia has multi-provider model that promotes a positive "competition" that facilitates access to funds for the development of new services and quicker adoption of local solutions. On the other hand, this situation may create undesired situations of inequality of services or distribution of resources. Another negative aspect is the difficulty to scale up solutions that are successful, or the ability to guarantee interoperability and communication between providers in the network.

3.7 Conclusions

Integrated care embodies the paradigmatic shift from reactive disease management to proactive, patient-centered care, where service provision is designed and harmonized taking into account needs and preferences of patients. Implementing integrated care requires organizational efforts aimed at ensuring equity while designing integrated care plans, that take into account the peculiarities of the different settings: capacity, resources, regulatory framework, technologies. Innovative approaches imply cultural changes in the way professional roles are envisaged, and re-designing the relationships between them. The challenges lie in the educational pathways, as well as in the Life-Long-Learning opportunities that should strengthen hands-on training opportunities among peers for all involved professionals, highlighting the needs for the soft skills required by collaborative approaches to problem solving. The potential generally provided by digital technologies for the provision of integrated person-centered and coordinated care is clear. As the COVID-19 pandemic has shown, it is incorrect to expect that digital technologies will automatically lead to better care [41]. The availability of practical and secure applications is crucial to verify the usability and benefit of digital technologies in integrated care, according to the context and the needs of the target populations [11].

References

1. Berwick DM, Nolan TW, Whittington J. The triple aim: care, health, and cost. Health Aff (Millwood). 2008;27(3):759–69. https://doi.org/10.1377/hlthaff.27.3.759.
2. Shaw S, Rosen R, Rumbold B. What is integrated care? An overview of integrated care in the NHS. London: The Nuffield Trust; 2011.
3. Rigby M, Koch S, Keeling D, Hill P, Alonso A, Maeckelberghe E. Developing a new understanding of enabling health and wellbeing in Europe: harmonising health and social care

delivery and informatics support to ensure holistic care. Strasbourg, France: European Science Foundation; 2013.

4. Communication from the Commission On effective, accessible and resilient health systems COM (2014) 215 final (4.4.2014).

5. WHO. Integrated care models: an overview. WHO Regional Office for Europe; 2016.

6. WHO. Policy brief 13. How can telehealth help in the provision of integrated care? WHO Regional Office for Europe; 2010.

7. Local Government Association. The journey to integrated care: learning from seven leading localities. LGA; 2016.

8. Dorling G, Fountaine T, McKenna S, Suresh B. The evidence for integrated care. McKinsey & Company; 2015.

9. Kubitschke L, Meyer I, Müller S. Kann e-Health einen Beitrag zu verstärkter Integration von Gesundheitsdienstleistungen und verbesserter Kooperation beteiligter Akteure leisten? Erfahrungen aus europäischen Pilotprojekten. In: Brandhorst A, Hildebrandt H, Luthe E-W, editors. Kooperation und Integration–das unvollendete Projekt des Gesundheitssystems. Springer; 2017.

10. Burney LE. Community organization: an affective tool. Am J Public Health Nations Health. 1954;44(1):1–6. https://doi.org/10.2105/ajph.44.1.1.

11. Lindner S, Kubitschke L, Lionis C, Anastasaki M, Kirchmayer U, Giacomini S, De Luca V, Iaccarino G, Illario M, Maddalena A, Maritati A, Conforti D, Roba I, Musian D, Cano A, Granell M, Carriazo AM, Lama CM, Rodríguez S, Guligowska A, Kostka T, Konijnendijk A, Vitullo M, García-Rudolph A, Solana Sánchez J, Maggio M, Liotta G, Tziraki C, Roller-Wirnsberger R, on behalf of VIGOUR consortium. Can integrated care help in meeting the challenges posed on our health care systems by COVID-19? Some preliminary lessons learned from the European VIGOUR project. Int J Integr Care. 2020;20(4):4. https://doi.org/10.5334/ijic.5596.

12. Dobrow M. Caring for people with chronic conditions: a health system perspective. Int J Integr Care. 2009;9:e08.

13. OECD. Improving health sector efficiency: the role of information and communication technologies, OECD Health Policy Studies. Paris: OECD Publishing; 2010. https://doi.org/10.178 7/9789264084612-en.

14. Kim KI, Gollamudi SS, Steinhubl S. Digital technology to enable aging in place. Exp Gerontol. 2017;88:25–31. https://doi.org/10.1016/j.exger.2016.11.013.

15. Kubitschke L, Cullen K. ICT & Ageing–European study on users, market and technologies. Brussels: European Commission; 2010. Final report. http://healthliteracycentre.eu/wp-content/uploads/2015/11/ICT-and-Ageing.pdf. Accessed Feb 22, 2022

16. Stellefson M, Dipnarine K, Stopka C. The chronic care model and diabetes management in US primary care settings: a systematic review. Prev Chronic Dis. 2013;10:E26.

17. Wagner EH, Austin BT, Von Korff M. Organizing care for patients with chronic illness. Milbank Q. 1996;74(4):511–44.

18. Bodenheimer T, Wagner EH, Grumbach K. Improving primary care for patients with chronic illness. JAMA. 2002;288(14):1775–9. https://doi.org/10.1001/jama.288.14.1775.

19. Maggio M, Barbolini M, Longobucco Y, Barbieri L, Benedetti C, Bono F, Cacciapuoti I, Donatini A, Iezzi E, Papini D, Rodelli PM, Tagliaferri S, Moro ML. A novel tool for the early identification of frailty in elderly people: the application in primary care settings. J Frailty Aging. 2020;9(2):101–6.

20. De Luca V, Bozzetto L, Giglio C, Tramontano G, Chiatti C, Gonidis F, Birov S, Beyhan O, Robinson S, Sanchez-Nanclares G, López-Acuña M, Fernandes A, Triassi M, Annuzzi G, Iaccarino G, Illario M. Satisfaction, self-management and usability: assessment of two novel it solutions for type 2 diabetes patients' empowerment. In: Proceedings of the 7th International Conference on Information and Communication Technologies for Ageing Well and e-Health–ICT4AWE; 2021. p. 130–6. https://doi.org/10.5220/0010395901300136.

21. Dayer L, Heldenbrand S, Anderson P, Gubbins PO, Martin BC. Smartphone medication adherence apps: potential benefits to patients and providers. J Am Pharm Assoc. 2003;53(2):172–81. https://doi.org/10.1331/JAPhA.2013.12202.

22. Wu F, Lin Y-C, Wu Y-H. CNN-based medical device design for the smart pillbox with face recognition. In: 2020 International Conference on Culture-oriented Science & Technology (ICCST); 2020. p. 607–11. https://doi.org/10.1109/ICCST50977.2020.00125.

23. Liguori G, American College of Sports Medicine (ACSM). ACSM's Guidelines for Exercise Testing and Prescription (2021).

24. Brouns B, van Bodegom-Vos L, de Kloet AJ, Tamminga SJ, Volker G, Berger MAM, Fiocco M, Goossens PH, Vliet Vlieland TPM, Meesters JJL. Effect of a comprehensive eRehabilitation intervention alongside conventional stroke rehabilitation on disability and health-related quality of life: A pre-post comparison. J Rehabil Med. 2021;53(3):jrm00161. https://doi.org/10.2340/16501977-2785.

25. Cano Porras D, Siemonsma P, Inzelberg R, Zeilig G, Plotnik M. Advantages of virtual reality in the rehabilitation of balance and gait: systematic review. Neurology. 2018;90(22):1017–25. https://doi.org/10.1212/WNL.0000000000005603.

26. Ge S, Zhu Z, Wu B, McConnell ES. Technology-based cognitive training and rehabilitation interventions for individuals with mild cognitive impairment: a systematic review. BMC Geriatr. 2018;18(1):213. https://doi.org/10.1186/s12877-018-0893-1.

27. Solana J, Cáceres C, García-Molina A, Opisso E, Roig T, Tormos JM, Gómez EJ. Improving brain injury cognitive rehabilitation by personalized telerehabilitation services: Guttmann neuropersonal trainer. IEEE J Biomed Health Inform. 2015;19(1):124–31. https://doi.org/10.1109/JBHI.2014.2354537.

28. Ascolese A, Kiat J, Pannese L, Morganti L. Gamifying elderly care: feasibility of a digital gaming solution for active aging. Digit Med. 2016;2016(2):157–62.

29. Cicirelli G, Marani R, Petitti A, Milella A, D'Orazio T. Ambient assisted living: a review of technologies, methodologies and future perspectives for healthy aging of population. Sensors. 2021;21(10):3549. https://doi.org/10.3390/s21103549.

30. van Bergen APL, Wolf JRLM, Badou M, et al. The association between social exclusion or inclusion and health in EU and OECD countries: a systematic review. Eur J Pub Health. 2019;29(3):575–82. https://doi.org/10.1093/eurpub/cky143.

31. Xie B, Charness N, Fingerman K, Kaye J, Kim MT, Khurshid A. When going digital becomes a necessity: ensuring older adults' needs for information, services, and social inclusion during COVID-19. J Aging Soc Policy. 2020;32(4–5):460–70. https://doi.org/10.1080/08959420.2020.1771237.

32. Reiser U, Jacobs T, Arbeiter G, et al. Care-O-bot ® 3–Vision of a Robot Butler. Your Virtual Butler. 2013;7407:97–116.

33. Kanamori M, Suzuki M, Oshiro H. Pilot study on improvement of quality of life among elderly using a pet-type robot. IEEE Int Conf Robot Autom. 2003:107–12.

34. Sung HC, Chang SM, Chin MY, Lee WL. Robot-assisted therapy for improving social interactions and activity participation among institutionalized older adults: a pilot study. Asia Pac Psychiatry. 2015;7(1):1–6. https://doi.org/10.1111/appy.12131.

35. Kouroubali A, Kondylakis H, Logothetidis F, Katehakis DG. Developing an AI-enabled integrated care platform for frailty. Healthcare. 2022;10:443. https://doi.org/10.3390/healthcare10030443.

36. Cain C, Frazer F, Kilaberia T. Identity work within attempts to transform healthcare: invisible team processes. Hum Relat. 2019;72(2):370–96.

37. Korica M, Molloy E. Making sense of professional identities: stories of medical professionals and new technologies. Hum Relat. 2010;63(12):1879–901.

38. Cano I, Dueñas-Espín I, Hernandez C, et al. Protocol for regional implementation of community-based collaborative management of complex chronic patients. NPJ Prim Care Respir Med. 2017;27(1):44. https://doi.org/10.1038/s41533-017-0043-9.

39. De Luca V, Tramontano G, et al. "One health" approach for health innovation and active aging in Campania (Italy). Front Public Health. 2021;9:658959. https://doi.org/10.3389/fpubh.2021.658959.
40. Santaeugènia S, Contel JC, Amblàs J. The journey from a chronic care program as a model of vertical integration to a national integrated health and care strategy in Catalonia. In: Amelung V, Stein V, Suter E, Goodwin N, Nolte E, Balicer R, editors. Handbook integrated care. Cham: Springer; 2021. https://doi.org/10.1007/978-3-030-69262-9_67.
41. Øvretveit J. Digital technologies supporting person-centered integrated care–a perspective. Int J Integr Care. 2017;17(4):6. https://doi.org/10.5334/ijic.3051.

Technologies in Long-Term Care and Nursing Homes

4

Gubing Wang, Armagan Albayrak, Francesco Mattace-Raso, and Tischa J. M. van der Cammen

4.1 Introduction

Long-term care is defined as a variety of services designed to meet a person's health and personal care needs which help people live as independently and safely as possible when they can no longer perform everyday activities on their own [1]. Depending on the needs and social context of the patient, long-term care can be provided in different places by different kinds of formal or informal caregivers, either at home or in an institutionalised setting, which from here on we will refer to as the nursing home. In all these fields, technology has an increasing role to play.

There is an increasing body of work on the development of technologies for facilitating integrated care for older adults [2]. According to the World Health Organisation (WHO), integrated care is "a concept bringing together inputs, delivery, management, and organisation of services related to diagnosis, treatment, care, rehabilitation, and health promotion" [3]. Integrated care focuses on the integration of care for mental and physical health, the integration of healthcare and social care, and the involvement of multiple stakeholders. The principles of integrated care are holistic and comprehensive, and therefore pre-eminently useful to address the challenges of long-term care. In this chapter, we would like

G. Wang
Department of Medical and Clinical Psychology, School of Social and Behavioural Sciences, Tilburg University, Tilburg, Netherlands

A. Albayrak · T. J. M. van der Cammen (✉)
Faculty of Industrial Design Engineering, Department of Human-Centered Design, Delft University of Technology, Delft, The Netherlands
e-mail: t.j.m.vandercammen@tudelft.nl

F. Mattace-Raso
Division of Geriatrics, Department of Internal Medicine, Erasmus MC, University Medical Center Rotterdam, Rotterdam, The Netherlands

to present the two most-researched geriatric syndromes, falls and impaired cognition (commonly referred to as dementia), as examples on what could be supported by technology to achieve integrated care for older adults in long-term care settings.

4.2 Technologies in Dementia Care

The technologies recently developed in dementia care can be categorised into two groups based on their primary users, i.e., people with dementia, or caregivers. When the primary users are people with dementia, their caregivers play a facilitating role in using the technology. Within this group, the technologies developed mainly address three types of needs that people with dementia usually have, which are: *physical needs*, *social needs*, and the *needs for being independent*.

The technological interventions targeting *physical needs* can be exemplified by Virtual Reality (VR), which is used to promote physical activity or rehabilitation [4] among people with dementia; or video games to help people with dementia maintain health in general [5].

The technological interventions addressing *social needs* have a wide range, such as social robots that act as artificial companions for people with dementia [6]; or video-conferencing tools for people with dementia to maintain social connection with family and friends [7]; another example is an m-health app developed to facilitate communication between people with dementia and their caregivers and to share memories together [8].

Most technological interventions on facilitating *independence* in people with dementia aim to reduce the risk and worry when people with dementia are alone. For instance, previously, the human-centred location tracking device allows people with dementia to travel outdoors, and their caregivers will keep an eye on where they are to prevent them from getting lost [9]. This function has recently been embedded as a feature in some technologies mentioned above, another example is the reminder feature of the social robot that can help people with dementia to remember when to take their medication [10].

Some technological interventions target two or all types of the three needs that are mentioned above, i.e., physical needs, social needs, and the needs for being independent. For example, a TV-based home support offers a reminding system, cognitive stimulations, and the measurement of vital parameters for people with dementia, and helps them with video-calling with healthcare professionals, family, and friends [11]. Sometimes the kind of effect of the technology on people with dementia also depends on how the technology is used in the context. For example, when the VR technology was applied in creating a virtual group cycling experience for people with dementia, it not only promoted physical activity but also social stimulation among the participants [12].

When the primary users are the caregivers, the technological interventions are designed to support them with caring tasks. Within this group, the difference between the technologies developed for informal caregivers and that for professional caregivers is huge.

For informal caregivers, one type of technology is on providing information about the dementia condition and offering a platform for peer support. For example, OneCare is developed as a phone app to offer information about the disease, medication, outpatient consultation management and to support communications with peers [13]. Social robots have also been envisioned to support ageing-in-place for people with dementia; they can give physical and cognitive support to the informal caregivers who are often under heavy workload [10].

For professional caregivers, the technologies focus mainly on how to streamline their workflow and reduce their workload. For instance, a pain assessment app was developed to replace the pen-and-paper approach that has been used by caregivers for pain management [14].

4.2.1 Effectiveness of the Technologies in Dementia Care

Regarding the effectiveness of these technological interventions we have introduced above, only two of them have been evaluated quantitatively, i.e., the VR-based rehabilitation [4], and the pain assessment app [14]. The other studies either evaluated the effectiveness of the intervention qualitatively, evaluated parameters other than effectiveness, or only reported the design process of the intervention without evaluation. This is partly because we have selected the most recently developed technological interventions as illustrative examples in this chapter, and these interventions are in their early stage of development. Most of the studies about these interventions are formative, and summative studies are usually conducted when the researchers and stakeholders are confident about the value of the intervention after a few rounds of formative studies. Besides, in comparison to medicine, it is more costly to evaluate the effectiveness of technological interventions quantitatively. Some research projects stopped at the formative stage due to a lack of funding and support. We hope that in the near future, researchers with the same goals will get together, to collaborate, and to evaluate these early-stage interventions further. In addition, qualitative evaluations of technological interventions are gaining recognition in the medical field. Technological interventions are usually developed in an agile manner with fast iteration cycles, which means it is unlikely that the effectiveness of these technological interventions will be evaluated in the same way as new medications or traditional therapies. For example, the sample size for evaluating technological interventions is usually smaller, and it is difficult to conduct randomised controlled trials or longitudinal studies. As a good start, descriptive studies, case studies, and qualitative studies of these technological interventions have been increasingly accepted by medical journals. We posit that new evaluation methods and consensus need to be agreed upon by researchers in the fields of medicine, technology, and design for facilitating the development of these technological interventions to be efficient and effective in the future.

A summary of the technologies on dementia care that have been mentioned so far and the evidence of their effectiveness (if any) can be found in Table 4.1. The evidence is listed as bullet points under each intervention, and for qualitative evaluations the evidence consists of selected quotes from these studies, given the space limit of this chapter.

In Table 4.1, the categorisations of these interventions are based on the type of primary users and the type of care settings (i.e., home care, nursing-home care).

Table 4.1 Recent technologies for dementia care and their effectiveness categorised by primary users and care settings

		People with dementia	Caregivers
Home care		TV-based home care support [11] • Patients "liked the contact list and appreciated having a pre-view of their camera", "reported to enjoy videoconferencing with their caregivers and healthcare professionals", "enjoy cognitive exercises especially those with 'no time limit'" mHealth app [8] • "Appeared useful in stimulating memory and cognitive function, aiding communication, and providing a sense of normalcy for people living with dementia and their carers" Video-conferencing [7] • Older adults "regard video-conferencing positively, and see it as a good way of communicating with family/friends" • "Video-conferencing is an unfamiliar technology for many older residents, and practice and staff assistance are required"	OneCare [13] • No evaluation conducted Social robot [10] • Caregivers "asserted the potential of the social assistive robot to relieve care burden and envisioned it as a next-generation technology for caregivers"
Nursing home care		Virtual group cycling experience [12] • Participants "reported the virtual cycling experience to be immersive and challenging and reminisced about cycling earlier in life" • The activity manager "observed that the virtual cycling experience was an overall positive experience and emphasised benefits of safety screening and preparation prior to the activities"	Pain assessment app [14] • Frontline staff reported lower levels of workload, lower levels of emotional exhaustion, lower levels of depersonalisation
		Social robot [6] • Evaluated parameters other than effectiveness Videogame [5] • Informal and professional caregivers "perceived a self-rated improvement in the physical and cognitive resources of the person with dementia". VR-based rehabilitation [4] • "Only seven dementia patients were happy to use the VR system. The remaining reported experiencing claustrophobia and did not complete the study" • "A significant increase in the scores of the emotional state of people with dementia in pre- and post-VR exercising exposures"	

There are several differences between the technologies adopted in the home care settings and those adopted in a nursing-home care setting. In the home care setting, a person with dementia (usually in the early to moderate stages) is mainly cared for by informal caregivers; while in the nursing-home care setting, a group of people with dementia (usually in the moderate to late stages) are mainly cared for by professional caregivers.

Depending on the care settings, the functionalities of the technologies regarding people with dementia as primary users could be different. First, since most people with dementia living at home are in the early to moderate stages of dementia, they can use more advanced technologies such as a mHealth app. In contrast, the technologies deployed in the nursing homes are mainly in the form of visuals and physical robots. Besides, technologies in the nursing-home care setting usually have a feature for group activities [15], sometimes the residents can provide social company to each other when the caregivers are busy with other tasks. For the technologies regarding caregivers as primary users, as mentioned before, their functionalities differ widely between informal caregivers and professional caregivers.

It is worth mentioning that the benefits of these technologies to people with dementia and their caregivers are intertwined. To explain, when the technologies primarily address the needs of people with dementia, people with dementia will require less help as a result, which will indirectly reduce the care burden in the caregivers; when the technologies primarily address the needs of the caregivers, the workload of the caregivers will be reduced as a result, which will allow them to have more time and energy to care for people with dementia. To conclude, these technologies, no matter which primary user they target, will contribute to the well-being of both people with dementia and their formal and informal caregivers.

Most technologies target either people with dementia or caregivers or both, and a limited number of technologies also support other stakeholders in dementia care. For example. in nursing homes, caring for people with dementia is a group effort. Recently, a digital platform was developed to fill this gap [16]. Specifically, it helps the care team to keep track of the health status of the residents and of their surrounding environment by means of analysing location data collected from people with dementia and the caregivers.

4.2.2 Reflections on Technologies for Dementia Care

Technology for dementia care is a broad topic, the review provided by this chapter is by no means exhaustive. There are a few review articles about this topic recently, while from different perspectives. A recent scoping review is on the use of technologies to promote meaningful engagement for adults with dementia in residential aged care, and centres on the technologies addressing the social needs of people with dementia [17]. A recent systematic review is on electronic assistive technology within supporting living environment for people with dementia, and is more focused on the autonomous needs of people with dementia [18]. A scoping review protocol indicates that the use of touch screen tablets for supporting social connections among people with dementia will be reviewed in the near future [19].

Lastly, the ethical issues raised by these technologies should be highlighted. Ethical consideration should be an integral part of the development process of new technologies, especially when the target group consists of vulnerable people. Since people with dementia have impaired cognition, special attention should be paid to aspects of privacy, and concerns of deception. Informed consent should be considered before and during the development of the technology.

4.3   Technologies in Falls Management

We categorised the technologies developed for addressing falls into four sequential groups, which are: prevention phase (before a fall happens), detection phase (when the fall is about to happen or is happening), consequence reduction phase (when the fall just happened), and treatment phase (after the fall has happened).

A variety of technological interventions have been developed for falls prevention. Video games have been designed for encouraging older adults to do exercise [20], which is an effective way for improving one's physical health. Another example is the Intelligent walker [21], which has sensors and actuators embedded to guide people with visual impairments to navigate the surroundings. Besides, DVD videos on falls education have been distributed to older adults to increase their awareness on falls prevention and to practice the recommendations in their daily lives [22]. An augmented reality prototype has been developed to allow falls prevention experts to superimpose proposed recommendations into the home environment of the older adult [23], which helps older adults to understand these recommendations and hence eases the discussion and evaluation of these recommendations. Smart home systems have been developed for facilitating older adults with activities of daily living, and a recent smart home system can help older adults with operating lights, windows, doors, and appliances; one rationale behind these functions is that taking over these tasks could reduce the risk of falls for older adults [24]. Moreover, researchers have also deployed CCTV cameras to capture the moments of falls for understanding why people fall. One study identified that the most frequent cause of falling was incorrect weight shifting, followed by trip or stumble, hit or bump, loss of support, collapse, and lastly, slipping [25]. It has also been found that falls occur more during standing and transferring than during walking [25]. Another study uncovered that the agreement between video analysis and incident reports on the cause of imbalance and activity while falling is below 50% [26]. These findings shed light on how to design for falls prevention.

Regarding falls detection, some fall alarms have been developed to inform caregivers that a fall might happen or is happening [21]. Fall alarms can be categorised as a technology for falls detection because the caregivers need to act quickly to stop the fall from happening. The alarm is usually triggered when the person is sitting up from the chair or bed, and caregivers have reported that sometimes they do not have enough time to intervene before the fall happens. To cope with this issue, voice-recorded messages, such as "Grandpa, please get back in your chair", can be played to the older adult when the alarm is triggered. This is more informative and less frightening to older adults than the sound of an alarm. Some recent fall alarms can also be individualised based on the needs of the patient. The fall alarms are oftentimes incorporated as a feature in the smart home system as well [27].

The third category is consequence reduction, which implies how to reduce the consequence of the fall when the fall has happened. Some fall alarms are developed to inform caregivers that a fall has just happened so that the caregivers can react quickly, and the older adult will receive pain relief and treatment in time [21]. Telecare has been applied to allow older adults to reach out to healthcare professionals, their families, or friends when there is a health-related accident. For example, when one falls, this person can push a wearable emergency button to send the helping signal to the people in his or her emergency contact list [28]. A hip protector is also developed to provide cushioning and spreading the impact when the person falls, which has been found to be effective in preventing hip fracture when they are worn [29]. However, their uptake by older adults is low, the reported reasons are: mild discomfort while wearing them; difficulty in putting them on and taking them off; poor fit; forgetfulness; and perceived lack of personal risk [29].

As for treatments after falls, the physical treatments older adults receive are similar to other types of therapeutic rehabilitation; for example, an innovative prototype software tool has been developed to visualise dynamic movement data when older adults undertake activities of daily living to guide the rehabilitation process [30]. Besides, some older adults will undertake psychological therapies to overcome the fear of falling after the incident, and mixed reality has been applied to facilitate these therapies [31].

These four categories are by no means mutually exclusive. For example, when the fall alarm detects a fall is about to happen, the caregiver will be notified and try to prevent the fall from happening. Despite these overlaps, these categories provide a structure for the readers to understand and remember the variety of technologies on falls management.

4.3.1 Effectiveness of the Technologies on Falls Management

Both formative and summative evaluations have been conducted for these technologies. The summative evaluations usually report the evidence of effectiveness for these interventions. The formative evaluations usually discuss the evaluation outcome on how to develop the intervention further. A summary of the technologies on falls management that have been mentioned so far and the evidence for their effectiveness (if any) can be found in Table 4.2. The evidence (or evaluation outcome) is listed as bullet points under each intervention.

Table 4.2 Recent technologies for falls management and their effectiveness categorised by phases

Prevention phase	Video games that encourage exercise [20] • The Wii (video game platform) was perceived to be easy to use, to provide a way to socialise with peers and to give opportunities to participate in activities in a new way. Intelligent walker [21] • No evaluation reported. DVD videos for falls education [22] • Patients in the treatment group were significantly more likely to report not falling at 3 months than patients in the control group. • The number of falls was lower for the treatment group, while the difference was not statistically significant. Augmented reality for home modification [23] • The use of this tool helps older adults with understanding the benefits of home modifications for falls prevention. Smart home [24] • Those in the intervention group reported a high degree of satisfaction with the technology. Videos for falls analysis [25] • No evaluation reported.
Detection phase	Fall alarms (part of smart home) [27] • The placement and sensitivity of the fall alarms should be carefully thought through. • Some caregivers report they do not have sufficient time to prevent the fall from happening after receiving the alarm.
Consequence reduction phase	Fall alarms (part of Telecare) [28] • An automatic fall detector was useful for older people who were unable or reluctant to use a pendant alarm following a fall. Telecare [28] • Some participants felt a greater sense of security and reassurance, yet confidence levels were not increased for others. Hip protector [29] • Their uptake by older adults is low, which could be due to mild discomfort while wearing them; difficulty in putting them on and taking them off; poor fit; forgetfulness; and perceived lack of personal risk.
Treatment phase	Software for visualisation of biomechanical data [30] • No evaluation reported. Mixed reality intervention on fear of falling [31] • Mixed reality has the potential to help older users perform physical exercises that could improve their health conditions. • More research on the effect of mixed reality falls prevention interventions should be conducted with special focus given to usability issues of mixed reality.

4.3.2 Reflections on Technologies for Falls Management

There are a few review articles on the use of technology on older adult falls prevention, and the most recent scoping review examined these technologies from the perspective of occupational therapy [32]. This review indicates that multifactorial programs in occupational therapy are useful for preventing and reducing falls. This is because the factors contributing to falls are diverse and their relations are complex. A multifactorial intervention includes the complex assessment of different components for addressing falls, such as activities of daily living, fall risk, environment, education, and fear of falling. However, most of the current technologies developed for addressing falls mainly offer single-component interventions. This reveals one direction for improving these current technologies in falls, that is, integrating them carefully to form a comprehensive support from falls prevention to treatment after falls.

To do so, more evidence about the effectiveness of each technological intervention is needed. Besides, with the increasing privacy awareness and ethical concerns over the years, some of the technologies applied for falls management might not be appropriate in the future. For instance, the use of CCTV cameras might be replaced by ambient intelligent or wearable sensors for capturing the behaviours of the older adults and the context that they are in before and during a fall incident.

4.4 Acceptance of Technology in Long-Term Care

Only a fraction of the technologies developed in long-term care for older adults have been successfully implemented in a real-life context. Researchers have been investigating what are the barriers and facilitators for technology adoption for older adults and their caregivers. A few theoretical models have been proposed and applied, such as the Technology Acceptance Model [33] and the Unified Theory of Acceptance and Use of Technology [34], to develop technologies that will be accepted by users. A few common determinants shared by these models are "perceived usefulness", "perceived ease of use", and "self-efficacy with technology". The weighting of these determinants for older adults has been different from their caregivers. For instance, a study has found that older adults with less education and not familiar with the Internet have a lower acceptance towards technology while caregivers are more likely to use the technology when they think the older adults could benefit from it [34].

It is also common for older adults and their caregivers to have conflicting needs and goals. As identified during the evaluation of a smart home system for dementia care [35], the person with dementia tends to use the alarm feature often even when there are no urgent events. This feature brings a sense of safety when the person with dementia is feeling insecure while has the risk of exhausting the caregivers. These tensions need to be addressed early-on during the development of the technology.

4.5 Future Directions of Technology in Long-Term Care

4.5.1 Chatbot as the Technology Interface

We would like to highlight chatbot as one of the future directions of technology in long-term care for older adults. A chatbot is a computer program that simulates and processes human conversation to facilitate humans on interacting with digital devices [36]. The chatbots communicate with users in either a written or spoken manner and make the users feel as if they were communicating with a real person.

Chatbot can be a useful tool on delivering e-health to older adults. They are more accessible than mobile apps, robots, and voice-enabled conversational agents due to the low cost, the prevalence of smartphone usage and the familiarity with text messaging among older adults.

A chatbot has been applied to facilitate older adults with reporting symptoms who receive chemotherapy at home [37]. This frees up time of the nurses, who had to administer questionnaires on symptoms reporting. Besides, the survey compliance rate and question completion rate were very high. Moreover, some conversations between participants and chatbot revealed serious health or care plan adherence issues, which were intervened timely in this study [37]. The researchers acknowledged that the caregivers might be able to identify the same issues with the traditional approach, while the additional benefit of the chatbot is that they are able to store the conversation record over a long time and the older adults can write to the chatbot at any time. This could reduce the recall bias and might help older adults to report less severe but underreported symptoms (e.g., constipation).

Chatbots have also been developed for improving the mental health of older adults. Older adults tend to experience anxiety and depression induced by social exclusion and loneliness. One study evaluated a chatbot built for tackling this issue [36]. This chatbot encourages emotional self-disclosure, checks on sleep, general wellness, and diet, provides games, to name a few of its features. It has been found that the human-like interactions created by the chatbot make older adults feel being cared for and accompanied, and sometimes even though older adults are reluctant to use the chatbot at the beginning, they started to chat with the chatbot after the chatbot has been regularly initiating conversations for a period of time. The anxiety and depression among older adults were reduced at the end of the study. This study also generated guidelines on how to design user-friendly interfaces to reduce the technology anxiety among older adults.

Chatbots have also been developed for people with dementia and their caregivers, yet their design is in its stage of infancy. Dementia is progressive, some advanced chatbots can learn from their users and adapt themselves timely. The more personalised and evidence-based the chatbots, the more support and benefits they can provide to older adults. Like social robots, chatbots raise the same ethical concern of deception, monitoring and tracking, as well as informed consent. These issues need to be discussed with older adults at the early stage of the chatbot development process. In general, the current research on chatbots for older adults is limited, and more research needs to be done to evaluate and refine the current guidelines on designing chatbots for older adults as well.

4.5.2 Achieve the P4Healthcare Vision

The vision that healthcare should be preventative, personalised, predictive and participatory (P4Healthcare) has been proposed as a set of guiding principles with the potential for improving the current healthcare delivery [38], which we posit could be operationalised and applied for long-term care for older adults.

A systematic review indicates that the P4 principles are embraced partially and non-systematically by the current technology-based interventions focusing on cognitive impairment [39]. We postulate that integrating appropriate technologies and design approaches could lead to a systematic application of the P4 principles in long-term care for older adults.

We present below a hypothetical case on how to integrate technology and design for achieving the P4Healthcare vision. Specifically, three design approaches are explored, which are: Co-design, Behavioural Design and Data-enabled Design, each can be facilitated by technology. The application of these three design approaches is intertwined, each has its emphasis:

- Co-design helps the research team to engage users as co-designers and understand their unmet needs. Technologies such as VR help older adults and their caregivers to experience what current technologies are like and spark their creativities. Besides, with VR, they can experience the designed scenario early-on, which can help them to provide more accurate feedback regarding their attitude towards the design. Co-design mainly taps into the Participatory aspect of the P4 vision.
- Behavioural Design is based on the application of theories and models of behaviours and behavioural change to design for desired behavioural change. For example, in healthcare, Behavioural Design has guided the design of e-health interventions to promote active lifestyles among older adults. These e-health interventions could monitor the physical activities of the users with built-in sensors in their smartphones so as to evaluate if they become more physically active, hence shed light on the effectiveness of the interventions. Lifestyle has a significant influence on one's health. An active lifestyle could prevent the initiation and progression of many chronic diseases. Behavioural Design mainly contributes to the Preventative aspect of the P4 vision.
- With the surge of big data and artificial intelligence, Data-enabled Design has been applied to guide the collection, visualisation and analysis of data needed for the development and evaluation of the interventions designed. Data-enabled Design has been applied to reveal insights at both the personal level and the environmental level. At the personal level, behavioural, emotional, and experiential data about a person could be collected and analysed. At the environmental level, temperature, sound, light, and air quality data about the living environment could be collected and analysed. The integration of insights about the personal and environmental level could allow users to receive personalised, context-aware notifications and predictions. Therefore, Data-enabled Design mainly contributes to the Predictive and Personalised aspects of the P4 vision.

4.5.3 Rethinking the Functions of the Nursing Home

After summarising the latest developments in technology, we think the nursing home could play an increasing role as a centre for testing and investigating the (effectiveness and effects of) new technologies for the care of older adults. But perhaps, even more importantly—in view of the growing number of senior citizens ageing at home—we think the nursing home is ideally placed to be the community hub for the care of the older citizen, and technology will be essential to achieve this role.

We acknowledge that the long-term care industry has been encouraged to focus on supporting ageing in place or in community-based settings rather than in typical nursing homes, although the need for 24/7 nursing home care will always remain for certain patients at the end of their long-term care journey. In addition to relocating some residents who were able to receive care at home, some nursing homes have acquired home-care agencies, hospices, and assisted-living facilities [40], and in doing so, they have expanded their services so that they are equipped to offer integrated care throughout the various parts of the long-term care journey. To illustrate, when a person is admitted to a nursing home, it will help the person to adapt to this new phase of long-term care better if this person has previous experience with this nursing home, for example, this person had received home-care services from this nursing home when he or she was still living at home. Besides, the nursing home already has information about this person and his/her preferences, so is equipped to provide personalised care. In Fig. 4.1, we illustrate the connections of the nursing

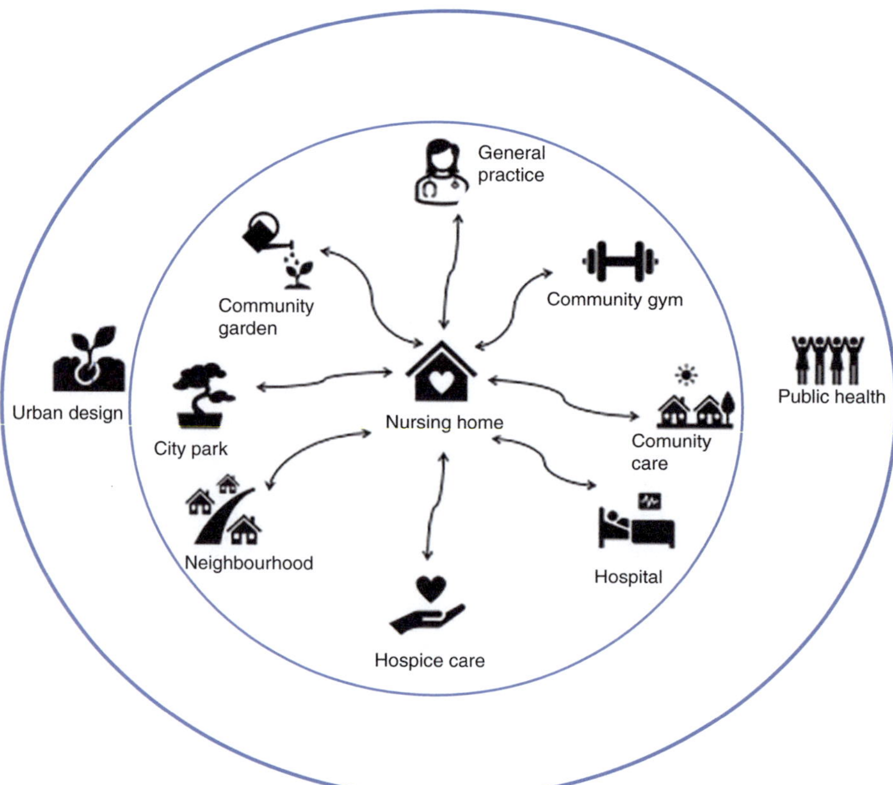

Fig. 4.1 The nursing home as the hub for elderly care where the dotted lines represent the technology-supported channels for communication and exchange of knowledge/expertise/data between the nursing home and its partners and vice versa

homes within the community, which could be both physical and digital, representing our vision of the long-term care journey.

4.6 Conclusions

In this chapter, we have discussed the role of technologies in long-term care and nursing homes, which is a broad field under development. Due to the limit of space, we have used examples to highlight the landscape of technology in long-term care for older adults, specifically focused on dementia care and falls management. The evidence of effectiveness of the technological interventions developed is limited so far, and we hope this chapter could bridge researchers from different disciplines to collaborate on improving long-term care for older adults with technology. We posit that technology is not the final solution, rather, it is a means to the end, which needs to be designed carefully to be ethical, appropriate, desirable, and sustainable.

For future directions, we see the emergence of the chatbot technology, among others; and suggest that design approaches should be applied to guide the technology development process for shaping technologies that provide long-term care to older adults that are preventative, personalised, participatory, and predictive. In the end, we encourage the potential of nursing homes to be explored further on their roles in facilitating long-term care. The readers are encouraged to explore this field with this chapter as a guide, and find more technologies, application areas and future directions.

References

1. "What Is Long-Term Care? | National Institute on Aging." https://www.nia.nih.gov/health/what-long-term-care. Accessed Aug 06 2021.
2. D. S. and E. Al. Integrated Care for Older Patients: geriatrics. In: Amelung V, Stein V, Suter E, Goodwin N, Nolte E, Balicer R, editors. Handbook integrated care. Springer International Publishing; 2021. p. 699–717.
3. WHO/Europe | Health services delivery–Integrated care models: an overview. 2016. https://www.euro.who.int/en/health-topics/Health-systems/health-services-delivery/publications/2016/integrated-care-models-an-overview-2016. Accessed Aug 06 2021.
4. Matsangidou M, et al. Dementia: i am physically fading can virtual reality help? physical training for people with dementia in confined mental health units, vol. 12188. LNCS; 2020.
5. Unbehaun D, et al. Social technology appropriation in dementia: investigating the role of caregivers in engaging people with dementia with a videogame-based training system; 2020. https://doi.org/10.1145/3313831.3376648.
6. Ke C, Lou VW-Q, Tan KC-K, Wai MY, Chan LL. Changes in technology acceptance among older people with dementia: the role of social robot engagement. Int J Med Inform. 2020;141:104241. https://doi.org/10.1016/j.ijmedinf.2020.104241.
7. Moyle W, Jones C, Murfield J, Liu F. 'For me at 90, it's going to be difficult': feasibility of using iPad video-conferencing with older adults in long-term aged care. Aging Ment Heal. 2020;24(2):349–52. https://doi.org/10.1080/13607863.2018.1525605.
8. O'Connor S. Co-designing technology with people with dementia and their carers: exploring user perspectives when co-creating a mobile health application. Int J Older People Nursing. 2020;15(3):e12288. https://doi.org/10.1111/opn.12288.
9. Robinson L, Brittain K, Lindsay S, Jackson D, Olivier P. Keeping in touch everyday (KITE) project: developing assistive technologies with people with dementia and their carers to

promote independence. Int Psychogeriatrics. 2009;21(3):494–502. https://doi.org/10.1017/S1041610209008448.

10. Arthanat S, Begum M, Gu T, LaRoche DP, Xu D, Zhang N. Caregiver perspectives on a smart home-based socially assistive robot for individuals with Alzheimer's disease and related dementia. Disabil Rehabil Assist Technol. 2020;15(7):789–98. https://doi.org/10.1080/17483107.2020.1753831.

11. Cortellessa G, et al. Co-design of a TV-based home support for early stage of dementia. J Ambient Intell Humaniz Comput. 2021;12(4):4541–58. https://doi.org/10.1007/s12652-020-01823-4.

12. D'Cunha NM, et al. Effects of a virtual group cycling experience on people living with dementia: a mixed method pilot study. Dementia. 2021;20(5):1518–35. https://doi.org/10.1177/1471301220951328.

13. Lobão MJ, et al. Solution to support informal caregivers of patients with dementia. Procedia Computer Science. 2021;181:294–301. https://doi.org/10.1016/j.procs.2021.01.149.

14. Zahid M, Gallant NL, Hadjistavropoulos T, Stroulia E. Behavioral pain assessment implementation in long-term care using a tablet app: case series and quasi-experimental design. JMIR Mhealth Uhealth. 2020;8(4):e17108. https://doi.org/10.2196/17108.

15. Anderiesen H. Playful Design for Activation: co-designing serious games for people with moderate to severe dementia to reduce apathy.," Ph.D Thesis. Delft, The Netherlands: Delft University of Technolgy; 2017.

16. Wang G, Albayrak A, Kortuem G, van der Cammen TJM. A digital platform for facilitating personalized dementia care in nursing Homes: formative evaluation study. JMIR Form Res. 2021;5(5):e25705. https://doi.org/10.2196/25705.

17. Neal I, Du Toit SHJ, Lovarini M. The use of technology to promote meaningful engagement for adults with dementia in residential aged care: a scoping review. Int Psychogeriatrics. 2020;32(8):913–35. https://doi.org/10.1017/S1041610219001388.

18. Daly Lynn J, et al. A systematic review of electronic assistive technology within supporting living environments for people with dementia. Dementia (London). 2019;18(7–8):2371–435. https://doi.org/10.1177/1471301217733649.

19. Hung L, et al. Use of touch screen tablets to support social connections and reduce responsive behaviours among people with dementia in care settings: a scoping review protocol. BMJ Open. 2019;9(11):e031653. https://doi.org/10.1136/bmjopen-2019-031653.

20. Glännfjord F, Hemmingsson H, Larsson Ranada Å. Elderly people's perceptions of using Wii sports bowling–a qualitative study. Scand J Occup Ther. 2017;24(5):329–38. https://doi.org/10.1080/11038128.2016.1267259.

21. Nelson A, et al. Technology to promote safe mobility in the elderly. Nurs Clin North Am. 2004;39(3):649–71. https://doi.org/10.1016/j.cnur.2004.05.001.

22. Potter P, Pion S, Klinkenberg D, Kuhrik M, Kuhrik N. An instructional DVD fall-prevention program for patients with cancer and family caregivers. Oncol Nurs Forum. 2014;41(5):486–94. https://doi.org/10.1188/14.ONF.486-494.

23. Lo Bianco M, Pedell S, Renda G. Augmented reality and home modifications: A tool to empower older adults in fall prevention. In: Proceedings 28th Australian Computer-Human Interaction Conference OzCHI 2016; 2016. p. 499–507. https://doi.org/10.1145/3010915.3010929.

24. Chase CA, Mann K, Wasek S, Arbesman M. Systematic review of the effect of home modification and fall prevention programs on falls and the performance of community-dwelling older adults. Am J Occup Ther. 2012;66(3):284–91. https://doi.org/10.5014/ajot.2012.005017.

25. Robinovitch SN, et al. Video capture of the circumstances of falls in elderly people residing in long-term care: an observational study. Lancet. 2013;381(9860):47–54. https://doi.org/10.1016/S0140-6736(12)61263-X.

26. Yang Y, Feldman F, Leung PM, Scott V, Robinovitch SN. Agreement between video footage and fall incident reports on the circumstances of falls in long-term care. J Am Med Dir Assoc. 2015;16(5):388–94. https://doi.org/10.1016/J.JAMDA.2014.12.003.

27. Arthanat S, Chang H, Wilcox J. Determinants of information communication and smart home automation technology adoption for aging-in-place. J Enabling Technol. 2020;14(2):73–86. https://doi.org/10.1108/JET-11-2019-0050.
28. Stewart LSP, McKinstry B. Fear of falling and the use of telecare by older people. Br J Occup Ther. 2012;75(7):304–12. https://doi.org/10.4276/030802212X13418284515758.
29. Garfinkel D, Radomislsky Z, Jamal S, Ben-Israel J. High efficacy for hip protectors in the prevention of hip fractures among elderly people with dementia. J Am Med Dir Assoc. 2008;9(5):313–8. https://doi.org/10.1016/j.jamda.2007.10.011.
30. Macdonald AS, Loudon D, Rowe PJ. Visualisation of biomechanical data to assist therapeutic rehabilitation. Gerontechnology. 2010;9(2) https://doi.org/10.4017/gt.2010.09.02.047.00.
31. Anna W, Chen A, Pripp H, Bergland A. The effect of mixed reality technologies for falls prevention among older adults: systematic review and meta-analysis. JMIR Aging. 2021;4(2):e27972. https://doi.org/10.2196/27972.
32. Del M, et al. Occupational therapy and the use of technology on older adult fall prevention: a scoping review, vol. 18; 2021. https://doi.org/10.3390/ijerph18020702.
33. Tsai T-H, Chang H-T, Chen Y-J, Chang Y-S. Determinants of user acceptance of a specific social platform for older adults: an empirical examination of user interface characteristics and behavioral intention. PLoS One. 2017;12(8):e0180102. https://doi.org/10.1371/JOURNAL.PONE.0180102.
34. de Veer AJE, Peeters JM, Brabers AE, Schellevis FG, Rademakers JJJ, Francke AL. Determinants of the intention to use e-health by community dwelling older people. BMC Health Serv Res. 2015;15(1):103. https://doi.org/10.1186/s12913-015-0765-8.
35. Wang G, Marradi C, Albayrak A, van der Cammen TJM. Co-designing with people with dementia: A scoping review of involving people with dementia in design research. Maturitas. 2019;127. Elsevier Ireland Ltd:55–63. https://doi.org/10.1016/j.maturitas.2019.06.003.
36. Ryu H, Kim S, Kim D, Han S, Lee K, Kang Y. Simple and steady interactions win the healthy mentality. Proc ACM Human-Computer Interact. 2020;4(CSCW2):1–25. https://doi.org/10.1145/3415223.
37. Piau A, Crissey R, Brechemier D, Balardy L, Nourhashemi F. A smartphone Chatbot application to optimize monitoring of older patients with cancer. Int J Med Inform. 2019;128:18–23. https://doi.org/10.1016/j.ijmedinf.2019.05.013.
38. Patou F, Maier A. Engineering value-effective healthcare solutions: a systems design perspective. In: Proceedings of the 21st International Conference on Engineering Design (ICED17), vol. 3; 2017. p. 31–41.
39. Patou F, Ciccone N, Thorpe J, Maier A. Designing P4 healthcare interventions for managing cognitive decline and dementia: where are we at? J Eng Des. 2020;2020(7):379–98. https://doi.org/10.1080/09544828.2020.1763272.
40. "Rethinking Care for Older Adults A Report on a Series of Convergence Conversations," A Report on a Series of Convergence Conversations, 2020. https://convergencepolicy.org/wp-content/uploads/2020/12/Rethinking-Care-for-Older-Adults_12-10-20.pdf. Accessed Sep 22 2021.

Part II

Specific Clinical Applications of Technologies in the Older People

Technologies and Frailty: A Multidimensional Approach

5

Alberto Cella, Marina Barbagelata, and Alberto Pilotto

5.1 Conceptual Models and Clinical Measures of Frailty

Geriatric frailty is a syndrome burdened with several negative clinical outcomes (falls, hospitalization, long-term care admission and mortality). Its early recognition can allow strategies to be put in place to prevent or contain its effects. Geriatric research in recent years has seen heated debate particularly in terms of its definition and pathophysiology: in the *Frailty Operative Definition-Consensus Conference Project* experts agreed on the importance of a more comprehensive definition of frailty that should include assessment of physical performance (gait speed and mobility), nutritional status, mental health, and cognition and that frailty can be modulated by diseases [1].

Different models of frailty, based on different theoretical constructs, capture different groups of older adults or different frailty pathways; similarly, the different assessment tools proposed for the measurement of frailty have shown a varying degree of reliability and clinical usefulness [2]. The two best-known models of frailty are the phenotype model, i.e., the physical frailty developed in the

A. Cella (✉)
Department of Primary Care, Local Health Agency, Savona, Italy
e-mail: a.cella@asl2.liguria.it

M. Barbagelata
Department of Geriatric Care, Orthogeriatrics and Rehabilitation, Galliera Hospital, Genoa, Italy

A. Pilotto
Department of Geriatric Care, Orthogeriatrics and Rehabilitation, Galliera Hospital, Genoa, Italy

Department of Interdisciplinary Medicine, "Aldo Moro" University of Bari, Bari, Italy

A. Pilotto, W. Maetzler (eds.), *Gerontechnology. A Clinical Perspective*, Practical Issues in Geriatrics, https://doi.org/10.1007/978-3-031-32246-4_5

Cardiovascular Health Study (CHS) [3] and the cumulative deficit model developed in the Canadian Study of Health and Aging (CSHA-Frailty Index) [4].

More recently, a novel conceptual model has emerged, the multidimensional model of frailty that can be better captured by the comprehensive geriatric assessment (CGA) and its derived Multidimensional Prognostic Index (MPI) [5]. This tool evaluates eight domains (Activities of Daily Living—ADL, Instrumental ADL—IADL, risk of pressure sores/mobility, cognition, nutritional status, comorbidity, polypharmacy, cohabitation status) and has been applied in different clinical settings, showing always excellent predictive accuracy of negative health outcomes [5]. Furthermore, some data seems to indicate the superiority of the MPI in predicting mortality compared to the most widespread models of physical frailty, i.e., the frailty phenotype and the cumulative deficit model [6, 7].

The problem of 'assembling' the most significant data of the domains that characterize frailty could be solved by the availability of more reliable and cheaper technologies, that could allow for an automated assessment and monitoring of all the constitutive dimensions of frailty in the daily life of older people overcoming the problem of partial and indirect evaluations as happens in a doctor's office.

5.2   Gerontechnologies and Frailty

The technologies usable in the context of digital healthcare and assistance for the elderly are very varied and have recently played a relevant role during the Covid-19 pandemic, for example, through web-based platforms, apps on mobile devices and video calls [8]. During the pandemic, some authors have also developed CGA models suitable for telemedicine programs that can be used through teleconferencing applications to evaluate the more vulnerable subjects [9]; for example, the development and implementation of a telephone-administered digital version of the MPI (TELE-MPI) for remote monitoring of community-dwelling older people could identify the frail subjects at higher risk for falls and psychotic symptoms in a home-based clinical setting [10]. The same assessment tool (TELE-MPI) made it possible to define the frailty trajectories of the elderly living in the community during 1 year of follow-up, suggesting that the negative effects of the COVID-19 pandemic were far beyond simple infection and disease, causing a significant deterioration of the multidimensional state of frailty in both infected and uninfected elderly subjects [11].

Furthermore, the widespread use of digital technologies to facilitate access to health and social care during the Covid-19 pandemic has offered a unique opportunity to better understand the usefulness and barriers and limitations of their use [12].

Information and communication technologies (ICTs) can be beneficial for older adults under many aspects: they favour direct interaction with people, contributing to the well-being and improving quality of life and social engagement. ICT use offers challenging activities that can empower individuals; many internet services can support autonomy in old age by facilitating the execution of many routine tasks through e-services (e.g., banking, shopping) and communication with social and health services.

'Internet-of-Things' (IoT) is the set of "web-enabled smart devices that use integrated systems, such as processors, sensors and communication hardware, to collect, send and act on data they acquire from their environments; the devices do most of the work without human intervention, although people can interact with them—for instance, to set them up and give them instructions or access the data" (see Chap. 1).

In a recent narrative review about wearable technologies and the role of the IoT, the authors identified different devices and different areas of application for the aged care [13]. In this study as many as 11 main areas of IoT applications have been identified in elderly healthcare: aged care monitoring, chronic disease monitoring, human activity recognition (HAR), specific clinical applications, emergency conditions, mental health, movement disorders, rehabilitation, preventive measures, accessibility to healthcare services and accessibility for caregiver. All these solutions could be applied in specific areas of healthcare and assistance for older people: ambient assisted living (AAL), monitoring health status, smart homes, fall prevention and alerts, therapeutic adherence, monitoring gait changes and physical performance, tele-rehabilitation, tele-care, tele-assistance, virtual assistive companion and robotic assistive technology. The researchers pointed out how these studies on IoT/wearable application were discussed more at a technological than a clinical level, highlighting the need for specific clinical studies, aimed not only at the effectiveness of the technologies but also at cost-benefit analyses [13].

A few years ago, a systematic review analysed the technologies used for these subjects within the following areas: prevention, care, diagnosis and treatment [14]. The authors used the following criteria: frail phenotype model for the diagnosis of physical frailty [3] and a model based on trials for the design of devices; the studies based on these models accounted for 55% and 45% of cases respectively. In the area of prevention, the results proved similar regarding the use of wireless sensors with cameras (35.71%), and KinectTM sensors (28.57%) to analyse movements and postures at risk of falling. In the area of care, the studies included in the review used various wireless motion, physiological and environmental sensors (46.15%), the so-called smart homes. In the area of treatment, the Nintendo® Wii™ console was the most used tool (37.5%) for improving balance and physical activity. The authors highlighted the need of narrowing the gap between technology, frail elderly, healthcare workers and caregivers to contribute with their different views to better target future research [14].

5.3   Clinical Studies on Technologies for Frail Older Adults

Looking at the evidence supporting the use of technology for the frail elderly, there are few clinical studies and few reviews on this topic, as proof of the poor attention to this population in the field of digital health. The main common characteristics of digital health interventions tested in clinical trials on frail people are shown in Table 5.1.

Table 5.1 Purpose, mode of delivery and content of digital health interventions in frail people (items listed in order of frequency of use in clinical trials, from N. Linn 2021—mod [15].)

Purpose	Mode of delivery	Content
• Assessing and monitoring health status • Communication • Care and support • Enhancing health status • Frailty detection • Fall prevention • Rehabilitation	• Sensor-based technologies • Other technology (including robots) • Videoconferencing • Mobile apps • Web-based technology • Game-based technology	• Feedback • Educational info/ training • Self/reporting • Reward • Goal setting

A recent review examined 105 studies that enrolled a total of 13,104 subjects described as frail, with varying degrees of cognitive ability and personal autonomy, and observed in different contexts (nearly 65% in community settings, just over 25% in clinical settings, while 7% did not report the setting); indeed, 46% of the studies on participants in need of long-term care services [15]. The classification of frailty was carried out with validated tools (mostly the frailty phenotype) in less than 50% of the studies; furthermore, the relative share of frail, pre-frail and non-frail subjects in each study sample was not always been clearly reported. The digital interventions were aimed at monitoring (43%), communication (39%), care and support (38%), assessing health status (35%) or improving health status (28%), frailty detection (29%), prevention of falls (11%) and rehabilitation (7%) [15]. The most used technologies were sensor-based technologies (56%), other technologies, such as robots and electronic pillbox (41%), video conferencing technology (17%), mobile applications (14%), technology web-based (14%) and game-based technology (6%). Regarding the outcome measured in these studies, evaluations in terms of usability and feasibility were reported in 54% of the studies, effectiveness in 30%, user experiences (e.g., satisfaction surveys) in 23%, diagnostic accuracy in 22% and cost analysis only in 7% [15].

The overall level of evidence from these studies was relatively low, given the paucity of randomized controlled trials (one exercise program based on a game system and another exercise program in a tablet and a night light to prevent falls); in some cross-sectional studies, positive results emerged in terms of assessing the frailty and risk of falling and fall detection [15].

Another recent systematic review about the use of technologies in the management of older frail people [16] confirmed that the frailty phenotype was the frailty model used by the majority of the included studies (14 out of 16). Three main classes of ICT technologies have been employed: (1) accelerometers and inertial sensors (to assess gait, balance, specific performance tasks, and movement and kinematic data); (2) dynamometer (to measure grip strength); (3) motion sensors (for the assessment of the physical activity). The included studies generally aimed at assessing frailty by using ICT technologies to sharpen gait analysis, standardize the measurement of physical activity, or integrate information from several devices to detect frailty.

ICTs have also been used to test the effects of rehabilitation interventions; in this application, multiparameter measurements derived from inertial sensors were more sensitive in detecting improvements after a physical rehabilitation programme than traditional clinical evaluation [17]. The use of a robotic platform has proved useful, through the analysis of the specific components of postural control, to identify the risk of falling after 1 year; in this way, it is possible to lay the foundations for a personalized robotic rehabilitation [18].

Some recent studies have focused in particular on the ability to refine the detection of the degree of multidimensional frailty through the use of ICT and Artificial Intelligence (AI) applications. In older patients admitted to geriatric wards the automatic calculation of the MPI on the basis of CGA data derived from the electronic clinical record (record-based MPI) accurately predicted mortality and re-admission rates in patients over the age of 75 [19]. In another study, machine learning applications were able to classify hospitalized older patients into different levels of multidimensional frailty (i.e., no frail, pre-frail or frail) and categorize their risk of mortality [20].

By contrast, very few intervention studies have implemented technological solutions in the field of frailty. In a systematic review [21] including 48 studies, only one was a Randomized Controlled Trial (RCT) specific for the frailty condition: the aim of the RCT was to evaluate the effect of a 12-month home Tele-monitoring to prevent frailty and death in older adults with clinical problems [22]. The technology used in the study was a Tele-monitoring system, consisting of a health guide placed at the patient's home along with other peripheral equipment for monitoring biometric parameters. This study showed that the home Telemonitoring did not decrease the rate of functional decline as measured by frailty status and mortality in older adults [22].

5.4   Living Labs and Multidimensional Frailty

Gerontechnology and digital automation have found a relevant field of application in the so-called Living Labs, indicating possible useful applications even for the frail elderly. The concept of Living Lab (LL) appeared in the 2000s, evolving from the definition of a particular research infrastructure (an environment that replicates a normal home in which services, automations and technologies are experimented) to that of a dynamic multi-stakeholder network aimed at fostering user-driven innovation in real-life contexts [23]. Even if the concept of LL is quite complex because it can refer to an environment, a methodology and a system, LLs are now considered one of the main actors in innovation management: the LL-based approach allows the identification of micro-level factors, related to the individual user, and macro-level factors, related to the stakeholder network existing in the ecosystem; hence a dynamic interaction between design, development and provision of services for users [23].

In this research context, the recent data from the LLs "MoDiPro" (Protected Discharge Model) and "Pro-Home Project" (co-funded by the Italian Ministry of Health) for older hospitalized patients at high risk of delayed discharge due to social and/or housing problems has shown that innovative solutions can be useful for the assessment and monitoring of elderly people through home automation, robotics, environmental solutions (RGB-D and depth cameras for body tracking) and wearable devices (smartwatches) (see Figs. 5.1 and 5.2) [24].

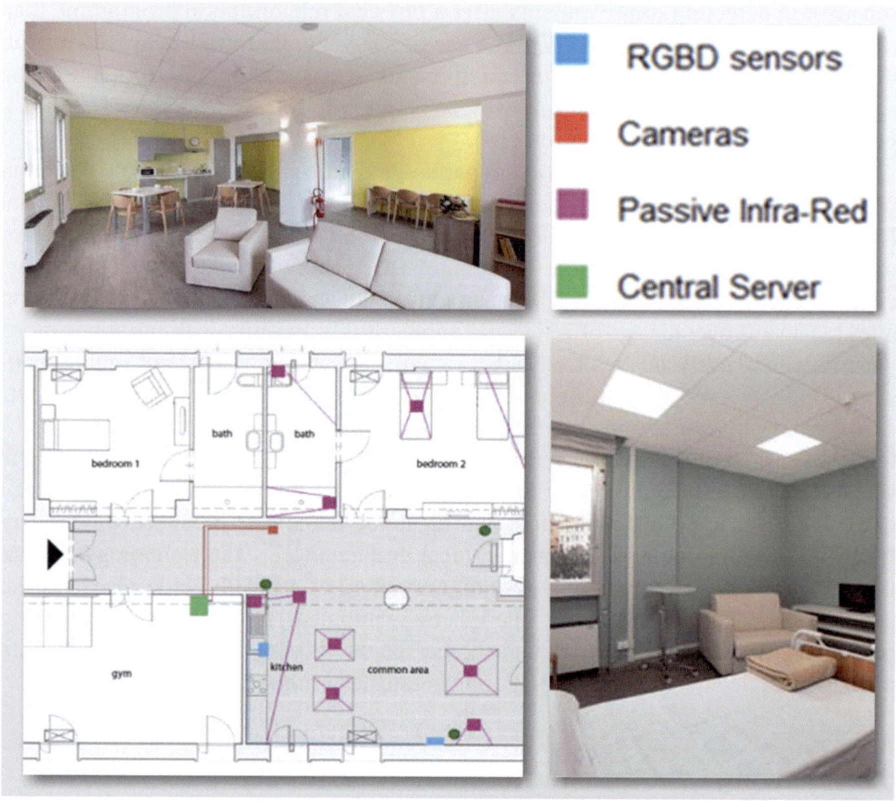

Fig. 5.1 Architectural and sensor design in the 'smart home' of the MODIPRO project [24]

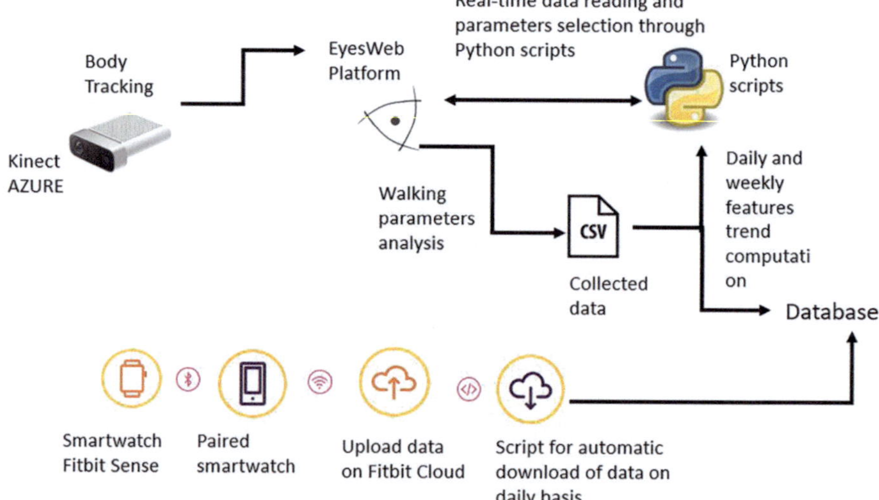

Fig. 5.2 Data flow and monitoring scheme in the Pro-Home Project [24]

Subjects admitted to the Living Labs can be assessed and monitored as regards movements, gait speed, basal and instrumental daily living activities, sleep quality and other functions (drinking, eating, taking medicines, leisure activities, etc.) but most of all as regards the degree of their multidimensional frailty [25]. In the LLs, digital technology and robotics have been combined, also to test the effects of rehabilitation interventions, demonstrating that multiparameter measurements derived from inertial sensors were more sensitive in detecting improvements after a physical rehabilitation program than traditional clinical evaluation [26]; it was also possible to calculate the individual risk of falling in an ecological context such as the home environment simulated by the LL [18].

5.5 Gerontechnology and Frail Older People with Dementia

The relationship between ageing, frailty and dementia is very complex. First, ageing is associated with both frailty and cognitive decline; second, frailty is known to be a predictor of all forms of dementia, especially in women. Despite inherent differences in ageing metrics that incorporate cognitive and physical function, they consistently capture mortality risk. The available data support the incorporation of cognitive and physical function for the stratification of mortality risk and suggest the possibility of adopting suitable metrics to grasp both the physical and cognitive dimension of frailty [27].

Data from a large epidemiological study (UK Biobank prospective cohort study) show that two parameters of the phenotypic model of frailty (low physical activity—in this study measured with an accelerometer—[28] and lower grip strength [29]) were associated with a higher risk of all-cause incident dementia, independently of major confounding factors.

Most ICT applications developed for both patients with dementia and primary caregivers are focused on in-home care and can help caregivers better manage situations in daily life and understand the disease process [30]. An aspect in which telemedicine can help in monitoring the disease over time is the evaluation of cognitive functions. Some data support the possibility of carrying out the remote administration of neuropsychological tests, particularly those that rely on verbal responses from participants [31]. Cognitive training solutions showed clear positive effects on objective and subjective cognitive functioning and promising effects on depression of subjects with cognitive impairment or dementia, while supportive web platforms for informal caregivers were indirectly beneficial for behavioural and psychological symptoms of dementia (BPSD) and were successful in increasing their self-efficacy [28]. Furthermore, a systematic review about cognitive telerehabilitation for neurodegenerative disease provides preliminary evidence suggesting that it may have comparable effects as conventional in-person cognitive rehabilitation [32].

Another relevant question is whether assistive technology (AT) can help people with dementia and their caregivers: limited evidence is available regarding the effectiveness of AT in improving the safety of demented people in the domestic setting (reducing fall-risk) and the available data are not conclusive about whether AT is effective in decreasing care home admission [33]. Moreover, there is no evidence that AT is effective in supporting people with dementia to manage their memory problems [34] or in maintaining an independent life [35].

5.6 Gerontechnology and Frail Older People Living in Aged Care Facilities

As we all know, nursing homes (NH) and other long-term care facilities constitute the care environment in which the greatest number of frail elderly subjects are found [36]. There is a growing number of technology-based interventions designed to support the health and quality of life of nursing home residents. The Covid-19 and the recommended social distancing policy have led to increased interest in relying on technology-based solutions; although these solutions have the potential to provide healthcare, there is limited evidence of the benefits and delivery options of technology-based interventions specifically designed for nursing home residents. A review of the literature on implementing health information technology (HIT) in NH found that these facilities often do not use a systematic process for HIT implementation, lack the necessary technology support and infrastructure, such as wireless connectivity, and make little investment in staff training [37]. Without an initial investment in the implementation and training of their workforce, nursing homes are unlikely to make potential HIT-related gains in productivity and quality of care support; to overcome the problem, policy makers should ensure greater incentives for preparation, infrastructure and training, with greater involvement of nursing home staff in design and implementation [35]. In this context, leadership practices that value innovation and employee empowerment appear to be the determining factor in bringing nursing homes to adapt to HIT implementation and streamline the implementation process.

5.7 The New Challenges of Gerontechnology

5.7.1 Digital Literacy

Digital literacy is one of the most important problems in the spread of gerontechnology: older age, lower education, lower income, belonging to an ethnic minority or living in a remote area are all associated with reduced access or use of eHealth resources (health information, communication with health professionals, health monitoring, use of medical records). Although the concept of eHealth literacy was introduced in 2006 [38], in most eHealth development studies digital literacy was not explicitly considered or evaluated [39]; moreover, it lacked a theoretical framework to inform eHealth planners on how to meet the needs of users, whose point of view was only marginally considered. It is clear that failure to address this problem leads to poor adoption of eHealth interventions and ineffective outcomes. As a result, older people (among other disadvantaged groups) are at risk of digital exclusion, leading to a potential widening of health inequalities. There is also a lack of adequate scientific evidence on how to assess the digital literacy of older people, the implications of digitalization for their treatment, and how healthcare professionals can benefit from this phenomenon [40]. However, a recent survey of the Italian Geriatrics Hospital and Community Society reported that there is significant interest in improving eHealth literacy in older adults and geriatric healthcare professionals [41].

5.7.2 Usability

eHealth system designers need to consider the age-related issues in cognition, perception and behaviour of geriatric patients while designing telemedicine applications and devices [42]. Indeed, the potential for e-Health to improve healthcare is largely dependent on its ease of use; for this reason, to determine the usability for any technology, rigorously developed and appropriate measures must be chosen.

The usability of technologies becomes even more complex in the case of frail elderly subjects. A population survey of people aged 65–98 living in Northern Finland showed that physical frailty was negatively associated with older people's ICT use regardless of age, education and opinions on the use of ICT, with relevant implications in the design of preventive and assistive technologies and interventions for the most compromised elderly [43].

One area that deserves specific investigation is that of consumer experience measurement tools, in order to assess whether the use of these technologies is making a measurable difference in the quality of care or patient experience [39]. Finally, it should be noted that there is currently a lack of psychometrically valid measures to assess the usability of eHealth technologies.

5.7.3 Ethical Issues

The most frequent ethical objections arise from the idea that people are, or should be, independent and self-determining. However, it has been observed that this point of view is not very applicable and useful in the debate on the use of ICT and AT for the frail elderly, especially when cognitive deficits are present: it seems more appropriate to adopt an ethical approach that considers individuals as social and reciprocal persons [44].

Two main ethical themes have been identified in a recent literature review in which surveillance and monitoring technologies were mainly investigated: (1) 'balance between the benefits of using gerontechnology and the fundamental rights of the elderly', that is, the issues of safety, privacy and autonomy; (2) "gerontechnology as a risk of insecurity for the elderly", including the fear of losing human contact and concern [45]. Respect for privacy, in particular, requires the definition of data ownership policies [42].

Finally, in times when health and social services are increasingly offered online, the digital divide may predispose people with low digital literacy and high needs for services to exclusion from them [42].

5.8   Conclusions

Important limitations emerge in the clinical research carried out so far on the use of technologies in frailty. First, most studies have focused on diagnosing frailty rather than experimenting with interventions to prevent or contain its effects. Secondly, considering the technology-based 'diagnosis' of frailty, there is no homogeneous clinical validation reference, although the adoption of the phenotypic model is prevalent. The latter model, however, explores only parameters related to physical function (exhaustion, low energy expenditure, poor grip strength, slowed walking speed) and nutritional status (unintentional weight loss), neglecting important dimensions of frailty, such as cognitive functions, socio-relational aspects, comorbidities, polypharmacy, etc. According to a comprehensive and multidimensional approach to frailty, the opportunities offered by ICT, machine learning or other aspects of AI should instead allow the exploration of all these aspects to define the most effective combination of data to identify frail people at an early stage and to monitor their changes over time [46].

We then need RCTs testing different application or models of eHealth compared to the usual care to define the best practices and which frail older subjects can be the target of ICT-based interventions able to guarantee their possibility of 'ageing-in-place', safe and with the best possible quality of life. Comparative studies on devices and different technologies in terms of usability, reliability and costs are also needed. Finally, cost-effectiveness and cost-benefit analyses will be essential in assessing the sustainability of these solutions in an ageing world with an ever-increasing number of frail people [47].

The development of innovative digital solutions must be considered with particular urgency for the frailest of the frail older subjects, i.e., the elderly population living in nursing homes as the Covid pandemic has dramatically highlighted.

References

1. Rodríguez-Mañas L, Féart C, Mann G, Viña J, Chatterji S, Chodzko-Zajko W, Gonzalez-Colaço Harmand M, Bergman H, Carcaillon L, Nicholson C, Scuteri A, Sinclair A, Pelaez M, Van der Cammen T, Beland F, Bickenbach J, Delamarche P, Ferrucci L, Fried LP, Gutiérrez-Robledo LM, Rockwood K, Rodríguez Artalejo F, Serviddio G, Vega E. FOD-CC group (Appendix 1). Searching for an operational definition of frailty: a Delphi method based consensus statement: the frailty operative definition-consensus conference project. J Gerontol A Biol Sci Med Sci. 2013;68(1):62–7. https://doi.org/10.1093/gerona/gls119.
2. Dent E, Martin FC, Bergman H, Woo J, Romero-Ortuno R, Walston JD. Management of frailty: opportunities, challenges, and future directions. Lancet. 2019;394(10206):1376–86. https://doi.org/10.1016/S0140-6736(19)31785-4.

3. Fried LP, Tangen CM, Walston J, Newman AB, Hirsch C, Gottdiener J, Seeman T, Tracy R, Kop WJ, Burke G, McBurnie MA. Cardiovascular health study collaborative research group. Frailty in older adults: evidence for a phenotype. J Gerontol A Biol Sci Med Sci. 2001;56(3):M146–56. https://doi.org/10.1093/gerona/56.3.m146.

4. Rockwood K, Song X, MacKnight C, Bergman H, Hogan DB, McDowell I, Mitnitski A. A global clinical measure of fitness and frailty in elderly people. CMAJ. 2005;173(5):489–95. https://doi.org/10.1503/cmaj.050051.

5. Pilotto A, Custodero C, Maggi S, Polidori MC, Veronese N, Ferrucci L. A multidimensional approach to frailty in older people. Ageing Res Rev. 2020;60:101047. https://doi.org/10.1016/j.arr.2020.101047. Epub 2020 Mar 21

6. Pilotto A, Rengo F, Marchionni N, Sancarlo D, Fontana A, Panza F, Ferrucci L, on behalf of the FIRI-SIGG Study group. Comparing the prognostic accuracy for all-cause mortality of the frailty instruments: a multicentre 1-year follow-up in hospitalized older patients. PLoS One. 2012;7(1):e29090 (1-9).

7. Cella A, Veronese N, Pomata M, Leslie Quispe Guerrero K, Musacchio C, Senesi B, Prete C, Tavella E, Zigoura E, Siri G, Pilotto A. Multidimensional frailty predicts mortality better than physical frailty in community-dwelling older people: a five-year longitudinal cohort study. Int J Environ Res Public Health. 2021;18(23):12435. https://doi.org/10.3390/ijerph182312435.

8. Golinelli D, Boetto E, Carullo G, Nuzzolese AG, Landini MP, Fantini MP. Adoption of digital Technologies in Health Care during the COVID-19 pandemic: systematic review of early scientific literature. J Med Internet Res. 2020;22(11):e22280. https://doi.org/10.2196/22280.

9. DiGiovanni G, Mousaw K, Lloyd T, Dukelow N, Fitzgerald B, D'Aurizio H, Loh KP, Mohile S, Ramsdale E, Maggiore R, Zittel J, Kadambi S, Magnuson A. Development of a tele-health geriatric assessment model in response to the COVID-19 pandemic. J Geriatr Oncol. 2020;11(5):761–3. https://doi.org/10.1016/j.jgo.2020.04.007. Epub 2020 Apr 17

10. Custodero C, Senesi B, Pinna A, Floris A, Vigo M, Fama M, Mastropierro V, Sabbà C, Prete C, Pilotto A. Validation and implementation of telephone-administered version of the multidimensional prognostic index (TELE-MPI) for remote monitoring of community-dwelling older adults. Aging Clin Exp Res. 2021;33(12):3363–9. https://doi.org/10.1007/s40520-021-01871-6. Epub 2021 May 18

11. Pilotto A, Custodero C, Zora S, Poli S, Senesi B, Prete C, Tavella E, Veronese N, Zini E, Torrigiani C, Sabbà C, Cella A, PRESTIGE Study Investigators. Frailty trajectories in community-dwelling older adults during COVID-19 pandemic: the PRESTIGE Study. Eur J Clin Investig. 2022;17:e13838. https://doi.org/10.1111/eci.13838.

12. Kunonga TP, Spiers GF, Beyer FR, Hanratty B, Boulton E, Hall A, Bower P, Todd C, Craig D. Effects of digital technologies on older People's access to health and social care: umbrella review. J Med Internet Res. 2021;23(11):e25887. https://doi.org/10.2196/25887.

13. Tun SYY, Madanian S, Mirza F. Internet of things (IoT) applications for elderly care: a reflective review. Aging Clin Exp Res. 2021;33(4):855–67. https://doi.org/10.1007/s40520-020-01545-9. Epub 2020 Apr 10

14. Mugueta-Aguinaga I, Garcia-Zapirain B. Is technology present in frailty? Technology a Back-up tool for dealing with frailty in the elderly: a systematic review. Aging Dis. 2017;8(2):176–95. https://doi.org/10.14336/AD.2016.0901.

15. Linn N, Goetzinger C, Regnaux JP, Schmitz S, Dessenne C, Fagherazzi G, Aguayo GA. Digital health interventions among people living with frailty: a scoping review. J Am Med Dir Assoc. 2021;22(9):1802–1812.e21. https://doi.org/10.1016/j.jamda.2021.04.012. Epub 2021 May 14

16. Gallucci A, Trimarchi PD, Abbate C, Tuena C, Pedroli E, Lattanzio F, Stramba-Badiale M, Cesari M, Giunco F. ICT technologies as new promising tools for the managing of frailty: a systematic review. Aging Clin Exp Res. 2021;33(6):1453–64. https://doi.org/10.1007/s40520-020-01626-9. Epub 2020 Jul 23

17. Ganea R, Paraschiv-Ionescu A, Büla C, Rochat S, Aminian K. Multi-parametric evaluation of sit-to-stand and stand-to-sit transitions in elderly people. Med Eng Phys. 2011;33(9):1086–93. https://doi.org/10.1016/j.medengphy.2011.04.015. Epub 2011 May 20

18. Cella A, De Luca A, Squeri V, Parodi S, Vallone F, Giorgeschi A, Senesi B, Zigoura E, Quispe Guerrero KL, Siri G, De Michieli L, Saglia J, Sanfilippo C, Pilotto A. Development and validation of a robotic multifactorial fall-risk predictive model: A one-year prospective study in community-dwelling older adults. PLoS One. 2020;15(6):e0234904.

19. Hansen TK, Shahla S, Damsgaard EM, Bossen SRL, Bruun JM, Gregersen M. Mortality and readmission risk can be predicted by the record-based Multidimensional Prognostic Index: a cohort study of medical inpatients older than 75 years. Eur Geriatr Med. 2021;12(2):253–61. https://doi.org/10.1007/s41999-021-00453-.

20. Woodman RJ, Bryant K, Sorich MJ, Pilotto A, Mangoni AA. Use of Multiprognostic index domain scores, clinical data, and machine learning to improve 12-month mortality risk prediction in older hospitalized patients: prospective cohort study. J Med Internet Res. 2021;23(6):e26139. https://doi.org/10.2196/26139.

21. Liu L, Stroulia E, Nikolaidis I, Miguel-Cruz A, Rios RA. Smart homes and home health monitoring technologies for older adults: a systematic review. Int J Med Inform. 2016;91:44–59. https://doi.org/10.1016/j.ijmedinf.2016.04.007. Epub 2016 Apr 19

22. Upatising B, Hanson GJ, Kim YL, Cha SS, Yih Y, Takahashi PY. Effects of home telemonitoring on transitions between frailty states and death for older adults: a randomized controlled trial. Int J Gen Med. 2013;6:145–51. https://doi.org/10.2147/IJGM.S40576. Epub 2013 Mar 14

23. Leminen S. Q&a. what are living labs?. Technology innovation. Manag Rev. 2015;5(9):29–35. https://doi.org/10.22215/timreview/928.

24. Patrone C, Cella C, Martini C, Pericu S, Femia R, Barla A, Porfirione C, Puntoni M, Veronese N, Odone F, Casiddu N, Rollandi GA, Verri A, Pilotto A. Development of a smart post-hospitalization facility for older people by using domotics, robotics, and automated telemonitoring. Geriatric Care. 2019;5(1) https://doi.org/10.4081/gc.2019.8122.

25. Martini C, Barla A, Odone F, Verri A, Cella A, Rollandi GA, Pilotto A. Data-driven continuous assessment of frailty in older people. Frontiers in Digit Humanities. 2018;5 https://doi.org/10.3389/fdigh.2018.00006.

26. Cella A, De Luca A, Squeri V, Parodi S, Puntoni M, Vallone F, Giorgeschi A, Garofalo V, Zigoura E, Senesi B, De Michieli L, Saglia J, Sanfilippo C, Pilotto A. Robotic balance assessment in community-dwelling older people with different grades of impairment of physical performance. Aging Clin Exp Res. 2020;32(3):491–503.

27. Cao X, Chen C, Zhang J, Xue QL, Hoogendijk EO, Liu X, Li S, Wang X, Zhu Y, Liu Z. Aging metrics incorporating cognitive and physical function capture mortality risk: results from two prospective cohort studies. BMC Geriatr. 2022;22(1):378. https://doi.org/10.1186/s12877-022-02913-y.

28. Petermann-Rocha F, Lyall DM, Gray SR, Gill JMR, Sattar N, Welsh P, Quinn TJ, Stewart W, Pell JP, Ho FK, Celis-Morales C. Dose-response association between device-measured physical activity and incident dementia: a prospective study from UK biobank. BMC Med. 2021;19(1):305. https://doi.org/10.1186/s12916-021-02172-5.

29. Esteban-Cornejo I, Ho FK, Petermann-Rocha F, Lyall DM, Martinez-Gomez D, Cabanas-Sánchez V, Ortega FB, Hillman CH, Gill JMR, Quinn TJ, Sattar N, Pell JP, Gray SR, Celis-Morales C. Handgrip strength and all-cause dementia incidence and mortality: findings from the UK biobank prospective cohort study. J Cachexia Sarcopenia Muscle. 2022;13:1514. https://doi.org/10.1002/jcsm.12857. Epub ahead of print.

30. Dequanter S, Gagnon MP, Ndiaye MA, Gorus E, Fobelets M, Giguère A, Bourbonnais A, Buyl R. The effectiveness of e-health solutions for aging with cognitive impairment: a systematic review. Gerontologist. 2021;61(7):e373–94. https://doi.org/10.1093/geront/gnaa065.

31. Brearly TW, Shura RD, Martindale SL, Lazowski RA, Luxton DD, Shenal BV, Rowland JA. Neuropsychological test administration by videoconference: a systematic review and meta-analysis. Neuropsychol Rev. 2017;27(2):174–86. https://doi.org/10.1007/s11065-017-9349-1. Epub 2017 Jun 16

32. Cotelli M, Manenti R, Brambilla M, Gobbi E, Ferrari C, Binetti G, Cappa SF. Cognitive telerehabilitation in mild cognitive impairment, Alzheimer's disease and frontotemporal

dementia: a systematic review. J Telemed Telecare. 2019;25(2):67–79. https://doi.org/10.117 7/1357633X17740390. Epub 2017 Nov 8

33. Brims L, Oliver K. Effectiveness of assistive technology in improving the safety of people with dementia: a systematic review and meta-analysis. Aging Ment Health. 2019;23(8):942–51. https://doi.org/10.1080/13607863.2018.1455805. Epub 2018 Apr 10

34. Van der Roest HG, Wenborn J, Pastink C, Dröes RM, Orrell M. Assistive technology for memory support in dementia. Cochrane Database Syst Rev. 2017;6(6):CD009627. https://doi. org/10.1002/14651858.CD009627.pub2.

35. Gathercole R, Bradley R, Harper E, Davies L, Pank L, Lam N, Davies A, Talbot E, Hooper E, Winson R, Scutt B, Montano VO, Nunn S, Lavelle G, Lariviere M, Hirani S, Brini S, Bateman A, Bentham P, Burns A, Dunk B, Forsyth K, Fox C, Henderson C, Knapp M, Leroi I, Newman S, O'Brien J, Poland F, Woolham J, Gray R, Howard R. Assistive technology and telecare to maintain independent living at home for people with dementia: the ATTILA RCT. Health Technol Assess. 2021;25(19):1–156. https://doi.org/10.3310/hta25190.

36. Veronese N, Custodero C, Cella A, Demurtas J, Zora S, Maggi S, Barbagallo M, Sabbà C, Ferrucci L, Pilotto A. Prevalence of multidimensional frailty and pre- frailty in older people in different settings: a systematic review and meta- analysis. Ageing Res Rev. 2021;72:101498. https://doi.org/10.1016/j.arr.2021.101498. Epub 2021 Oct 23

37. Ko M, Wagner L, Spetz J. Nursing home implementation of health information technology: review of the literature finds inadequate Investment in Preparation, infrastructure, and training. Inquiry. 2018;55:46958018778902. https://doi.org/10.1177/0046958018778902.

38. Norman CD, Skinner HA. eHealth literacy: essential skills for consumer health in a networked world. J Med Internet Res. 2006;8(2):e9. https://doi.org/10.2196/jmir.8.2.e9.

39. Cheng C, Beauchamp A, Elsworth GR, Osborne RH. Applying the electronic health literacy lens: systematic review of electronic health interventions targeted at socially disadvantaged groups. J Med Internet Res. 2020;22(8):e18476. https://doi.org/10.2196/18476.

40. Oh SS, Kim KA, Kim M, Oh J, Chu SH, Choi J. Measurement of digital literacy among older adults: systematic review. J Med Internet Res. 2021;23(2):e26145. https://doi. org/10.2196/26145. Erratum in: J Med Internet Res. 2021 Mar 3;23(3):e28211. Erratum in: J Med Internet Res 2021 Jun 15;23(6):e30828

41. Cella A, Volta E, Demurtas J, Zaccaria R, Ceci M, Pilotto A, Boccardi V, Castagna A, Custodero C, Vetta F, Barbagelata M, Veronese N, Pilotto A. The use of e-health and digital technologies in the Italian geriatric practice: a survey of the Italian geriatric society (SIGOT). Geriatric Care. 2021;7:10301. https://doi.org/10.4081/gc.2021.10301.

42. Narasimha S, Madathil KC, Agnisarman S, Rogers H, Welch B, Ashok A, Nair A, McElligott J. Designing telemedicine systems for geriatric patients: a review of the usability studies. Telemed J E Health. 2017;23(6):459–72. https://doi.org/10.1089/tmj.2016.0178. Epub 2016 Nov 22

43. Keranen NS, Kangas M, Immonen M, et al. Use of information and communication technologies among older people with and without frailty: a population-based survey. J Med Internet Res. 2017;19:e29. https://doi.org/10.2196/jmir.5507.

44. Zwijsen SA, Niemeijer AR, Hertogh CM. Ethics of using assistive technology in the care for community-dwelling elderly people: an overview of the literature. Aging Ment Health. 2011;15(4):419–27. https://doi.org/10.1080/13607863.2010.543662.

45. Sundgren S, Stolt M, Suhonen R. Ethical issues related to the use of gerontechnology in older people care: a scoping review. Nurs Ethics. 2020;27(1):88–103. https://doi. org/10.1177/0969733019845132. Epub 2019 May 21

46. Zampino M, Polidori MC, Ferrucci L, O'Neill D, Pilotto A, Gogol M, Rubenstein L. Biomarkers of aging in real life: three questions on aging and the comprehensive geriatric assessment. Geroscience. 2022;7:1–12. https://doi.org/10.1007/s11357-022-00613-4.

47. Pilotto A, Boi R, Petermans J. Technology in geriatrics. Age Ageing. 2018;47:771–4.

Technologies in Mobility Disorders

6

Andrea Pilotto, Cinzia Zatti, Alessandro Padovani,
and Walter Maetzler

6.1 Mobility Alterations in Normal Aging

Mobility is defined as the ability to independently move around in the environment; it is a strong prognostic marker for disability and mortality in the general population, and it is a key contributor to quality of life, especially in older age. The digital assessment of mobility has been recently recognized as pivotal endpoint for pharmacological and non-pharmacological interventions [1]. The normal aging process has been associated with several changes in mobility, including the global speed and ability to move but also specific modifications of gait and balance, two of the most basic aspects of mobility [2].

Two abilities are essential to walking: (i) locomotion, i.e., the ability to initiate and to maintain rhythmic stepping and (ii) balance, that is the ability to assume the upright posture and to maintain it in response to changes required by walking. These are separate but interrelated components of gait [2]. Walking is a learned activity acquired during the first year(s) of life and refined until the age of seven. The walking pattern and the gait parameters remain then stable during the entire adulthood until old ages when significant changes of gait and balance occur and age-related diseases can also occur [2, 3]. Several components of gait have been demonstrated

A. Pilotto (✉) · C. Zatti · A. Padovani
Department of Clinical and Experimental Sciences, Neurology Unit, University of Brescia, Brescia, Italy

Laboratory of Digital Neurology and Biosensors, University of Brescia, Brescia, Italy

Department of continuity of care and frailty, Neurology Unit, ASST Spedali Civili of Brescia, Brescia, Italy
e-mail: andrea.pilotto@unibs.it

W. Maetzler
Department of Neurology, University Hospital Schleswig-Holstein and Kiel University, Kiel, Germany

to change with these diseases, including gait velocity, gait phases, walking posture, joint motion, and step length [4]. The reasons are heterogeneous and include diminished range of motion, reduced cerebral and vestibular function, reduced visual acuity, diminished cardiopulmonary function, and reduced muscle strength [5].

6.1.1 Gait Pattern Changes in Normal Ageing

Decreased walking speed is the most consistent change in the elderly, with a reduction by about 1% per year from the age of 60 years onwards. As already mentioned above, walking speed is an important prognostic indicator of general health and thus received much attention in translational research even before a systematic use of digital technology for the assessment of gait has been possible [5].

Classically, the gait cycle can be measured from one to the subsequent strike of the same foot. A single gait cycle can be subdivided into two phases, namely stance phase—the time that a foot is on the ground, and swing phase—the time that the foot is in the air. When both feet are simultaneously in the stance phase, this is called the double limb support phase (normally about 20% of the gait cycle). When only one foot is in the support phase, one speaks of the single limb support phase. Running is defined as having 0% double limb support phase, which differentiates it from walking (>0% double limb support phase during the gait cycle). During normal aging we usually observe a slightly increased duration of the global gait cycle—especially of the double limb support phases—necessary for increase of stability.

6.1.2 Balance Alterations in Normal Ageing

The ability to stand and maintain posture strongly depends on an effective interaction between the center of mass and the base of support [6]. Aging leads to an alteration of this interaction between the center of mass and the base of support. The posture in the elderly is usually characterized by thoracic kyphosis and loss of lumbar lordosis. This often leads to an increased area of the base of support, modest knee flexion, and forward inclination of the trunk. The postural stability thus diminishes, which is further influenced by deteriorating neural, sensory, and musculoskeletal systems [6–8]. Moreover, there is often an increase in the hip flexion angle to compensate for these changes.

Due to these changes in mobility and equilibrium, many elderlies have a greater risk of falls.

Different explanations are proposed for these changes: on one side, if balance, the ability to control the center of mass during movement, is impaired, older persons may shorten single support time to reduce instability; on the other side, muscle weakness may decrease power reducing velocity and shorten step length [5, 9–11]. Other alterations that can occur with increasing age are increased stiffness and tremor. The mechanistic basis for these signs is still not well understood, but it seems to be multifactorial, with factors including an age-associated decline in dopaminergic nigrostriatal activity, and the accumulation of vascular pathology in the brain [12].

Impaired gait and balance changes, rigidity, bradykinesia, and tremor are defined as mild Parkinsonian signs (MPS), which can occur regularly in the elderly without having a "real" neurological diagnosis [12]. However, MPS are associated with an increased risk of developing neurodegenerative disorders, namely Parkinson's disease (PD) and Alzheimer's disease (AD).

6.1.3 Mobility Alterations in Common Diseases of the Elderly

Several age-related pathological conditions, including frailty, lead to dysfunctions of gait and other components of movement, and, consequently, to reduced general mobility. For example, heart failure and pulmonary problems can impact general muscle power and energy. In these conditions, decreased gait speed probably represents one of the most important prognostic parameters for (increased) morbidity and mortality. Other examples are neurological disorders that are highly prevalent in the elderly—including both central and peripheral nervous system diseases. These diseases usually present a set of different signs and symptoms—most of them shared between different disorders, whereas some specific features and gait alterations are specific for some conditions. Step time asymmetry, for example, is an important element suggestive for the presence of a pathological alteration of gait. However, this sign is unspecific, as it can be present in Parkinson's disease but also in an asymmetric paresis or in neuromuscular disorders and orthopedic conditions.

Other parameters of gait often affected by neurological disorders are gait speed and step length. This makes it difficult to define a cut-off between physiological and pathological states. For gait speed, however, some rough cut-offs have been proposed: <1 m/s is considered abnormal [7, 13], <0.8 m/s is associated with limited ambulatory capacity, and <0.4 m/s is associated with dependency in ADL [1, 14]. These cut-offs are important as prognostic markers in elderly persons, as they seem relevantly associated with disability and frailty.

6.1.4 Neurodegenerative Conditions: Parkinsonism and Cognitive Disorders

The evaluation of mobility is pivotal for the diagnosis of parkinsonism- which is clinically defined by bradykinesia, combined with either rigidity or tremor. Parkinsonism is almost always associated with gait impairment. Parkinson's disease (PD) is the most common form of parkinsonism, affecting about 1% of people aged >60 years of age. Mobility evaluation is central for the diagnosis, monitoring, and prognosis of PD patients. Nigrostriatal dopamine depletion is the core pathophysiological finding of PD and dopaminergic treatment is pivotal for improving motor

Table 6.1 Typical gait changes in common geriatric syndromes and disorders

Limp or antalgic gait	Due to inflammatory muscular or skeletal diseases, such as arthritis or due to traumas. Characterized by lifting and lowering the foot with ankle fixed.
Hemiparetic gait	Due to spasticity, a semicircular outward movement can often be observed during the swing phase of the affected leg. In addition, there is often paresis of the distal leg muscles with foot drop.
Stepping walk	Seen in patients with weakness of foot dorsiflexion, e.g., due to herniated disc L5 or paresis of the peroneal nerve. Patients lift the leg particularly in the knee joint so that the foot does not drag on the floor.
Ataxic gait	Most commonly seen in cerebellar disease, but also in diseases with severe involvement of the sensory nerves. Patients show wide-based, irregular, and arrhythmic gait. Even while standing still, the patient's body may swagger back and forth and from side to side.
Parkinsonian gait	Presents most often slow and small steps. Patient may have difficulties initiating steps, and problems stopping a walk thereby even increasing step frequency (festination; often followed by freezing of gait episodes).
Magnetic gait	Typically seen in Normal Pressure Hydrocephalus. During the swing phase, the leg is always relatively close to the ground, which has led to the term "magnetic gait".
"Exhausted" gait	Associated with decreased velocity of gait and increased risk of falling, e.g., due to loss of muscle strength and increased (physical) fatigue. Can be observed (especially in advanced stages of) cardiovascular and respiratory disorders

performance, including mobility. Other forms of Parkinsonism are atypical Parkinsonian disorders, including progressive supranuclear palsy and multisystem atrophy among others. These diseases are classically characterized by even more severe affection of mobility, as can be observed in PD. Unfortunately, response to dopaminergic treatment is often reduced or even not observable.

The diagnosis of PD and other Parkinsonian disorders is still based on clinical diagnostic criteria, with or without dopaminergic imaging. Implementation of mobile health technology can improve the diagnostic process and add important insights into the pathophysiology but also measure the response to pharmacological and non-pharmacological treatment at different disease stages.

Alterations of gait and mobility are observable also in other neurological disorders and conditions that are age-associated and often highly prevalent in geriatric patients. Some typical examples are shown in Table 6.1.

6.2 Role of Mobile Health Technologies in Identifying Gait and Mobility Alterations

Mobile health technologies can support clinical assessment, or even overcome at least some limits of clinical assessment by providing quantitative data from a standard assessment of gait, turning, and further mobility aspects. Lots of different technologies, able to target different gait parameters, have been proposed.

A digital analysis of gait enables the quantification of the different phases of gait [15–17]. The parameters most commonly evaluated in a standard gait analyses are

Table 6.2 Mobile health technology parameters

Time Parameters:
– **Step time**: Time between heel strike of one leg and heel strike of the contralateral leg.
– **Stride time**: Time between two consecutive heel strikes / toe offs of the same foot.
– **Stance time**: Time during which one leg and foot are bearing most or all of the body weight.
– **Swing time**: Time during which the foot is not touching the ground.
– **Double limb support phase**: Phase in which both feet are in contact with the floor at the same time.
Step Length: Distance between the point of initial contact of one foot and the point of initial contact of the opposite foot.
Variability: Fluctuations of gait measured between steps
Asymmetry: Difference between right and left side
Balance Parameters:
– **Antero-posterior and latero-lateral acceleration**
– **Surface**
Turning Parameters:
– **Angle of turn**
– **Velocity of turn**

gait speed, total step time, time of the stance and swing phases, double limb support, and the variability between the different gait cycles. Even space characteristic can be evaluated, in particular step length. Other gait parameters frequently evaluated are asymmetry and variability. Another interesting component of gait, which can be evaluated from digital health technology, is turning. Turning requires a more complex synchronization of the different components of gait, compared to straight walking. Altered turning has been associated with freezing and hesitations in Parkinsonian disorders, and with increased risk of falls in the elderly in general. Table 6.2 gives an overview of regularly extracted parameters from digital technologies.

6.2.1 Different Instruments and Technology for Evaluating Gait and Mobility

The gold standard of the analyses of movement still relies on 3D motion capture systems, which consists of high-quality cameras, and force plates. These devices are validated for specific tasks and provide quantitative, granular and objective gait and balance parameters for adequate evaluation. With these parameters one can evaluate different positions of the limbs in the space in high time and space resolutions, which allows to draw—at least cautious—supportive conclusions concerning diagnosis, course, and treatment response of/within a disease [18].

These assessments are currently only applied in specific mobility labs, as they are expensive, and require space and experienced personnel [18]. Moreover, these assessments allow, per definition, only an assessment under stationary conditions ("supervised assessment"). For several diseases, especially for Parkinsonism, the supervised evaluation is however reductive, since the patient is influenced by the presence of an observer and the performance is altered. Moreover, the evaluation is time limited, confined to at most some hours, usually during the day and at specific hours. As physical performance is depending on the local environment of the person and is also time-dependent, the collection of mobility parameters in the real life over longer time periods may add relevant information to clinical assessment and management.

In the last decade mobile health technologies have been developed to allow such real-life measurements. Mobile health technologies include wearable or portable devices but also digital application, body-worn or even consumer-market (e.g., smartphone) devices [19]. These technologies are less expensive than gold standard assessment machines as mentioned above, and they do not need specific space and dedicated staff. Another advantage of these devices is the possibility to register potentially unlimited amount of data in different times during the day, week, month, and year. In summary, patients can be evaluated with such technology in their normal life, removing also the influence of an external observer on data production and collection. From a research point of view there is an additional advantage: increased temporal and spatial resolution reduces the sample size required to evaluate the effect of therapeutic strategies [18–21].

Another important advantage of mobile health technology is the general increase of devices that allow data collection, e.g., by using also commercially available devices for the collection of unsupervised data [20]. The large diffusion of smartwatches and devices registering physical activity already enables their use for evaluating basic movements and changes in mobility. In the next future, such devices might be used as screening tools to catch people deserving specific medical attention in relation to neurological and neuromuscular diseases or prognostic tools for elderly people. The next section will discuss these different aspects that can be addressed with mobile health technology in more detail.

6.3 Role of Mobile Health Technology in Mobility Disorders

Mobile health technologies can provide at least additional, complementary information concerning the evaluation of age-related diseases. This can refer to diagnosis, prognosis, and evaluation of treatment response.

6.3.1 Mobile Health Technology as Diagnostic Tools

Mobile health technologies, including both device-based clinical tests conducted in a supervised environment by the clinical professional team, and those that are self-administered by patients, can improve sensitivity, accuracy, and reproducibility of diagnoses in age-related diseases, capturing the full complexity of motor and non-motor features [22]. They may even allow an earlier diagnosis, and detect occult diseases [23]. In addition, mobile health technologies can help in differential diagnosis [24]. Smartphones and smartwatches could soon be used as screening tools to identify people deserving more specific and more exhaustive assessment [21]. One of the most studied disorders in this respect is PD, as subtle mobility changes have been shown to appear years before the clinical diagnosis. From the patients' point of view, mobile health technologies can be an instrument to engage them and to enable remote monitoring, reducing the need of outpatient visits saving time and money without reducing the quality of care, and, consecutively, leading to a real democratization of health. Moreover, the use of home monitoring can facilitate adherence to trials [19].

However, some hurdles have to be overcome before mobile health technologies can be used on large scale in clinical management of age-related disorders and in the development of new treatments. First and foremost, a consensus on the type and the scope of measures is needed [24]. One particular shortcoming in current research with mobile health technologies is that often these devices are developed to target specific aspects of a disease, without having the global picture and without considering the patients' needs [20]. For example, the evaluation of finger tapping through specific devices can be useful in research and for the diagnosis of a specific disease, but is of low interest in the long-term monitoring and in the evaluation of disabilities [21]. Moreover, the different sensors reveal usually low compatibility between each other, preventing the possibility of comparing data across different devices, studies, and datasets.

Another hurdle is that monitoring patients in their ecological environment makes interpretation of data more complex: for example, if a device and an algorithm find that a person showed slowness of movement during a specific time of a day, interpretation of this finding may still be challenging. This person may indeed have had suffered from a medication off phase as part of their fluctuations in the frame of dopaminergic treatment. However, it may have been due to fatigue or fear of falling [21]. Therefore, removing noise out of the data is essential. Not surprisingly only 25% of all trials currently performed in this area use mobile health technologies in an ecological environment [19]. This may also be explained, at least partly, by the lack of regulatory approval of these devices [23].

A fundamental aspect for the successful future development of the field toward clinical applicability is thus to define useful and generally acceptable standards and systems. The CTTI recommendations may be an important first step in this direction [25, 26].

6.4   Parkinson's Disease as Paradigm of Mobility Disorder in the Elderly

PD is one of the most important diseases for the application of mobile health technologies, as mobility limitations occur early in the course of the disease, can be treated with medication and allied health, and progress during the course of the disease. Several studies showed that PD patients present with reduced gait velocity, reduced step length, increased double limb support time and decreased single support time, and often with festination. Some of these gait alterations may be present already in the prodromal phases of the disease. Moreover, several studies showed already the applicability and value of mobile health technologies in evaluating the response to pharmacological and non-pharmacological treatment strategies. During early phases of PD, dopaminergic treatment is highly efficacious for gait alterations, bradykinesia, and rigidity. During the advanced phases of the disease, some patients can develop an abnormal response to dopaminergic treatment with ON and OFF phases during the so-called motor fluctuations. OFF periods are those parts of the day in which patients manifest with particularly severe PD symptoms. On the contrary, ON periods refer to the time in which patients regain movement control and the only appreciable movement alteration can be dyskinesia [27]. Several studies evaluated mobile health technologies for the detection of changes of mobility between ON and OFF phases—in order to use mobile health technologies as monitoring tools for treatment in addition to commonly used diaries [28].

Specific mobility alterations can also occur, such as freezing of gait, that is a disabling phenomenon characterized by brief episodes of inability to step or by extremely short steps that typically occur on initiating gait or on turning while walking [29].

6.4.1 Use of Mobile Health Technology in Trials and as Target of Treatment

Currently, the most-often used instruments for PD assessment are the Movement Disorder Society-sponsored version of the Unified Parkinson's disease rating scale (MDS-UPDRS), to evaluate the presence, severity, and progression of PD symptoms, and the Hoehn and Yahr scale to evaluate disease progression [18, 30, 31]. Levodopa treatment appears to improve gait and balance parameters, however not all gait and balance parameters seem to be dopamine-responsive [23]. Therefore, clinicians and researchers are moving from single parameters of the movement to more complex, even multi-component parameters to measure mobility, as these may also be more related to quality of life [1].

In summary, technology is already very important for measuring mobility and its limitations, e.g., due to age-associated diseases. Furthermore, it can be assumed that this implementation of technology, especially mobile health technologies, for diagnostics as well as determination of progression and treatment response will continue to increase in the course of the next few years. This is primarily due to the fact that these devices make it possible for the first time to record objective and detailed parameters on real-life mobility.

References

1. Simon U, Jaeger SU, Wohlrab M, Schoene D, et al. Mobility endpoints in marketing authorisation of drugs: what gets the European medicines agency moving? Age Ageing. 2022;51(1):afab242. https://doi.org/10.1093/ageing/afab242.
2. Nutt JG, Marsden CD, Thompson PD. Human walking and higher-level gait disorders, particularly in the elderly. Neurology. 1993;43(2):268–79.

3. Paróczai R, Bejek Z, Illyés Á. Kinematic and kinetic parameters of healthy elderly people. Periodica Polytechnica Mechanical Engineering. 2005;49(1):63–70.

4. Rantakokko M, Mänty M, Rantanen T. Mobility decline in old age. Exerc Sport Sci Rev. 2013;41(1):19–25.

5. Ko SM, Haussdorf JM, Ferrucci L, et al. Age-associated differences in the gait pattern changes of older adults during fast-speed and fatigue conditions: results from the Baltimore longitudinal study of ageing. Age Ageing. 2010;39:688–94.

6. McGibbon CA. Toward a better understanding of gait changes with age and disablement: neuromuscular adaptation. Exerc Sport Sci Rev. 2003;31(2):102–8.

7. Maki BE, McIlroy WE. Postural control in the older adult. Clin Geriatr Med. 1996;12(4):635–58.

8. Cruz-Jimenez M. Normal changes in gait and mobility problems in the elderly. Phys Med Rehabil Clin N Am. 2017;28(4):713–25.

9. Chamberlin ME, et al. Does fear of falling influence spatial and temporal gait parameters in elderly persons beyond changes associated with normal aging? J Gerontol A Biol Sci Med Sci. 2005;60(9):1163–7.

10. Judge JO, Davis RB 3rd, Ounpuu S. Step length reductions in advanced age: the role of ankle and hip kinetics. J Gerontol A Biol Sci Med Sci. 1996;51(6):M303–12.

11. Murray MP, Kory RC, Clarkson BH. Walking patterns in healthy old men. J Gerontol. 1969;24(2):169–78.

12. Louis ED, Bennett DA. Mild parkinsonian signs: an overview of an emerging concept. Mov Disord. 2007;22(12):1681–8.

13. Brach JS, et al. Challenging gait conditions predict 1-year decline in gait speed in older adults with apparently normal gait. Phys Ther. 2011;91(12):1857–64.

14. Fritz S, Lusardi M. White paper: "walking speed: the sixth vital sign". J Geriatr Phys Ther. 2009;32(2):46–9.

15. Morfis P, Gkaraveli M. Effects of aging on biomechanical gait parameters in the healthy elderly and the risk of falling. Anthropol Sci. 2007;115:67–72.

16. Pirker W, Katzenschlager R. Gait disorders in adults and the elderly: a clinical guide. Wien Klin Wochenschr. 2017;129(3–4):81–95.

17. Mielke MM, et al. Assessing the temporal relationship between cognition and gait: slow gait predicts cognitive decline in the Mayo Clinic study of aging. J Gerontol A Biol Sci Med Sci. 2013;68(8):929–37.

18. Matias R, et al. A perspective on wearable sensor measurements and data science for Parkinson's disease. Front Neurol. 2017;8:677.

19. Artusi CA, et al. Implementation of Mobile health Technologies in Clinical Trials of movement disorders: underutilized potential. Neurotherapeutics. 2020;17(4):1736–46.

20. Godinho C, et al. A systematic review of the characteristics and validity of monitoring technologies to assess Parkinson's disease. J Neuroeng Rehabil. 2016;13:24.

21. Guo Y, et al. Sample size and statistical power considerations in high-dimensionality data settings: a comparative study of classification algorithms. BMC Bioinformatics. 2010;11:447.

22. Espay AJ, et al. Technology in Parkinson's disease: challenges and opportunities. Mov Disord. 2016;31(9):1272–82.

23. Odin P, et al. Viewpoint and practical recommendations from a movement disorder specialist panel on objective measurement in the clinical management of Parkinson's disease. NPJ Parkinsons Dis. 2018;4:14.

24. Espay AJ, et al. A roadmap for implementation of patient-centered digital outcome measures in Parkinson's disease obtained using mobile health technologies. Mov Disord. 2019;34(5):657–63.

25. Coran P, et al. Advancing the use of mobile technologies in clinical trials: recommendations from the clinical trials transformation initiative. Digit Biomark. 2019;3(3):145–54.

26. Sánchez-Ferro Á, et al. New methods for the assessment of Parkinson's disease (2005 to 2015): a systematic review. Mov Disord. 2016;31(9):1283–92.

27. Pérez-López C, et al. Assessing motor fluctuations in Parkinson's disease patients based on a single inertial sensor. Sensors (Basel). 2016;16(12)

28. Erb MK, et al. mHealth and wearable technology should replace motor diaries to track motor fluctuations in Parkinson's disease. NPJ Digit Med. 2020;3:6.
29. Nutt JG, et al. Freezing of gait: moving forward on a mysterious clinical phenomenon. Lancet Neurol. 2011;10(8):734–44.
30. Bächlin M, et al. Wearable assistant for Parkinson's disease patients with the freezing of gait symptom. IEEE Trans Inf Technol Biomed. 2010;14(2):436–46.
31. Maetzler W, Klucken J, Horne M. A clinical view on the development of technology-based tools in managing Parkinson's disease. Mov Disord. 2016;31(9):1263–71.

Digital Technologies in Cognitive Disorders

7

Alessandro Padovani and Andrea Pilotto

7.1 Cognitive Disorders in the Elderly

Dementia is one of the most common diseases in the world and is destined to increase its rates, due to the progressive ageing of the population. The World Health Organization indicates that about 50 million people worldwide are now living with dementia, with a growth rate of ten million new cases every year and an estimated proportion of the general population aged 60 and over with dementia between 5–8%. Cognitive deficits due to neurodegeneration are one of the major causes of disability and dependency in older people with potentially serious consequences also for the caregivers and with severe implications for society and economy [1]. Alzheimer's disease (AD) is the most common form of neurodegenerative dementia characterized by accumulation of both amyloid and tau pathology in the brain. The second most common cognitive disorder of aging population is vascular cognitive impairment and dementia, secondary to cerebrovascular events including both ischemic and hemorrhagic stroke [2]. Other common neurodegenerative disorders include dementia with Lewy bodies (DLB), characterized by a combination of parkinsonism, fluctuating cognition and hallucinations [3], and frontotemporal dementia (FTD), defined by prominent behavioral or language dysfunction [4]. Pharmacological and non-pharmacological interventions can improve the trajectories of AD and other cognitive disorders since the early stages and might even prevent progression in prodromal or at-risk stage [5, 6].

Considering the exponential spread of the availability and use of new technologies and devices in everyday life, it could be useful to take advantage of them to reach more people in an easy and home-based setting.

A. Padovani · A. Pilotto (✉)
Department of Clinical and Experimental Sciences, Neurology Unit, University of Brescia, Brescia, Italy
e-mail: andrea.pilotto@unibs.it

In fact, there is an urgent need to track cognitive changes in early symptomatic or even presymptomatic stages of AD and other cognitive disorders. The landscape of cognitive testing in supervised and unsupervised conditions is rapidly changing as technology advances [7].

## 7.2	Digital Testing: Different Setting and Techniques for Different Purposes

The increasing percentage of patients affected by dementia calls for the need to a wider and more effective cognitive screening in healthcare in order to identify early signs of cognitive neurodegeneration worthy of a more meticulous analysis which could possibly lead to early intervention. Mild cognitive impairment (MCI) has been defined as a stage between the expected age-associated cognitive decline and the more serious decline observed in dementia. At this stage, subjects present mild cognitive alterations with no impairment in daily living activities. Several studies showed that subjects with MCI have a higher risk of developing dementia and that they might benefit from preventive pharmacological and non-pharmacological strategies [8].

The longitudinal evaluation of these subjects using more efficient and less demanding cognitive assessment is thus an urgent need for clinicians and researchers who are dealing with a growing number of at-risk subjects.

Very important characteristic of new Digitized Cognitive Assessment (DCA) is the ability to provide accurate measurement of new variables, such as reaction time for individual tasks within a test battery and frequency of errors, with the option to adapt the difficulty of the exercises online, in order to avoid ceiling or floor effects.

Cognitive assessment using digital technology offers new opportunities to overcome the limitations of current classical paper-and-pencil assessments. One issue in traditional neuropsychological testing is the test/retest effect and the need of neuropsychologists or trained specialists who apply the assessment.

The digital assessment can be applied in different settings: in the clinic even together with "classical" paper and pencil neuropsychology assessment or at home. In addition to this, the assessment can be applied in supervised conditions, i.e., applied and explained by trained specialists or in unsupervised conditions in self-administered test.

The supervised digital assessment is usually applied for a specific diagnostic or prognostic purpose and might provide information about specific cognitive domains in a similar way compared to classical pen and pencil neuropsychological tests. These digital assessments are of high interest for the development of specific tests or optimizing a global evaluation in clinic but often need a rater and could not be used for self-reported evaluation of the subject (see next section for details).

The unsupervised self-administered assessment, conversely, can capture similar proxies of cognitive dysfunction and could be used—especially in internet-based platforms—as screening tool to identify subjects at risk of dementia or to track cognitive changes over time. The major limitations are related to the higher attrition rate and the lack of control of conditions of testing (see section 4 for details).

7.3   Digital Testing in the Clinic

The first digital assessments developed during the last two decades were electronic versions of paper and pencil traditional tests such as the Montreal Cognitive Assessment (MoCA). Clinical trial data management companies have adapted traditional cognitive measures to be administered as electronic clinical outcome assessments such as the Pearson's Q-interactive for Wechsler Adult Intelligence Scale.

Automatic recording mitigates common error sources and could thus represent an important instrument for clinicians in the next future, as they have demonstrated a fair correlation with traditional neuropsychological assessment.

Several different computerized cognitive tests have been developed to detect cognitive deficits and cognitive decline. These may include stand-alone apps and programs as well as web-based apps that can be completed either on personal computers (PC) or tablets. For AD and MCI in general, several specific tests have been developed including CANTAB, Cogstate, and NIH toolbox (Table 7.1, adapted and updated from [7]), which are discussed in the following.

7.3.1   CANTAB

The CANTAB battery (Fig. 7.1) is a language-independent and culturally neutral battery applied in several studies focusing on brain aging and dementia [9, 10]. The assessment was originally developed in the 1980s by the University of Cambridge, and is now commercially provided by the company Cambridge Cognition. CANTAB tests have demonstrated sensitivity in detecting changes in neuropsychological performance and include tests of working memory, learning, and executive function; visual, verbal, and episodic memory; attention, information processing and reaction time, decision making and response control social and emotion recognition. Administration of CANTAB was initially on PC but is now available also on mobile (tablet-based) devices, in shorter versions and with special focuses on specific domains. The battery has been applied in large cohorts of subjects at risk for AD, particularly using the Verbal Recognition Test, including measures of memory

Table 7.1 Principal cognitive tests and platforms

Computer-Based	Tablet-Based	Smartphone-Based	Novel Platform
	CANTAB	ARC	Analysis of voice
	NIH-toolbox	M2C2	Ocular movement
	Cogstate	PACC5	Virtual reality
ORCA-LLT (through a web browser)			
BRANCH (through a web browser)			
BoCA			

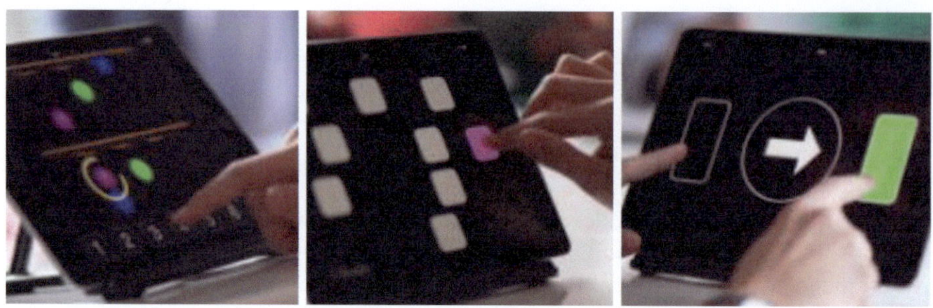

Fig. 7.1 CANTAB, display example. (adapted from CANTAB website, https://www.cambridgecognition.com/cantab/)

recall and recognition. In this test, the participants are shown a sequence of words on a touchscreen. Subsequently, the subjects are asked to recall the words, and the task ends with a recognition task. Bischoff and coauthors showed an association between higher Amyloid-β1–42 and memory recall and recognition measures in younger adults, whereas the effect weakened in older people [11].

7.3.2 Cogstate

Cogstate, one of most used platforms, was specifically designed to mitigate the effects of language and culture on cognitive assessment [12, 13], Darby et al. 2012). The battery was originally developed for personal computer but is now also available for tablets. The measures are mainly extracted from tasks using the universal stimulus set of common playing cards. Using different paradigms, the test can provide accurate measures evaluating response time, working memory, and continuous visual memory. The new versions of the assessment include further non-card playing tasks. An important strength of Cogstate is the design specifically developed as reliable measurement of change over time through randomized alternative versions to reduce confounding practice effects. The battery was originally designed to be administered by an examiner, but there have been recent efforts for the implementation of a remote administration version. A new unsupervised version with fair diagnostic performance is now also available (see below).

The Cogstate test batteries are used in several ongoing studies and clinical trials, such as the Anti-Amyloid Treatment in Asymptomatic Alzheimer's Disease (A4) study and the Alzheimer's Disease Neuroimaging Initiative 3 (ADNI3) or the Dominantly Inherited Alzheimer Network-Trials Unit (DIAN-TU) [11].

7.3.3 NIH Toolbox

The National Institutes of Health Toolbox Cognitive Battery (TBCB) was developed and approved by more than 80 institutions in order to provide an easy-to-use and low-cost standard for a brief cognitive test in different settings [14]. The battery includes seven different tests adapted to a digital platform, designed by an expert panel. The tests evaluate episodic and working memory, attention, processing speed, executive functions, and language. Both computer and tablet versions are available and have been validated against standard neuropsychological measures [15] The battery has been regularly used in studies and trials investigating early phases of AD, and have been compared against established cognitive composite scores [16].

7.4   Unsupervised Digital Cognitive Assessment

The large and still growing number of aged people that are able to use smartphones and digital technology opens a wide range of new opportunities of digital technology use in an unsupervised setting even continuously for months or years [7]. Improved ecological validity and everyday life applicability of smartphone-based measures is timely. Researchers, patients, caregivers, and even regulatory institutions (such as FDA, EMA) now underlined the importance of patient-reported outcomes with clinically relevant impact on well-being [17] for both diagnostic and prognostic purposes.

Indeed, the last decade showed a dramatic increase in smartphone-based applications specifically designed for cognitive assessment in unsupervised settings for older populations [18]. The strengths of smartphone-based cognitive assessment for detection and tracking subtle cognitive changes in the aging population are obvious. This way of testing enables frequent assessment with potentially more sensitive cognitive paradigms compared to classical neuropsychological testing [19]. This kind of assessment is also largely scalable, allowing a remote assessment in a much larger populations compared to samples acquired through in-clinic and supervised assessments. Thus, unsupervised cognitive testing might be used for large population screenings in order to identify at-risk subjects for cognitive impairment.

With mobile technology, cognitive assessment can be performed in a familiar environment and may thus increase ecological validity (i.e., generalizability to the real-life scenarios) of the assessment.

The assessment in familiar environment may also reduce the "white-coat effect" (i.e., different performances observed on tasks in a medical environment, compared to the usual environment) and reduce the time and costs for a frequent re-evaluation (e.g., for clinical trials). Furthermore, several digital cognitive tools provide alternative versions able to track subtle changes of cognition and response to pharmacological and non-pharmacological intervention, omitting learning effects.

Several important challenges should be also mentioned, specifically related to validity of measures (i.e., ensuring alignment between smartphone-based vs gold-standard cognitive assessment data), and reliability of testing (higher variability observed in tasks when the tested subjects are in free-living conditions and not under a defined and structured task setting). Also, privacy issues are relevant in this context and should be considered for any relevant outcome measure or automatically delivered information—especially when the own mobile phone of the subjects is used for testing. Moreover, the feasibility of studies and trials depending on repeated testing could be limited by increased attrition rates and low compliance—especially in those participants with cognitive deficits. The adherence in short studies is quite promising if the subjects are well-instructed [20]. Daily testing and assessment are more difficult, but preliminary studies indicate an adherence of 80–90% in young adults with low rate of missing data over an observation period of at least 6 days [21]. In patients with MCI or mild dementia, however, many studies using remote assessments indeed reported a limited participant engagement. As a general observation, higher response and retention rate have been observed in trials that included also supervised assessment and when monetary compensation was provided [21].

The use of tests using mobile devices should enable more frequent testing, resulting in more reliable and informative longitudinal data [22] and potentially more cost-effective assessment using self-administration [7]. The self-administered and remote testing, however, has also generated new challenges for the interpretation of findings. Unsupervised remote digital assessments require systems to ensure the individual assigned to a remote assessment is the individual taking that assessment and that no additional inputs/help by caregivers or other persons are provided. Furthermore, the human cognitive performances can be easily impacted by mood, stress, or time of day [22]. To avoid this, several studies assessed cognition by adopting shorter assessments, but several times per day.

Despite the advances in the field, only few large studies and trials on neurodegenerative disorders have been applying unsupervised cognitive testing several times. In the next section, we will provide more specific details for the most often used tests and assessments so far. Further work is required to fully establish whether more "ecologic" unsupervised testing is more closely associated with neurodegenerative markers than "classical in-clinic assessment" which is still considered the gold standard for the assessment of cognitive performance.

7.4.1 Specific Unsupervised Digital Cognitive Tests Used in Older Subjects

The Mobile Monitoring and Cognitive Change (M2C2) test has been specifically developed to test cognitive performance over time and has been validated in younger people. A fair validity against the supervised in-clinic assessment has been observed [22]. Moreover, the application of the test up to five times per day and for 14 consecutive days showed a high reliability for the same subjects, thus confirming the validity of this design.

Another interesting tool is the Preclinical Alzheimer Cognitive Composite −5 (PACC5), developed by the team conducting the Harvard Aging Brain Study [23]. In subjects at risk for AD, the authors revealed a diminished practice effect in cognitive tests repeated for three months in subjects with higher burden of amyloid—thus suggesting that continuously-delivered cognitive testing might increase the sensibility for the detection of cognitive decline by showing different trends in longitudinal individualized data.

A web-based version of memory for face-and-name pairs (FNAME)—called the Boston Remote Assessment for Neurocognitive Health (BRANCH)—was designed to reduce costs of assessment and time for longitudinal evaluation [24]. These tasks are particularly sensitive to memory changes that should characterize AD-related pathology and are thus of high interest for prodromal and clinical AD studies.

Recently, a digital alternative to the MoCA called Boston Cognitive Assessment (BoCA) has been presented [25]. BoCA is a completely self-administered smartphone- and computer-based test able to track global cognitive function with subtests exploring different domains with a high test-retest reliability. It has already been proposed as an important research application for large screening or longitudinal follow-up studies.

For the assessment of cognition in the general population, the Many Brains Project has been suggested. It is aiming at evaluating cognitive changes in the aging population using normative data obtained from the TestMyBrain.org website. Even if the numbers of people tested include millions of people, the diagnostic accuracy and reproducibility of such assessments still need further validation versus normal in-house testing and in subjects at risk for different forms of cognitive decline [26].

A different approach based on learning ability was proposed with the Online Repeatable Cognitive Assessment Language Learning Test (ORCA-LLT). In this assessment, designed for older adults, subjects are asked to learn the English word equivalents of 50 Chinese characters for 25 min per day. The researchers found that the learning curve in persons with positive Amyloid β status (an early AD marker) was different from those with negative PET, with relatively little overlap between the groups [27]. Another interesting application called "Mezurio" was developed by the Oxford University Big Data Institute and is now included in several ongoing longitudinal studies focusing on early and preclinical AD. The application includes several game-like tests able to assess episodic memory, language, executive function with different degree of recall delays potentially associated with different degrees of risk of cognitive changes [28]. This example suggests that the use of game-like tests to assess cognitive function is one of the most promising approaches to increase retainment and long-term compliance of subjects. The so-called Sea Hero, for example, is a virtual reality-based game able to track visuospatial and memory function. It is already used by several millions of people in different countries. First results suggest that the ability of such games to detect cognitive changes is comparable with traditional tests but further research, especially in cohorts at risk for the development of cognitive decline and dementia, is needed before these tools can be implemented in clinical trial batteries and routine clinical management [29].

7.5 Digital Cognitive Training

Cognitive training is increasingly being applied for prevention of cognitive decline in research and clinical setting, and commercial training packages are on the market. 'Cognitive training' is defined as an intervention consisting of repeated practice on standardized exercises, targeting a specific cognitive domain or domains, for the purpose of benefiting cognitive function [30]. In cognitively healthy older adults, it is intended to reduce age-related cognitive decline and thus maintain cognitive function, to prevent or delay the development of neurodegenerative cognitive decline [31]. Computer-based cognitive training (CCT), including exercises, virtual reality, and gaming, offers highly accessible, low-cost, standardized interventions. Several randomized clinical trials and meta-analyses demonstrated significant benefit in specific domains and composite scores of cognitive functions in older adults, whereas in MCI some studies even found a reduced rate of incident dementia [30]. Additionally, some clinical trial results indicate that computerized and online cognitive training in adults without dementia may improve daily functioning and psychological well-being [32].

The unifying theoretical premise behind digital cognitive training is that it will increase cognitive reserve by stimulating neuroplasticity and thereby maintaining or even improving cognitive function. It has also been suggested that cognitive stimulation may result in the development of compensatory networks according to which cognitive performance is maintained, thus masking or preventing clinical manifestation of neurocognitive disease [33]. In a recent Cochrane review on randomized clinical trials for cognitive interventions, researchers found still a lot of inconsistencies between different trials. Overall, evidence on the efficacy of cognitive training on cognitive function is relatively low, although especially longer trials suggest some beneficial effect on memory [30]. Of note, the most important lifestyle intervention trials such as the so-called FINGER trail [5, 34] are now including cognitive training as part of a multidimensional approach, demonstrating the general efficacy and applicability of such interventions even in a large population. The main limitation of gaming and interventions is still the high attrition rate for long longitudinal trials, especially in those subjects who are at higher risk of developing dementia [34, 35]. Compared to traditional cognitive training, CCT allows the level of challenge to be more easily individualized and adapted as a result of training progression. Further, CCT is easily scalable, and training data can be automatically recorded (Kuider 2012). For these reasons, several cognitive training applications are now moving from standard cognitive training to adaptive versions able to optimize the levels of difficulty of a task based on the cognitive capabilities of the user. A very interesting approach is the application of such training and application to track cognitive changes over time, as recently suggested in old adults and subjects at risk for dementia in small trials [35, 36]. The integration of such assessments and trainings represents an important challenge but also a big opportunity, as it can represent an innovative intervention strategy for clinicians and at the same time a way to track cognitive changes and monitor the response to general management in clinical settings.

7.6 Promising New Digital Technologies to Track Cognitive Changes and Activities of Daily Living

A growing body of evidence indicates that features other than cognitive disorders, such as sensory and motor changes, play an important role in defining patients with cognitive decline. Mobile and wearable digital technology assessing changes within mobility and daily function have the great potential to overcome at least some limitations of cognitive testing and represent a growing area of interest for researchers.

Impairment of mobility is a core feature of cognitive disorders. Moreover, longitudinal observations found that reduction of gait speed could be observed even more than 10 years before a clinical diagnosis of MCI [37]. A growing number of technologies have been developed to quantify gait parameters and changes in fine motor control in both supervised and unsupervised settings (see Chap. 6) in both supervised and unsupervised settings [38]. The ability of new algorithms to quantify the amount and quality of mobility at home will dramatically change in the next future by opening a new window of observation in the home environment of healthy subjects and those with cognitive disorders [38, 39]. The evaluation of daily mobility and the correlation with cognitive function and behavioral changes—including apathy, depression, and even irritability or agitation—are still a growing field of research, as only few studies focused on non-cognitive measures in cognitive disorders so far [40].

Other interesting areas of assessment are based on analyses on voice, ocular movement, and even fine motor dexterity that enable researchers to have important information even when only using application-based assessments [40]. Also, sleep and autonomic dysfunction could now be evaluated using small sensors and mobile applications.

A wider use of data coming from phones and mental health applications could generate important data for a deeper understanding for the daily relevance of cognitive deficits and the complex relationship between behavioral, cognitive, and motor domains. Further research is still needed in this area, as the use of GPS sensors and metrics coming from daily personal mobile-phones application (e.g., evaluating the amount of use of specific applications and the interactions with other people) definitively need an adequate regulation and the development of specific privacy policies concerning personal data.

Digital phenotyping including these non-cognitive areas in neurodegenerative conditions is still in its infancy as research groups have yet to establish a clear link between these activities and the cognitive domains of interest. Nevertheless, a safe and accurate assessment of daily life functions in cognitive disorders in the new "digital era" will relevantly change the scenario of any diagnostic and prognostic evaluation and stimulate the development of new interventions based on more ecologically-valid parameters with a higher impact on well-being and quality of life.

References

1. Padovani A, Pilotto A. Looking at the burden of neurological disorders in Europe. Lancet Public Health. 2020;5(10):e523.
2. van der Flier WM, Skoog I, Schneider JA, Pantoni L, Mok V, Chen CLH, Scheltens P. Vascular cognitive impairment. Nat Rev Dis Primers. 2018;4:18003. https://doi.org/10.1038/nrdp.2018.3.
3. McKeith IG, et al. Diagnosis and management of dementia with Lewy bodies. Neurology. 2017;89:88–100.
4. Miller B, Llibre Guerra JJ. Frontotemporal dementia. Handb Clin Neurol. 2019;165:33–45.
5. Kivipelto M, et al. The Finnish geriatric intervention study to prevent cognitive impairment and disability (FINGER): study design and progress. Alzheimers Dement. 2013;9:657–65.
6. Scarmeas N, Anastasiou CA, Yannakoulia M. Nutrition and prevention of cognitive impairment. Lancet Neurol. 2018;17(11):1006–15.
7. Öhman F, et al. Current advances in digital cognitive assessment for preclinical Alzheimer's disease. Alzheimers Dement (Amst). 2021;13(1):e12217.
8. Qarni T, Salardini A. A multifactor approach to mild cognitive impairment. Semin Neurol. 2019;39(2):179–87.
9. Fray PJ, Robbins TW, Sahakian BJ. Neuropsychiatric applications of CANTAB. Int J Geriatr Psychiatry. 1996;11(4):329–36.
10. Juncos-Rabadán O, et al. Do the Cambridge neuropsychological test automated battery episodic memory measures discriminate amnestic mild cognitive impairment? Int J Geriatr Psychiatry. 2014;29(6):602–9.
11. Bischof GN, et al. Amyloid deposition in younger adults is linked to episodic memory performance. Neurology. 2016;87(24):2562–6.
12. Maruff P, Thomas E, Cysique L, et al. Validity of the CogState brief battery: relationship to standardized tests and sensitivity to cognitive impairment in mild traumatic brain injury, schizophrenia, and AIDS dementia complex. Arch Clin Neuropsychol. 2009;24(2):165–78.
13. Fredrickson J, et al. Evaluation of the usability of a brief computerized cognitive screening test in older people for epidemiological studies. Neuroepidemiology. 2010;34(2):65–75.
14. Hodes RJ, et al. NIH Blueprint for Neuroscience Research. The NIH toolbox: setting a standard for biomedical research. Neurology. 2013;80(11 Suppl 3):S1.
15. Weintraub S, Dikmen SS, Heaton RK, et al. Cognition assessment using the NIH toolbox. Neurology. 2013;80(11 Suppl 3):S54–64.
16. Buckley RF, et al. Computerized cognitive testing for use in clinical trials: a comparison of the NIH toolbox and CogState C3 batteries. J Prev Alzheimers Dis. 2017;4(1):3–11.
17. Pillemer F, et al. Direct release of test results to patients increases patient engagement and utilization of care. PLoS One. 2016;11(6):1–9.
18. Koo BM, Vizer LM. Mobile technology for cognitive assessment of older adults: a scoping review. Innov Aging. 2019;3(1):1–14.
19. Samaroo AH, et al. P1-466: diminished practice effects on a monthly computerized and home-administered face-name associative memory exam are predictive of elevated pet amyloid in normal older adults. Alzheimers Dement. 2019;15:P447.
20. Perin S, et al. Unsupervised assessment of cognition in the healthy brain project: implications for web-based registries of individuals at risk for Alzheimer's disease. Alzheimer's Dement Transl Res Clin Interv. 2020;6(1):1–11.
21. Pratap A, et al. Indicators of retention in remote digital health studies: a cross-study evaluation of 100,000 participants. npj Digit Med. 2020;3(1):1–10.
22. Sliwinski MJ, Mogle JA, Hyun J, Munoz E, Smyth JM, Lipton RB. Reliability and validity of ambulatory cognitive assessments. Assessment. 2018;25(1):14–30.
23. Jutten, et al. Monthly at-home computerized cognitive testing to detect diminished practice effects in preclinical Alzheimer's disease. Front Ageing Neuroscie. 2022;13:800–15.

24. Rentz DM, et al. Face-name associative memory performance is related to amyloid burden in normal elderly. Neuropsychologia. 2011;49(9):2776–83.
25. Vyshedsky A, et al. Boston cognitive assessment (BOCA)—a comprehensive self-administered smartphone- and computer-based at-home test for longitudinal tracking of cognitive performance. BMC Neurol. 2022;22(1):92.
26. Passell E, et al. Digital cognitive assessment: results from the TestMyBrain NIMH research domain criteria (RDoC) field test battery report. Digital Cognitive Assessment; 2019.
27. Lim YY, Baker JE, Bruns L, et al. Association of deficits in short-term learning and Aβ and hippoampal volume in cognitively normal adults. Neurology. 2020;95(18):e2577–85.
28. Lancaster C, Koychev I, Blane J, Chinner A, Wolters L, Hinds C. Evaluating the feasibility of frequent cognitive assessment using the Mezurio smartphone app: observational and interview study in adultswith elevated dementia risk. JMIR Mhealth Uhealth. 2020;8(4):e16142.
29. Coutrot A, et al. Virtual navigation tested on a mobile app is predictive of real-world wayfinding navigation performance. PLoS One. 2019;14(3):e0213272.
30. Gates NJ, et al. Computerised cognitive training for maintaining cognitive function in cognitively healthy people in late life. Cochrane Database Syst Rev. 2019;3:CD012277.
31. Petersen RC, et al. Practice guideline update summary: mild cognitive impairment. Neurology. 2018;90(3):126–35.
32. Rebok GW, et al. 2014 ten-year effects of the advanced cognitive training for independent and vital elderly cognitive training trial on cognition and everyday functioning in older adults. J Am Geriatr Soc. 2014;62(1):16–24.
33. Grady C. The cognitive neuroscience of ageing. Nat Rev Neurosci. 2012;13(7):491–505. https://doi.org/10.1038/nrn3256. PMID: 22714020.
34. Kivipelto, et al. Lifestyle interventions to prevent cognitive impairment, dementia and Alzheimer disease. Nat Rev Neurol. 2018;14(11):653–66.
35. Li, et al. The effect of cognitive training in older adults: be aware of CRUNCH. Neuropsychol Dev Cogn B Aging Neuropsychol Cogn. 2020;27(6):949–62.
36. Walton CC, et al. Design and Development of the Brain Training System for the Digital "Maintain Your Brain" Dementia Prevention Trial. JMIR Aging. 2019;2(1):e13135. https://doi.org/10.2196/13135.
37. Buracchio, et al. The trajectory of gait speed preceding mild cognitive impairment. Arch Neurol. 2010;67:980–6.
38. Warmerdam E, et al. Long-term unsupervised mobility assessment in movement disorders. Lancet Neurol. 2020;19(5):462–70.
39. Mikolizak AS, et al. Connecting real-world digital mobility assessment to clinical outcomes for regulatory and clinical endorsement-the Mobilise-D study protocol. PLoS One. 2022;17(10):e0269615.
40. Kourtis, et al. Digital biomarkers for Alzheimer's disease: the mobile/ wearable devices opportunity. NPJ Digit Med. 2019;2:9. https://doi.org/10.1038/s41746-019-0084-2. Epub 2019 Feb 21
41. Cummings J, et al. Alzheimer's disease drug development pipeline: 2022. Alzheimers Dement (N Y). 2022;8(1):e12295.

Technologies to Assess Psycho-Behavioural Symptoms

8

Kirsten Emmert and Walter Maetzler

8.1 Definition and Relevance of Psycho-Behavioural Symptoms, with Focus on Older Adults

Psycho-behavioural symptoms, such as depressive and manic symptoms, anxiety, delirium, lack of impulse control, fatigue and sleep disturbances, have a major influence on physical health [1] and quality of life (QoL), [2, 3], especially in older adults. For example, the mental component of health-related QoL (HRQoL) is a predictor of functional disability in older adults independent from the physical components [4]. The impact of these psycho-behavioural symptoms on society is severe. Major depressive disorder (MDD) alone is estimated to cause a loss of 7.5 million Disability Adjusted Life Years in older adults [5]. Psycho-behavioural symptoms should therefore be considered as an essential part of health in all treatment decisions.

These symptoms are associated with physiological reactions of the body, changes in mobility and social participation, which can potentially, or already demonstrably, be measured with digital technology.

8.2 Digital Technology that Is most Probably Relevant for Assessment of Psycho-Behavioural Symptoms

Technology can help to monitor psychological symptoms and their dynamics over time in an unobtrusive way. One particular advantage of such technology is that extreme data points (e.g. extremely low mood) can be detected that may not be apparent during a doctor's visit or when looking at mean values [6].

K. Emmert (✉) · W. Maetzler
Department of Neurology, University Medical Centre Schleswig-Holstein, Campus Kiel and Kiel University, Kiel, Germany
e-mail: k.emmert@neurologie.uni-kiel.de

A. Pilotto, W. Maetzler (eds.), *Gerontechnology. A Clinical Perspective*, Practical Issues in Geriatrics, https://doi.org/10.1007/978-3-031-32246-4_8

While technology can also help to actively collect data, e.g. with questionnaires, voice recording or neuropsychological testing, we focus here on passive data collection, as it can be applied more broadly and with minimal burden especially to older persons. In the following, some of the most important physiological reactions of the body, as well as a short overview of how mobility and social participation can be measured (e.g. in combination with physiological reactions) are presented, together with the digital technologies that can assess these reactions.

8.2.1 Physiology

8.2.1.1 Heart Rate and Heart Rate Variability

The heartbeat is generated by auto-rhythmic cell bundles in the sinoatrial node, which constantly receives neural input, most importantly from the medulla [7, 8]. In a stressful situation, healthy adults usually show a fast and consistent increase in heart rate (HR) [9].

Heart rate variability (HRV) measures changes to the intervals between consecutive heartbeats [10] and can be calculated from an electrocardiogram (ECG) or, in a less accurate way, using photoplethysmography (PPG). In health, these so-called inter-beat intervals (IBIs) vary in a complex manner to allow a rapid adjustment to changing external and internal circumstances. HRV measures can be grouped into time-domain (observed variability within a certain period), frequency-domain (absolute or relative signal energy within component bands), and non-linear metrics (quantification of unpredictability and complexity of a series of IBIs), [5]. There is a complex influence of autonomic, cardiovascular, central nervous, endocrine, and respiratory systems as well as baroreceptors and chemoreceptors on HRV on the short-term with effects in the very-low to high HRV spectrum frequencies [8].

8.2.1.2 Breathing Rate

Breathing is important for gas exchange and acid–base balance regulation [11, 12]. A normal breathing rate (BR) during rest ranges between 12 and 20 breaths/min [13]. Changes in BR can indicate the presence of pathologies such as adverse cardiac events or pneumonia as well as emotional stress, cognitive load, temperature change, physical effort, or fatigue after exercise [11]. It is often measured indirectly by extracting a respiratory waveform from ECG or PPG signals but data with better quality can usually be obtained by using strain sensors or IMUs placed at the chest and abdomen [11, 14, 15].

8.2.1.3 Skin Temperature

Skin temperature reflects a number of physiological changes such as cutaneous vasodilatation as well as secretion and evaporation of sweat [16, 17]. Skin temperature is usually measured by either thermocouples, thermistors or infrared sensors. Traditional thermistors and thermocouples need wires that connect the sensor to a body-worn data storage system. Infrared sensors, semiconductor temperature sensor or telemetry-based sensors offer wireless alternatives [16, 18].

8.2.1.4 Galvanic Skin Response/Electrodermal Activity

Electrodermal activity (EDA) assesses the change in electrical conductance of the skin, which is tightly linked to sweat production [19]. As sweat glands are innervated by the sympathetic nervous system, it can be used as an approximation for sympathetic nervous system arousal [20]. However, EDA is also influenced by central mechanisms such as movements, thermoregulatory sweating, affective processes, orientation and attention [19]. To measure EDA two electrodes can be placed on parts of the skin that are relatively close to each other, such as, e.g. neighbouring digits of the hand.

8.2.1.5 Electroencephalography (EEG)

Electroencephalogram (EEG) measures electrical activity on the scalp, which reflects activity of the surface layer of the brain. Specifically, EEG mainly records oscillations as the sum of excitatory and inhibitory post-synaptic potentials that are generated by cortical pyramidal neurons of the cerebral cortex [21]. EEG is a wide field of research and the EEG setups vary considerably, depending on the intended purpose. The most commonly used setup is the international 10–20 system, which distributes electrodes between Nasion (top of the nasal bones) and Inion (tip of the external occipital protuberance) as well as front to back at distances of 10% followed by four times 20% and again 10% of the total distance [21]. For standard applications the use of at least 25 electrodes is recommended, although high-density scalp EEG arrays with 64–256 electrodes are also often used in a research setting to allow a more granular source localization [22]. Mobile devices such as EEG headbands are usually simplified versions, with fewer electrodes, often focusing on frontal regions as there is less hair impacting data acquisition.

8.2.2 Movement and Mobility

Human movement and mobility assessments are mainly performed with body-worn inertial measurement units (IMU), force plates or optical motion capture systems. Due to ease-of-use and the lack of location boundness, IMUs are the most convenient method to capture movement in older adults. IMUs usually include triaxial accelerometers, gyroscopes and magnetometers to measure accelerations, angular velocities and the earth magnetic field each in three degrees of freedom [23]. Sensor fusion algorithms that need data from at least the accelerometers and the gyroscopes can be used to estimate the orientation and location of body-worn sensors over time [24, 25]. Smartphones also include IMUs and can hence be used for movement and mobility tracking. For further information on how mobility can be tracked in older adults, see Chap. 6.

8.2.3 Social Participation

Smartphones offer a new way to passively track social interactions. Apps can quantify social communication based on social media use, call and text messaging frequencies and social exploration based on environmental data derived from techniques such as GPS [26–28]. In addition, Bluetooth sensing can be used to detect if similar sensors on others' smartphones are near to determine if the person is currently alone or in company [29]. This way, different data types collected by a smartphone app may be combined to calculate a "sociability score" [26].

8.2.4 Combined Devices

In practice, several of these assessment methods may be combined in one device. For example, current smartwatches often include movement sensors as well as PPG technology.

8.3 How Is this Digital Technology Used to Examine the most Relevant Psycho-Behavioural Symptoms?

In this section, we focus on a selection of psycho-behavioural symptoms based on relevance for geriatric patients and describe how current technology can be used to assess them. This selection is not meant to be exhaustive and does not include cognitive (dys-)function, which is discussed in Chap. 7. The presented technology is usually not used for diagnosis, but rather to monitor disease course and therapeutic effects.

8.3.1 Depressive Symptoms

Depressive symptoms are frequent in older adults and usually assessed using patient-reported outcome (PRO) such as the Beck's Depression Inventory, Patient Health Questionnaire (PHQ)-9 or the Geriatric Depression Scale-15 (GDS-15, developed especially for use in older adults). Wearables promise a less intrusive way to monitor depressive symptoms on the long term. Technology to assess depressive symptoms has previously mainly been tested in confirmed diseases like MDD.

A systematic review of studies looking at HR and HRV during stress suggests that a hypo-reactivity during stress exists in MDD [7]. HR increases after stressful stimuli, and the HRV in the high-frequency (HF) band seems to be decreased [7]. Similarly, EDA seems to be reduced in depression, as demonstrated in a study with 50 depressed patients [30]. Another meta-analysis of 18 studies showed that HRV was reduced in patients with MDD and depression severity seemed to be negatively correlated with HRV [31].

The amount of physical activity, specifically the amount of moderate-to-vigorous-intensity physical activity, as measured by IMUs for seven days on the right hip, was negatively associated with rates of depression [32] in 2764 participants with a mean age of 45.7 years. In a study focusing on older adults, 29 participants (mean age 74 years) suffering from late-life depression (LLD) as measured with the Montgomery-Åsberg Depression Rating Scale score showed reduced physical activity (mean acceleration magnitude, measured with wrist-worn IMU). The strongest effect was seen in the morning [33]. Compared to controls, patients had slower fine motor movements ('jerk'), defined as the mean of the first derivative of acceleration magnitude [33].

Recent studies combined different measures to increase accuracy of prediction models [34]. One study using a multimodal wristband found that skin temperature, sleep time (IMU-derived), and correlation of those modalities were the most important features for depression prediction accuracy [35]. Another study using a wristband that included peripheral skin temperature, HR, IMU-derived parameters, sleep characteristics using actigraphy and EDA measurements in combination with a smartphone, showed moderate-to-high correlation, ranging from 0.46 to 0.7 between the developed model and clinician-rated depression scores [36]. The most predictive features in the model were related to mobile phone use, activity level, skin conductance (EDA), and HRV. Time spent talking, assessed with a microphone, was negatively correlated with depressive symptoms [37]. Several studies have tried to use EEG to detect depressive symptoms [38–40]. While the method seems promising, a lot of future research is needed as there is currently no clear consensus on which EEG measures are most predictive for depressive symptoms.

In conclusion, depressive symptoms seem to interact with various physiological processes such as HR during stress, HRV, activity level and EDA. Future research is needed to confirm which combination of these features is most promising to estimate depressive symptoms with clinically relevant accuracy.

8.3.2 Manic Symptoms

Manic phases are characterized by unreasonable euphoria or irritation, increased energy or agitation, thought disorder and increased speech [41]. Compared to depressive symptoms, the association between individual digital measures and manic symptoms is less clear, therefore most studies looked at a combination of different digital measures.

One study found that a model using location, distance travelled, conversation frequency, and non-stationary duration could predict social rhythm metric reasonably well in patients with bipolar disorder (BD) [42]. A similar study found physical activity (smartphone IMU) and especially location (using GPS tracking) to have a high recognition accuracy for BD state [43]. Another study found that manic symptoms are predicted by lower physical activity (smartphone IMU) and higher social communication [44]. One study using light exposure, number of steps, sleep data such as sleep length, quality and onset as well as a cosinor analysis of HRV as variables to predict the mood state was successful identifying sleep length, quality and steps during bedtime as the most important features for manic episode detection [45].

In sum, the evidence for the usefulness of individual digital measures to track manic symptoms is currently low, although some studies show that a combination of mobility and social interaction measures may be promising.

8.3.3 Anxiety

Anxiety, a feeling of fear, dread, and inner turmoil, is commonly characterized by sympathetic activation and vagal deactivation accompanied by faster and shallower breathing [46].

Acute anxiety can be artificially induced by a stressful situation, such as needing to deliver a speech, and is accompanied by an increase in HR in healthy adults [47]. One meta-analysis found that high-frequency (HF) HRV is often reduced in anxiety disorders [48]. A review that looked at ECG features in different anxiety disorders found a decrease in HRV. Low frequency (LF) and HF signal energy were most commonly used as features, followed by R-peak to R-peak intervals (RR) [49]. From six studies looking at panic disorder, three found that LF is useful to detect panic disorder symptoms [50–52], two found a connection between panic disorder symptoms and HF [50, 53] while two studies found no effect at all [54, 55]. For patients with social anxiety disorder several different HRV measures including HF were useful to differentiate them from healthy controls [56]. One study looking at HF also found an effect on social anxiety symptoms [53]. Four studies looked at general anxiety disorder and did not find any consistent link between ECG features and anxiety symptoms [53, 57–59].

One study with 32 healthy female participants showed that an anxiety-inducing task produced cooling on the hands and a slight warming on the face, showing that skin temperature may be differently influenced by anxiety [60]. However, a systematic review on body temperature in anxiety disorders showed equivocal results, with no clear indication that anxiety symptoms are linked to changes in skin temperature [61].

A study with 42 healthy participants showed that an anxious state is associated with an increased BR and increased EDA (specifically non-specific skin conductance reaction rate), compared to a neutral state [62]. Looking at cardiovascular features, pulse wave amplitude was also able to differentiate between the different states, though the effect size was lower. Standard HRV features did not show an effect [62].

A study on 98 young women showed that those with higher anxiety tended to have less variability in inspiratory time [63]. Studies in patients with panic disorder showed hyperventilation and increased tidal volume variability even when not in an acute panic attack [64].

In conclusion, anxiety symptoms seem to be related to an increase in BR and EDA. In addition, the majority of studies report a decrease in HRV mostly in the HF band.

8.3.4 Delirium

Delirium is characterized by idiopathic acute and fluctuating disturbances of attention and global cognitive dysfunction. Cognitive changes may include impairment of perception, memory and reasoning [65, 66]. So far, relatively few studies looked at the usefulness and efficacy of mobile technology-derived parameters in delirium, with most of these studies using IMUs.

A systematic review of delirium research with IMUs found that delirium was accompanied by decreased physical activity, including a high number of immobility minutes during the day as well as reduced amount of sleep and increased physical activity during the night [67]. One study looking at HRV in 37 patients developing delirium associated with hip fracture showed a decrease in the LF and an increase in the HF band [68].

8.3.5 Lack of Impulse Control, Addiction and Craving

Lack of impulse control means a person has trouble controlling emotions or behaviours. Impulse control disorders (ICD) include kleptomania, intermittent explosive disorder, trichotillomania, compulsive sexual behaviour and pyromania. In addition, substance abuse, compulsive buying and pathological gambling have also been related to an impaired impulse control [69, 70].

A meta-analysis looking at 24 articles with 26 studies examining task-based self-control in healthy adults showed that there is some support for the association of higher HRV with better impulse control. However, the overall effect size was small [71]. A review suggests that participants with low levels of resting HRV had difficulties in emotional, cognitive, and physiological regulation, possibly caused by the lack of inhibitory neural processes in these individuals [72]. One study with 98 students found that those with higher HF HRV power were less likely to act impulsively (measured using the consumer impulsiveness scale) when compared to students with lower HF HRV power [73]. Similarly, a trial found that disinhibited eaters had a reduced overall HRV, which was related to greater blood glucose excursions, emphasizing that lack of impulse control seems to be linked to a reduced HRV [74]. A similar trend was observed in young males with internet gaming disorders (IGD, [75]). Compared to 27 healthy controls, the 21 participants with IGD showed significant reductions in HF HRV power while playing online games, particularly during high attention periods and the last 5 min of the games, compared with baseline values, possibly linked to diminished executive control during online gaming. A follow-up study also showed decreased functional connectivity, among others between the right dorsolateral prefrontal cortex and the right inferior frontal gyrus, a functional network that is involved in cognitive control [76]. Participants with substance use disorder (SUD) showed a decreased resting HRV [77, 78]. In particular, low resting HF HRV power was associated with drug and alcohol symptom severity [79]. One study made use of this link by trying to increase HRV through biofeedback [80]. Twenty-one young men rhythmically stimulated their HRV by paced breathing at a frequency of about 0.1 Hz. There was no significant effect, although on a descriptive level, HRV biofeedback showed a higher reduction in alcohol and drug craving compared to those receiving only the treatment as usual (mean reduction on Penn Alcohol Craving Scale 5.5 points versus 3.7 points).

Interestingly, a study using the Go/NoGo task as a test for impulse control found that the presence of an ICD in patients with Parkinson's disease (PD; $n = 10$ vs. $n = 23$ PD patients without ICD, $n = 26$ healthy controls) was linked to a deterioration of the NoGo N2 and P3 peak amplitudes at fronto-central electrodes in the EEG [81], indicating that portable EEG might also be suitable to measure impulse control.

Overall, there is a consensus that a lack of impulse control is associated with decreased resting HRV, particularly in the HF band, while other digital measures have not been explored systematically for impulse control.

8.3.6 Fatigue

Pathological fatigue as a symptom can be described as *"an unpleasant physical, cognitive, and emotional symptom described as a tiredness not relieved by common strategies that restore energy. Fatigue varies in duration and intensity, and it reduces, to different degrees, the ability to perform the usual daily activities"* [82]. Fatigue often occurs in chronic diseases and is considered one of the most debilitating symptoms by those affected [83–86]. Fatigue is a particular suitable target for digital assessments, as fatigue levels often fluctuate from day to day or even within a day, making a continuous passive monitoring very attractive.

A recent review compared different fatigue monitoring approaches [87]. For mental fatigue and vigilance tasks EEG was used most frequently, followed by mobility assessment, HRV and EDA. This makes sense as EEG is regarded as the gold standard for vigilance monitoring [88]. Physical fatigue was mostly assessed with mobility-related parameters and HRV [87]. The majority of studies used a short-term, task-based design so that a transfer of the result to a natural setting is not possible without some restrictions. One long-term study looking at different classification approaches for multimodal data from 405 recording days of 27 participants showed initial promising results with mobility (energy expenditure, activity counts, and steps), HRV and BR as the most important parameters to predict fatigue [89]. Another pilot study with 7 days of data from each of the 13 participants showed that mobility and HRV data can be combined in deep learning models for the detection of fatigue [90]. These studies suggest that multimodal data are beneficial to measure fatigue in real-world settings.

The majority of studies with patients suffering from chronic diseases seem to support these results. A study on 49 participants with multiple sclerosis (MS) showed that IMU-based spatio-temporal gait parameters could predict fatigue with stride time, maximum toe clearance, heel strike angle, and stride length as the most important (together 67% contribution to the predictions made by the Random Forest model) components [91]. While one study with 101 persons with MS showed only weak correlations between fatigue and several gait parameters when using an electronic walkway [92], other studies rather support the link between gait parameters, such as velocity, cadence and stride length, and fatigue in MS [93, 94] and systemic lupus erythematosus [95]. A study with 45 chronic fatigue syndrome/myalgic encephalomyelitis patients showed that HRV time- and frequency-domain measurements were correlated with fatigue [96].

In conclusion, mobility and HRV, particularly in combination, seem to be promising digital parameters for the assessment of (the severity of) fatigue. For mental fatigue, EEG is currently the most well-established method.

8.3.7   Sleep

Sleep disturbances are common in (old) patients with chronic diseases [97] as well as in healthy older adults [98]. For example, 64% of PD patients reported at least one sleep-related disorder [99], such as insomnia or rapid eye movement (REM) behaviour disorder. Insomnia seems to have a severe impact on HRQoL [100]. In addition, many aspects of sleep are correlated with mental health status [101]. In a meta-analysis of randomized controlled trials, interventions to improve sleep led to a significant medium-sized effect on mental health, depression, anxiety, and rumination [102]. The analysis even suggests a dose-response relationship (greater improvements in sleep quality led to greater improvements in mental health).

However, measuring sleep quality and disturbances is not easy as sleep is a complex physiological state [103]. Currently, it is commonly tracked with wearables, in-bed sensors, contactless sensors (e.g. a radio frequency-based sensing device that can be placed on the bedside table) or smartphones [104]. Common parameters for mobile sleep monitoring include movement, EEG (often simplified using headbands developed for this purpose), HRV, EDA and skin temperature. The devices are usually compared to the gold standard polysomnography (PSG). PSG combines the use of EEG, ECG, electromyogram, electrooculogram, thoracic movement (chest/abdomen belts) and oximetry in a sleep lab [105]. Recordings are manually reviewed and scored by a sleep expert making it a good but complicated and expensive sleep assessment that cannot simply be performed at home. Even PSG does not represent all biochemical, physiological and mobility aspects of sleep. Due to the complexity of sleep and the different sleep disorders that disturb sleep in very different ways, a one-size-fits-all solution to measuring sleep is unlikely to be successful. Research is still at the beginning of finding individual key parameters for different sleep disturbances and disorders.

Common sleep problems in older adults include increased sleep latency and decreased sleep time, a more fragmented sleep, daytime sleepiness, obstructive sleep apnoea and restless legs syndrome (RLS, 98). Not all of these sleep disturbances share common pathophysiological processes [103, 106]. Therefore, different combinations of measures may be needed to capture the symptoms accurately. For example, RLS should obviously include movement tracking of the lower limbs while sleep staging may be more important to capture fragmented sleep and might also be used to explain subsequent excessive daytime sleepiness. Here, we briefly present sleep quantity and quality measures before exploring sleep movement parameters.

Usually, several different sensors are combined, e.g. in a smartwatch and used to classify sleep. However, commercially available multisensory wristbands showed a rather low accuracy for classification of sleep stages, in particular slow wave sleep and wake state, compared to PSG [104, 107]. In addition, studies demonstrated that performance under free-living conditions was acceptable for coarse quantitative measures such as total sleep time but not good for more granular parameters, such as sleep efficiency [108, 109]. Moreover, predictive performance was lower for patients, such as people suffering from insomnia [110]. In contrast, EEG headbands seem to be better at detecting slow wave power in particular [111] and sleep stages in general [112, 113]. However, the headbands often rely on electrodes over frontal regions thereby being prone to data corruption by ocular and muscle artefacts [112, 114].

Movement monitoring during sleep with mobile sensors cannot only contribute to sleep staging but also reveal periodic leg movement [115], which may be useful for patients with RLS, periodic limb movement disorder or REM sleep disorder, which is characterized by a persistent muscle tone and subsequent physical acting out of dreams during REM sleep. Movement sensors can also be used to monitor breathing effort, which may be of use in sleep apnoea and other diseases characterized by sleep-disordered breathing [116]. A study looking at movements during sleep of normal weight and obese people found that obesity affected sleep with fewer transitions and lower values of root mean square transition accelerations during the night [117]. One study showed that sleep problems can even cause differences in daytime movement [118]. Older women with subthreshold insomnia walked slower and showed an increased coefficient of variance of the stance phase during fast walking, compared to healthy older women.

In conclusion, current wearables are able to relatively reliably track sleep time and sleep movements, however sleep staging is not always reliable. EEG headbands currently seem to be a promising alternative to gain more insights into sleep architecture of older adults although further validation is needed.

8.4 Opportunities, Challenges and Relevant Questions for Future Research

As can be seen from this broad overview of the literature on digital technology, many wearables and phone apps offer ways to passively monitor psycho-behavioural symptoms. However, results are often inconsistent between studies, possibly due to methodological differences and the lack of standard parameters, for example, when looking at HRV. Therefore, more standardized research, more validation studies and more meta-analyses are needed to determine the most promising digital parameters. A first attempt at an overview of most relevant parameters based on the literature is presented in Table 8.1.

Another challenge in the field of digital medicine is translating these new findings into changes in clinical care. While some of the technology used is commercially available and has standardized output parameters (although usually not

Table 8.1 Main digital parameters used to capture psycho-behavioural symptoms

	Physiological measure(s)	Mobility measure(s)	Social participation measure(s)
Depressive symptoms	Decrease in HRV VS band and hypo-reactivity during stress depressed persons [7], possibly also reduced EDA [30]	Decreased physical activity (reduced mean acceleration magnitude [33]) or decreased amount of moderate-to-vigorous-intensity physical activity [32])	Little evidence, possibly reduced mobile phone use [36], decreased time spent talking [37].
Manic symptoms	Little evidence, possibly reduced sleep length and quality [45]	Little evidence, possibly increased distance travelled [42] and increased number of steps [45]	Little evidence, possibly increased social communication [44].
Anxiety	Decrease in HRV (mostly HF power [48]), faster, shallower breathing [46], possibly also increased EDA [62]	–	–
Delirium	Little evidence, possibly increased HF HRV power and decreased LF HRV power [68]	Little evidence, possibly decrease in mobility during day and increase during night [67]	–
Lack of impulse control & addiction	Decreased resting HRV [71]	–	–
Fatigue	Decreased overall HRV [87, 89], mental fatigue/vigilance: EEG metrics such as EEG power spectrum density [88]	Decreased spatio-temporal gait parameters such as stride length [91, 93]	–
Sleep	Decreased deep sleep time: Sleep staging based on EEG [111–113], decreased sleep time: Sleep detection with multisensoric smartwatches [104, 107–109]	Fewer transitions, lower transition acceleration measured by IMUs [117], presence of periodic leg movement and increased breathing effort: ballistocardiography sensor mat [115, 116]	–

optimized for clinical use), other technology is not available for sale and might require technical knowledge to manage the preparation before use as well as the data transfer and analysis. Therefore, technology and data use should be simplified. In addition, standards for the data format and orientation of sensors should be established and applied to all sensors to unify data reporting. Lastly, more intervention trials with digital technology are needed to assess how well wearables or apps can capture disease changes and facilitate interpretation of measures.

Looking at the presented literature, most research focuses on physiological and movement measures, while research about digital measures of social participation is limited. When trying to place the research in the WHO's International Classification of Functioning, disability and health (ICF) model, most was performed in the body functions and structures and activities domains, while participation (in societal roles), personal features and environmental factors are rarely explored. This is unfortunate, as a review in patients with PD found that the participation domain included factors showed the highest strength of association with HRQoL [119]. For fatigue a strong association with social participation has been demonstrated as well [120]. Therefore, future research should focus on the important domain of social participation and how digital technology can assess parameters from this domain. Table 8.1. gives a brief overview of the most prominent digital measures that past studies investigated.

8.5 Conclusion

New digital technology shows great promise to enable a continuous, unobtrusive monitoring of psycho-behavioural symptoms, which may increase diagnosis accuracy and facilitate treatment monitoring. For some of the psycho-behavioural symptoms, such as depressive symptoms and sleep disturbances, a relevant body of research investigating the association between symptoms and digitally extracted parameters exists. However, less is known about such associations for manic symptoms, delirium and lack of impulse control. Therefore, more validation work is needed especially for the latter symptoms. Nevertheless, digital technology can already provide a lot of useful information, although the development seems far away from implementation in routine clinical use.

References

1. Ohrnberger J, Fichera E, Sutton M. The relationship between physical and mental health: a mediation analysis. Soc Sci Med. 2017;195:42–9.
2. Celik SS, Celik Y, Hikmet N, Khan MM. Factors affecting life satisfaction of older adults in Turkey. Int J Aging Hum Dev. 2018;87(4):392–414.
3. Baranowski CJ. The quality of life of older adults with epilepsy: a systematic review, vol. 60. Seizure: W.B. Saunders; 2018. p. 190–7.
4. Tomioka K, Shima M, Saeki K. Mental component of health-related quality of life is an independent predictor of incident functional disability among community-dwelling older people: a prospective cohort study. Qual Life Res. 2021;30(7):1853–62.

5. Prince MJ, Wu F, Guo Y, Gutierrez Robledo LM, O'Donnell M, Sullivan R, et al. The burden of disease in older people and implications for health policy and practice. The Lancet. 2015;385:549–62.
6. Ebner-Priemer UW, Reichert M, Tost H, Meyer-Lindenberg A. Wearables for context-triggered assessment in psychiatry, vol. 90. Nervenarzt: Springer Medizin; 2019. p. 1207–14.
7. Schiweck C, Piette D, Berckmans D, Claes S, Vrieze E. Heart rate and high frequency heart rate variability during stress as biomarker for clinical depression. A systematic review. Psychol Med [Internet]. 2018;49(2):200–11. https://www.cambridge.org/core/article/heart-rate-and-high-frequency-heart-rate-variability-during-stress-as-biomarker-for-clinical-depression-a-systematic-review/FA90B43DA846B6F88AC14EFBFD7EB01A
8. Shaffer F, McCraty R, Zerr CL. A healthy heart is not a metronome: an integrative review of the heart's anatomy and heart rate variability [Internet]. Front Psychol. 2014;5. https://www.frontiersin.org/article/10.3389/fpsyg.2014.01040
9. Kudielka BM, Buske-Kirschbaum A, Hellhammer DH, Kirschbaum C. Differential heart rate reactivity and recovery after psychosocial stress (TSST) in healthy children, younger adults, and elderly adults: the impact of age and gender. Int J Behav Med. 2004;11(2):116–21.
10. Shaffer F, Ginsberg JP. An overview of heart rate variability metrics and norms [Internet]. Front Public Health. 2017;5. https://www.frontiersin.org/article/10.3389/fpubh.2017.00258
11. Nicolò A, Massaroni C, Schena E, Sacchetti M. The importance of respiratory rate monitoring: from healthcare to sport and exercise. Sensors (Switzerland). 2020;20:1–45. MDPI AG
12. Loughlin PC, Sebat F, Kellett JG. Respiratory rate: the forgotten vital sign—make it count! Jt Comm J Qual Patient Saf. 2018;44:494–9.
13. Yuan G, Drost NA, McIvor RA. Respiratory rate and breathing pattern. McMaster Univ Med J. 2013;10(1):23–5.
14. Massaroni C, Di Tocco J, Bravi M, Carnevale A, Lo PD, Sabbadini R, et al. Respiratory monitoring during physical activities with a multi-sensor smart garment and related algorithms. IEEE Sensors J. 2019;20(4):2173–80.
15. Siqueira A, Spirandeli AF, Moraes R, Zarzoso V. Respiratory waveform estimation from multiple accelerometers: an optimal sensor number and placement analysis. IEEE J Biomed Heal Informatics. 2019;23(4):1507–15.
16. Taylor NAS, Tipton MJ, Kenny GP. Considerations for the measurement of core, skin and mean body temperatures. J Thermal Biol. 2014;46:72–101.
17. Gagge A, Gonzalez R. Mechanisms of heat exchange: biophysics and physiology. Compr Physiol. 2011;
18. van Marken Lichtenbelt WD, Daanen HAM, Wouters L, Fronczek R, Raymann RJEM, Severens NMW, et al. Evaluation of wireless determination of skin temperature using iButtons. Physiol Behav. 2006;88(4–5):489–97.
19. Posada-Quintero HF, Florian JP, Orjuela-Cañón AD, Chon KH. Electrodermal activity is sensitive to cognitive stress under water [Internet]. Front Physiol. 2018;8. https://www.frontiersin.org/article/10.3389/fphys.2017.01128
20. Critchley HD. Review: electrodermal responses: what happens in the brain. Neurosci [Internet]. 2002;8(2):132–42. https://doi.org/10.1177/107385840200800209.
21. Feyissa AM, Tatum WO. Chapter 7–Adult EEG. In: Levin KH, PBT-H C, editors. Clinical neurophysiology: basis and technical aspects [Internet]. Elsevier; 2019. p. 103–24. https://www.sciencedirect.com/science/article/pii/B9780444640321000072.
22. Seeck M, Koessler L, Bast T, Leijten F, Michel C, Baumgartner C, et al. The standardized EEG electrode array of the IFCN. Clin Neurophysiol [Internet]. 2017;128(10):2070–7. https://www.sciencedirect.com/science/article/pii/S1388245717304832
23. Nez A, Fradet L, Marin F, Monnet T, Lacouture P. Identification of noise covariance matrices to improve orientation estimation by Kalman filter. Sensors (Switzerland). 2018;18(10)
24. Pham MH, Warmerdam E, Elshehabi M, Schlenstedt C, Bergeest L-M, Heller M, et al. Validation of a lower back "wearable"-based sit-to-stand and stand-to-sit algorithm for

patients with Parkinson's disease and older adults in a home-like environment. Front Neurol [Internet]. 2018;9:652. https://www.frontiersin.org/article/10.3389/fneur.2018.00652/full

25. Seel T, Raisch J, Schauer T. IMU-based joint angle measurement for gait analysis. Sensors. 2014;14:6891.

26. Eskes P, Spruit M, Brinkkemper S, Vorstman J, Kas MJ. The sociability score: app-based social profiling from a healthcare perspective. Comput Human Behav [Internet]. 2016;59:39–48.

27. Torous J, Kiang MV, Lorme J, Onnela JP. New tools for new research in psychiatry: a scalable and customizable platform to empower data driven smartphone research. JMIR Ment Heal. 2016;3(2)

28. Torous J, Onnela J-P, Keshavan M. New dimensions and new tools to realize the potential of RDoC: digital phenotyping via smartphones and connected devices [Internet]. Vol. 7, Translational Psychiatry. 2017. p. e1053. Boston, MA: Department of Psychiatry, Beth Israel Deaconess Medical Center, Harvard Medical School. http://europepmc.org/abstract/MED/28267146

29. Yan Z, Yang J, Tapia EM. Smartphone Bluetooth based social sensing. In: Proceedings of the 2013 ACM conference on pervasive and ubiquitous computing adjunct publication (UbiComp '13 adjunct) [Internet]. New York, NY: Association for Computing Machinery; 2013. p. 95–8. https://doi.org/10.1145/2494091.2494118.

30. Ward NG, Doerr HO. Skin conductance: a potentially sensitive and specific marker for depression. J Nerv Ment Dis. 1986;174(9):553–9.

31. Kemp AH, Quintana DS, Gray MA, Felmingham KL, Brown K, Gatt JM. Impact of depression and antidepressant treatment on heart rate variability: a review and meta-analysis. Biol Psychiatry. 2010;67(11):1067–74.

32. Vallance JK, Winkler EAH, Gardiner PA, Healy GN, Lynch BM, Owen N. Associations of objectively-assessed physical activity and sedentary time with depression: NHANES (2005–2006). Prev Med (Baltim). 2011;53(4–5):284–8.

33. O'Brien JT, Gallagher P, Stow D, Hammerla N, Ploetz T, Firbank M, et al. A study of wrist-worn activity measurement as a potential real-world biomarker for late-life depression. Psychol Med. 2017;47(1):93–102.

34. Lee S, Kim H, Park MJ, Jeon HJ. Current advances in wearable devices and their sensors in patients with depression. Front Psychiatry. 2021;12:672347.

35. Tazawa Y, Ching LK, Yoshimura M, Kitazawa M, Kaise Y, Takamiya A, et al. Evaluating depression with multimodal wristband-type wearable device: screening and assessing patient severity utilizing machine-learning. Heliyon. 2020;6(2):e03274.

36. Pedrelli P, Fedor S, Ghandeharioun A, Howe E, Ionescu DF, Bhathena D, et al. Monitoring changes in depression severity using wearable and Mobile sensors. Front Psych. 2020;11

37. Berke EM, Choudhury T, Ali S, Rabbi M. Objective measurement of sociability and activity: mobile sensing in the community. Ann Fam Med. 2011;9(4):344–50.

38. Čukić M, Stokić M, Simić S, Pokrajac D. The successful discrimination of depression from EEG could be attributed to proper feature extraction and not to a particular classification method. Cogn Neurodyn. 2020;14(4):443–55.

39. Čukić M, López V, Pavón J. Classification of depression through resting-state electroencephalogram as a novel practice in psychiatry: review. Journal of Medical Internet Research. 2020;22. JMIR Publications

40. Shah RV, Grennan G, Zafar-Khan M, Alim F, Dey S, Ramanathan D, et al. Personalized machine learning of depressed mood using wearables. Transl Psychiatry. 2021;11(1)

41. Martino DJ, Valerio MP, Parker G. The structure of mania: an overview of factorial analysis studies. Eur Psychiatry. 2020;63(1):e10.

42. Abdullah S, Matthews M, Frank E, Doherty G, Gay G, Choudhury T. Automatic detection of social rhythms in bipolar disorder. J Am Med Informatics Assoc [Internet]. 2016;23(3):538–43. https://doi.org/10.1093/jamia/ocv200.

43. Grünerbl A, Muaremi A, Osmani V, Bahle G, Oehler S, Tröster G, et al. Smartphone-based recognition of states and state changes in bipolar disorder patients. IEEE J Biomed Heal informatics. 2014;19(1):140–8.

44. Beiwinkel T, Kindermann SP, Maier A, Kerl C, Moock J, Barbian G, et al. Using smartphones to monitor bipolar disorder symptoms: a pilot study. JMIR Ment Heal. 2016;3(1)

45. Cho CH, Lee T, Kim MG, In HP, Kim L, Lee HJ. Mood prediction of patients with mood disorders by machine learning using passive digital phenotypes based on the circadian rhythm: prospective observational cohort study. J Med Internet Res. 2019;21(4)

46. Kreibig SD. Autonomic nervous system activity in emotion: a review. Biological Psychol. 2010;84:394–421.

47. Murakami H, Ohira H. Influence of attention manipulation on emotion and autonomic responses. Percept Mot Skills. 2007;105(1):299–308.

48. Chalmers JA, Quintana DS, Abbott MJA, Kemp AH. Anxiety disorders are associated with reduced heart rate variability: a meta-analysis. Front Psychiatry. 2014;5(JUL):5.

49. Elgendi M, Menon C. Assessing anxiety disorders using wearable devices: challenges and future directions. Brain Sci. 2019;9. MDPI AG

50. Chang HA, Chang CC, Tzeng NS, Kuo TBJ, Lu RB, Huang SY. Decreased cardiac vagal control in drug-naive patients with panic disorder: a case-control study in Taiwan. Asia Pac Psychiatry. 2013;5(2):80–9.

51. McCraty R, Atkinson M, Tomasino D, Stuppy WP. Analysis of twenty-four hour heart rate variability in patients with panic disorder. Biol Psychol [Internet]. 2001;56(2):131–50.

52. Cohen H, Benjamin J, Geva AB, Matar MA, Kaplan Z, Kotler M. Autonomic dysregulation in panic disorder and in post-traumatic stress disorder: application of power spectrum analysis of heart rate variability at rest and in response to recollection of trauma or panic attacks. Psychiatry Res [Internet]. 2000;96(1):1–13.

53. Pittig A, Arch JJ, Lam CWR, Craske MG. Heart rate and heart rate variability in panic, social anxiety, obsessive-compulsive, and generalized anxiety disorders at baseline and in response to relaxation and hyperventilation. Int J Psychophysiol. 2013;87(1):19–27.

54. Petrowski K, Herold U, Joraschky P, Mück-Weymann M, Siepmann M. The effects of psychosocial stress on heart rate variability in panic disorder. 2010.

55. Lavoie KL, Fleet RP, Laurin C, Arsenault A, Miller SB, Bacon SL. Heart rate variability in coronary artery disease patients with and without panic disorder. Psychiatry Res. 2004;128(3):289–99.

56. Alvares GA, Quintana DS, Kemp AH, Van Zwieten A, Balleine BW, Hickie IB, et al. Reduced heart rate variability in social anxiety disorder: associations with gender and symptom severity. PLoS One. 2013;8(7):e70468.

57. Thayer JF, Friedman BH, Borkovec TD. Autonomic characteristics of generalized anxiety disorder and worry. Biol Psychiatry [Internet]. 1996;39(4):255–66.

58. Lyonfields JD, Borkovec TD, Thayer JF. Vagal tone in generalized anxiety disorder and the effects of aversive imagery and worrisome thinking. Behav Ther [Internet]. 1995;26(3):457–66.

59. Hammel JC, Smitherman TA, McGlynn FD, Mulfinger AMM, Lazarte AA, Gothard KD. Vagal influence during worry and cognitive challenge. Anxiety, Stress Coping [Internet]. 2011;24(2):121–36. https://doi.org/10.1080/10615806.2010.490912.

60. Rimm-Kaufman S, Kagan J. The psychological significance of changes in skin temperature. Motiv Emot. 1996;20:63–78.

61. Fischer S, Haas F, Strahler J. A systematic review of thermosensation and thermoregulation in anxiety disorders. Front Phys. 2021;12

62. Blechert J, Lajtman M, Michael T, Margraf J, Wilhelm F. Identifying anxiety states using broad sampling and advanced processing of peripheral physiological information. Biomed Sci Instrum. 2006;42:136–41.

63. Van Diest I, Thayer JF, Vandeputte B, Van de Woestijne KP, Van den Bergh O. Anxiety and respiratory variability. Physiol Behav. 2006;89(2):189–95.

64. Roth WT. Physiological markers for anxiety: panic disorder and phobias. Int J Psychophysiol [Internet]. 2005;58(2):190–8.

65. American Psychiatric Association. Diagnostic and statistical manual of mental disorders: DSM-5™. 5th ed. Arlington, VA: American Psychiatric Publishing; 2013. p. 947.

66. Fong TG, Tulebaev SR, Inouye SK. Delirium in elderly adults: diagnosis, prevention and treatment. Nat Rev Neurol. 2009;5:210–20.
67. Davoudi A, Manini TM, Bihorac A, Rashidi P. Role of wearable accelerometer devices in delirium studies. Crit Care Explor. 2019;1(9):e0027.
68. Ernst G, Watne LO, Rostrup M, Neerland BE. Delirium in patients with hip fracture is associated with increased heart rate variability. Aging Clin Exp Res [Internet]. 2020;32(11):2311–8. https://doi.org/10.1007/s40520-019-01447-5.
69. Rogers RD, Moeller FG, Swann AC, Clark L. Recent research on impulsivity in individuals with drug use and mental health disorders: implications for alcoholism, vol. 34. Alcoholism: Clinical and Experimental Research. NIH Public Access; 2010. p. 1319–33.
70. Grant JE, Levine L, Kim D, Potenza MN. Impulse control disorders in adult psychiatric inpatients. Am J Psychiatry [Internet]. 2005;162(11):2184–8. https://doi.org/10.1176/appi.ajp.162.11.2184.
71. Zahn D, Adams J, Krohn J, Wenzel M, Mann CG, Gomille LK, et al. Heart rate variability and self-control-a meta-analysis. Biological Psychol. 2016;115:9–26.
72. Thayer JF, Lane RD. Claude Bernard and the heart–brain connection: further elaboration of a model of neurovisceral integration. Neurosci Biobehav Rev [Internet]. 2009;33(2):81–8.
73. Kittaneh A, Williams D, Bernardi A, Ejigu S, Koenig J, Thayer J. The relationship between resting heart rate variability and consumer impulsivity: a focus on consumer temptation. 2016.
74. Young HA, Watkins H. Eating disinhibition and vagal tone moderate the postprandial response to glycemic load: a randomised controlled trial. Sci Rep. 2016;6
75. Hong SJ, Lee D, Park J, Namkoong K, Lee J, Jang DP, et al. Altered heart rate variability during gameplay in internet gaming disorder: the impact of situations during the game. Front Psychiatry. 2018;9(SEP)
76. Lee D, Park J, Namkoong K, Hong SJ, Kim IY, Jung YC. Diminished cognitive control in Internet gaming disorder: a multimodal approach with magnetic resonance imaging and real-time heart rate variability. Prog Neuro-Psychopharmacol Biol Psychiatry. 2021;111
77. Brody S, Krause C, Veit R, Rau H. Cardiovascular autonomic dysregulation in users of MDMA ('ecstasy'). Psychopharmacology. 1998;136(4):390–3.
78. Malpas SC, Whiteside EA, Maling TJB. Heart rate variability and cardiac autonomic function in men with chronic alcohol dependence. Br Heart J. 1991;65(2):84–8.
79. D'Souza JM, Wardle M, Green CE, Lane SD, Schmitz JM, Vujanovic AA. Resting heart rate variability: exploring associations with symptom severity in adults with substance use disorders and posttraumatic stress. J Dual Diagn. 2019;15(1):2–7.
80. Eddie D, Kim C, Lehrer P, Deneke E, Bates ME. A pilot study of brief heart rate variability biofeedback to reduce craving in young adult men receiving inpatient treatment for substance use disorders. Appl Psychophysiol Biofeedback. 2014;39(3–4):181–92.
81. Lin YP, Liang HY, Chen YS, Lu CH, Wu YR, Chang YY, et al. Objective assessment of impulse control disorder in patients with Parkinson's disease using a low-cost LEGO-like EEG headset: a feasibility study. J Neuroeng Rehabil. 2021;18(1):109.
82. Mota DDCF, Pimenta CAM. Self-report instruments for fatigue assessment: a systematic review. Res Theory Nurs Pract. 2006;20(1):49–78.
83. Arends S, Meiners P, Moerman R, Kroese F, Brouwer E, Spijkervet F, et al. Physical fatigue characterises patient experience of primary Sjögren's syndrome. Clin Exp Rheumatol. 2016;35:255.
84. Ng W-F, Bowman SJ. Primary Sjögren's syndrome: too dry and too tired. Rheumatology [Internet]. 2010;49(5):844–53. https://doi.org/10.1093/rheumatology/keq009.
85. Chavarría C, Casanova MJ, Chaparro M, Barreiro-de Acosta M, Ezquiaga E, Bujanda L, et al. Prevalence and factors associated with fatigue in patients with inflammatory bowel disease: a multicentre study. J Crohn's Colitis [Internet]. 2019;13(8):996–1002. https://doi.org/10.1093/ecco-jcc/jjz024.
86. Chong R, Albor L, Wakade C, Morgan J. The dimensionality of fatigue in Parkinson's disease. J Transl Med [Internet]. 2018;16(1):192. http://www.ncbi.nlm.nih.gov/pubmed/29996887

87. Adão Martins NR, Annaheim S, Spengler CM, Rossi RM. Fatigue monitoring through wearables: a state-of-the-art review. Front Phys. 2021;12:790292.

88. Zhang X, Li J, Liu Y, Zhang Z, Wang Z, Luo D, et al. Design of a fatigue detection system for high-speed trains based on driver vigilance using a wireless wearable EEG. Sensors (Switzerland). 2017;17(3)

89. Luo H, Lee PA, Clay I, Jaggi M, De Luca V. Assessment of fatigue using wearable sensors: a pilot study. Digit Biomarkers. 2020;4(Suppl 1):59–72.

90. Bai Y, Guan Y, Ng W-F. Fatigue assessment using ECG and Actigraphy sensors. In: Proceedings of the 2020 international symposium on wearable computers (ISWC '20) [Internet]. New York, NY: Association for Computing Machinery; 2020. p. 12–6. https://doi.org/10.1145/3410531.3414308.

91. Ibrahim AA, Küderle A, Gaßner H, Klucken J, Eskofier BM, Kluge F. Inertial sensor-based gait parameters reflect patient-reported fatigue in multiple sclerosis. J Neuroeng Rehabil. 2020;17(1)

92. Kalron A. The correlation between symptomatic fatigue to definite measures of gait in people with multiple sclerosis. Gait Posture. 2016;44:178–83.

93. Sacco R, Bussman R, Oesch P, Kesselring J, Beer S. Assessment of gait parameters and fatigue in MS patients during inpatient rehabilitation: a pilot trial. J Neurol. 2011;258(5):889–94.

94. Motta C, Palermo E, Studer V, Germanotta M, Germani G, Centonze D, et al. Disability and fatigue can be objectively measured in multiple sclerosis. PLoS One. 2016;11(2):e0148997.

95. Mahieu MA, Ahn GE, Chmiel JS, Dunlop DD, Helenowski IB, Semanik P, et al. Fatigue, patient reported outcomes, and objective measurement of physical activity in systemic lupus erythematosus. Lupus. 2016;25(11):1190–9.

96. Escorihuela RM, Capdevila L, Castro JR, Zaragozà MC, Maurel S, Alegre J, et al. Reduced heart rate variability predicts fatigue severity in individuals with chronic fatigue syndrome/myalgic encephalomyelitis. J Transl Med [Internet]. 2020;18(1):4. https://doi.org/10.1186/s12967-019-02184-z.

97. Ballou S, Alhassan E, Hon E, Lembo C, Rangan V, Singh P, et al. Sleep disturbances are commonly reported among patients presenting to a gastroenterology clinic. Dig Dis Sci. 2018;63(11):2983–91.

98. Gulia KK, Kumar VM. Sleep disorders in the elderly: a growing challenge. Psychogeriatrics. 2018;18:155–65. Blackwell Publishing

99. Barone P, Antonini A, Colosimo C, Marconi R, Morgante L, Avarello TP, et al. The PRIAMO study: a multicenter assessment of nonmotor symptoms and their impact on quality of life in Parkinson's disease. Mov Disord. 2009;24(11):1641–9.

100. Duncan GW, Khoo TK, Yarnall AJ, O'Brien JT, Coleman SY, Brooks DJ, et al. Health-related quality of life in early Parkinson's disease: the impact of nonmotor symptoms. Mov Disord. 2014;29(2):195–202.

101. Del Rio João KA, de Jesus SN, Carmo C, Pinto P. Sleep quality components and mental health: study with a non-clinical population. Psychiatry Res. 2018;269:244–50.

102. Scott AJ, Webb TL, Martyn-St James M, Rowse G, Weich S. Improving sleep quality leads to better mental health: a meta-analysis of randomised controlled trials. Sleep Med Rev. 2021;60:101556.

103. Swick TJ. Parkinson's disease and sleep/wake disturbances. Frauscher B, editor. Park dis [Internet]. 2012, 2012 205471. doi:https://doi.org/10.1155/2012/205471.

104. De Zambotti M, Cellini N, Goldstone A, Colrain IM, Baker FC. Wearable sleep technology in clinical and research settings. Med Sci Sports Exerc. 2019;51(7):1538–57.

105. Bianchi MT. Sleep devices: wearables and nearables, informational and interventional, consumer and clinical. Metabolism [Internet]. 2018;84:99–108. https://www.sciencedirect.com/science/article/pii/S0026049517302822

106. Wetter TC, Beitinger PA, Beitinger ME, Wollweber B. In: Monti JM, Pandi-Perumal SR, Möhler H, editors. Pathophysiology of sleep disorders BT–GABA and sleep: molecular, functional and clinical aspects. Basel: Springer; 2010. p. 325–61. https://doi.org/10.1007/978-3-0346-0226-6_15.

107. Chinoy ED, Cuellar JA, Huwa KE, Jameson JT, Watson CH, Bessman SC, et al. Performance of seven consumer sleep-tracking devices compared with polysomnography. Sleep. 2021;44(5)
108. Gruwez A, Libert W, Ameye L, Bruyneel M. Reliability of commercially available sleep and activity trackers with manual switch-to-sleep mode activation in free-living healthy individuals. Int J Med Inform. 2017;102:87–92.
109. Mantua J, Gravel N, Spencer RMC. Reliability of sleep measures from four personal health monitoring devices compared to research-based actigraphy and polysomnography. Sensors (Switzerland). 2016;16(5)
110. Kang SG, Kang JM, Ko KP, Park SC, Mariani S, Weng J. Validity of a commercial wearable sleep tracker in adult insomnia disorder patients and good sleepers. J Psychosom Res. 2017;97:38–44.
111. Lucey BP, Mcleland JS, Toedebusch CD, Boyd J, Morris JC, Landsness EC, et al. Comparison of a single-channel EEG sleep study to polysomnography. J Sleep Res. 2016;25(6):625–35.
112. Casciola AA, Carlucci SK, Kent BA, Punch AM, Muszynski MA, Zhou D, et al. A deep learning strategy for automatic sleep staging based on two-channel eeg headband data. Sensors. 2021;21(10)
113. Arnal PJ, Thorey V, Debellemaniere E, Ballard ME, Hernandez AB, Guillot A, et al. The dreem headband compared to polysomnography for electroencephalographic signal acquisition and sleep staging. Sleep. 2020;43(11)
114. Dora C, Biswal PK. An improved algorithm for efficient ocular artifact suppression from frontal EEG electrodes using VMD. Biocybern Biomed Eng [Internet]. 2020;40(1):148–61.
115. Rauhala E, Virkkala J, Himanen SL. Periodic limb movement screening as an additional feature of Emfit sensor in sleep-disordered breathing studies. J Neurosci Methods. 2009;178(1):157–61.
116. Tenhunen M, Rauhala E, Virkkala J, Polo O, Saastamoinen A, Himanen SL. Increased respiratory effort during sleep is non-invasively detected with movement sensor. Sleep Breath. 2011;15(4):737–46.
117. Soangra R, Krishnan V. Wavelet-based analysis of physical activity and sleep movement data from wearable sensors among obese adults. Sensors (Switzerland). 2019;19(17)
118. Lee T, Lee M, Youm C, Noh B, Park H. Association between gait variability and gaitability decline in elderly women with subthreshold insomnia stage. Int J Environ Res Public Health. 2020;17(14):1–15.
119. van Uem JMT, Marinus J, Canning C, van Lummel R, Dodel R, Liepelt-Scarfone I, et al. Health-related quality of life in patients with Parkinson's disease–a systematic review based on the ICF model. Neurosci Biobehav Rev [Internet]. 2016;61:26–34. http://www.ncbi.nlm.nih.gov/pubmed/26645499
120. Murphy SL, Kratz AL, Whibley D, Poole JL, Khanna D. Fatigue and its association with social participation, functioning, and quality of life in systemic sclerosis. Arthritis Care Res. 2021;73(3):415–22.

Technologies to Prevent Falls and Their Consequences

9

Kayla Bohlke, Anisha Suri, Ervin Sejdcic,
and Clemens Becker

9.1 Introduction to Falls and Technology

Falls and injurious falls remain an important problem for older people. According to the World Health Organization (WHO) report, from 2021 this is a problem which is likely to worsen over the coming years. The number of falls and fall injuries will increase as the world's population ages. In this chapter, we focus on falls from older people still living in the community. In the first part, we will give a short overview over the burden of falls, the most common risk factors and the clinical progress that has been achieved over the past two decades in fall prediction, detection, and prevention. In the second section of the chapter, we will discuss the role and potential of technological solutions in this relevant field. We will discuss the upcoming hybrid solutions for the management of falls and fall prevention strategies. Often the notion of a fall may seem common sense. However, lay and clinical perspectives differ. The most adopted definition of a fall was proposed by the European Thematic Network ProFaNE (Prevention of Falls Network Europe). This group chose an inclusive definition of falls as 'an unexpected event in which the participant (person) comes to

K. Bohlke
Department of Bioengineering, Swanson School of Engineering, University of Pittsburgh, Pittsburgh, PA, USA

A. Suri
Department of Electrical and Computer Engineering, Swanson School of Engineering, University of Pittsburgh, Pittsburgh, PA, USA

E. Sejdcic
The Edward S. Rogers Department of Electrical and Computer Engineering, Faculty of Applied Science and Engineering, University of Toronto, Toronto, ON, Canada

T North York General Hospital, Toronto, ON, Canada

C. Becker (✉)
Unit Digitale Geriatrie, Universitätsklinikum Heidelberg, Heidelberg, Germany
e-mail: Clemens.Becker@rbk.de

rest on the ground, floor, or lower level.' [1]. Injurious falls are falls as described above which result in physical or psychological injury: categorized as minor (e.g. bruises, abrasions not requiring medical/healthcare treatment), moderate (e.g. wounds, bruises, etc. requiring medical/healthcare attention), or serious (e.g. fractures, head or internal injuries requiring emergency room or inpatient treatment) [2]. Fall rates are reported in a number of different ways in the literature, which can make interpretation of findings problematic. For clarity, data are best summarized by providing information in terms of *number of falls*; number of persons who are *non-fallers*, number of persons who are *fallers*, and number of *frequent fallers* (2+ falls in the period), *fall rate* per person year at risk and, in trials, *time to first fall*. Many studies do not follow this approach and at times this makes comparing results across studies difficult. As well as their physical consequences in terms of injuries, falls have a number of psychological consequences, most often referred to under the term of *'fear of falling'*. In brief, fear of falling is seen as an increase in anxiety or concern about activities that may result in falls and injuries and it can be measured in a number of ways using either single-item measures or scales such as the Short Falls Efficacy-Scale International (Short FES-I) [3]. The relationship between fear and falls is not straightforward. It is not the case that having a fall simply leads to increased fear, since some people are unrealistically confident and not fearful despite being regular fallers; and others are afraid of falling despite not having themselves fallen. What is clear is that fear of falling can lead to restriction of activity, which in itself is a negative consequence, as activity reduction can lead to loss of muscle and balance function, increasing risk of falling. In summary, falls are a major concern for health and social services since they are a major predictor of loss of independence and admission to care, to say nothing of the injuries that result and require medical attention.

9.2   Falls of Community-Dwelling Older People

Most studies of community-dwelling older people reveal that 20–33% of those aged over 65 years fall each year but estimates of 40% are not uncommon. The rate of falls (and recurrent fallers) increases with age 65 + from about 20% to 30–40% aged 80+. Rates are higher in the old-old (40 + %) and highest in the oldest-old (60%). Some 25–50% of fallers are 'multiple fallers' experiencing two or more falls per annum. The data on fall rates differ quite widely in the literature, because of differences in methodology for collecting the data (e.g. retrospective versus prospective designs; see [4] and differences in the underlying population.

Ethnic and socioeconomic differences have been noted in fall rates. For example, the risk appears higher among Whites compared with Hispanics and African Americans, and Chinese ethnic groups. However, there remains a poor understanding of the relationship between ethnicity and falls, which all too often confabulates ethnic origin with other issues such as poverty, living conditions, access to services, and 'migrant effects'. The consequences of falls are more easily quantified than falls themselves, especially the most serious consequences, since they result in need for medical attention and admission to hospital, and data are routinely collected by health services on the number of injuries treated. Hence one way to see the 'tip of the iceberg' of fall events is to consider fall-related injuries and fracture rates, especially hip fracture rates. It is generally accepted that 40–60% of falls result in no injury, 30–50% in minor injury, 5% in fractures (including about 1% being hip fracture) and 5–6% in other major injury.

9.3 Risk Factors for Falls and How to Identify Them

Falls are events that can be caused by numerous intrinsic factors. Acute onset of disease in various systems may present with falls necessitating hospital admissions. Examples include stroke, epilepsy, syncope from various causes, and postural hypotension. Often, it is the interaction between the person and an over-demanding environment that causes a fall. Personality traits such as risk-taking behaviour (e.g. climbing on unstable chairs) may influence the likelihood of falls. Intrinsic predisposing factors assessed might rapidly change. Fall risk should be considered using dynamic rather than static models. Most current fall prediction tools have acceptable sensitivity but lack sufficient specificity (meaning tools identify many people who go on to fall correctly, but they also identify too many people who do not go on to fall). In general, some 15% of falls are caused by an external event that would make most people fall; another 15% or so have a single identifiable cause such as syncope, while the remaining 70% or so have multiple interacting causal factors [5]. The first large systematic review and meta-analysis [6] of risk factors for falls among community-dwelling older people identified a plethora of risk factors, but restricted analysis to those which were reported on in at least five papers. There is a consistent rise in falls and recurrent falls with age and a 30% increase in risk for both falling and being a recurrent faller for women compared to men. However, it is perhaps the modifiable risk factors that are more important to focus on. Cognitive impairment is associated with more than twice the risk of falling and more than three times the risk of being a recurrent faller. Being depressed, having poor self-reported health, and being afraid of falling are all highly associated with falling. A number of medical conditions are associated with falls, particularly Parkinson's disease is nearly tripling the risk for recurrent falling.

9.4 The Role of Environmental Risk Factors

Environmental risk factors include factors in a person's living environment, whether at home or outdoors, that in conjunction with a person's intrinsic factors increase fall risk (Fig. 9.1). Home is a 'dangerous' place; most falls occur indoors at home, although of course this is where most community-dwelling older people spend most of their time. During the day the kitchen, living room, and halls/corridors and at night bedrooms, and corridors to toilets are scenes of most falls. Common hazards in the home are loose carpets and rugs, lack of supports, electrical cables and pets,

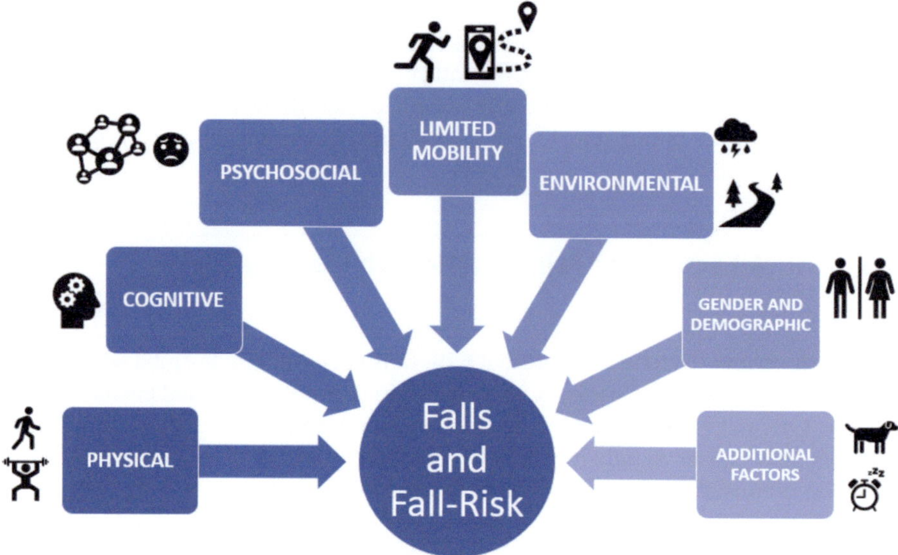

Fig. 9.1 Fall risk as a multi-factorial problem

and these can be identified by a number of different assessment tools [7, 8]. Outdoors, uneven pavements or steps, surface cracks, slippery surfaces, are common culprits. Environmental temperature is also associated with fall risk, since falls appear to increase during winter months. This has often been attributed to risk of walking on snowy and icy surfaces, however this phenomenon is also observed in subtropical climate, and may indicate that lower extremes of the temperature range to which older people are acclimatized represent a risk in itself.

9.5 Clinical Screening and Assessment for Community-Dwelling Older Persons

The most recent global guideline on fall prevention (Montero-Odasso 2022) recommends that physicians should proactively and at least annually ask about falls [9–11]. The CDC provides a self-complete checklist for older people to help them identify and discuss risk with their doctor [12]. If an older person presents for any condition the doctor or healthcare professional should ask if they have had a fall within the last 12 months, and should ask about the circumstances (frequency, context, and characteristics). Older people reporting a fall, or considered at risk, or presenting with an injurious fall should then undertake simple gait/balance tests and consideration be given to their potential to benefit from intervention such as strength and balance training.

A number of websites provide up-to-date guidance on clinical assessment tests and interventions [11–13]. There are a number of algorithms available to help healthcare professionals to conduct a falls assessment, for example, the CDC STEADI algorithm and AGS/BGS algorithm [9, 14]. If patients present with an injurious fall they should be carefully interviewed and assessed (see the videos at [15]). In general, the tests that are feasible in the clinical setting do not require extensive training, give objective information which will influence management, and are quick to administer. As part of the assessment, a medical history should be taken, including questions on falls history and the patient's subjective balance confidence as well as simple functional mobility tests as recommended in the various guidelines. Clear instruction and recording sheets for these standard tests are available at a number of falls websites including ([16, 17].

The BMJ has a number of videos [15] demonstrating how to clinically assess older people for fall risk in different settings. There are also new online fall risk assessments such as the Farseeing Fall Risk Assessment Tool (FFrat) [18] which permit inclusion of a wide range of clinical variables in calculation of a risk score and the App from the European Prevention of Falls Network for Dissemination [17] which links risk to a management plan. Assessment should always result in action, be it referral to another service, or changes in medication, and so on.

9.6 Assessment in Fall Clinics and Other Geriatric Services

Since there are many factors predisposing to falls, assessments for high-risk persons should ideally be carried out in one place by a multidisciplinary team, covering the well-established domains of comprehensive geriatric assessment: physical, functional, psychological, nutritional, and social domains. An example of a structured assessment requiring equipment is the physiological profile assessment (PPA) [19]. This tool consists of physiological assessments rather than disease-oriented ones, assuming that many disease processes will manifest as impairment in one or more of the test domains. These include visual contrast sensitivity, proprioception, quadriceps strength, reaction time, and postural sway on a compliant surface. In the original sample 75% of fallers were correctly identified by this method and a web-based falls risk calculator has been developed in Australia [20] which provides classification into five risk categories from very low to marked.

Assessment includes ascertaining the circumstances of the fall which often points to the likely cause. Environmental factors and 'risky' behaviours should be elicited, if necessary, with proxy information. History and physical examination is targeted towards detection of abnormalities in vision, cognition, cardiovascular, neurological, and musculoskeletal systems. Common diseases encountered include cataracts, postural hypotension, cardiac arrhythmias, stroke, Parkinson's disease, lower limb osteoarthritis, and recent fragility fractures. Action taken in the clinic may consist of medication adjustments, referrals to other specialists such as ophthalmologists, occupational, and physiotherapists. Cardiological and neurological testing should be initiated when the fall history is unclear and/or the injury indicates a loss of protective mechanisms (e.g. head trauma). Bone health assessment should also be considered.

9.7 Gap Analysis of Current Strategies

Given the development and uptake in consumer electronics such as mobile devices, it is a bit of a surprise that the use of technology in research of falls has been limited up to now. The other side of the coin is that the results of fall prediction, detection and prevention are still not satisfactory with classical clinical models based on the cascade of epidemiology, risk factor identification and elimination. One major barrier is the time demand to follow patients, the enormous task of fall reporting and the effort to recruit large number of participants into studies around the additional or substitutional effects of technology. We have identified at least four areas where technology can make a significant contribution in this field. However, we expect that this often be a complementary component to enhance or augment clinical approaches and less frequently a tech-only approach. The most promising areas are the improvement of fall prediction using body-worn sensors leading to a better stratification, personalization and monitoring of interventions, the use of body-worn sensors and ambient sensing to detect falls and reduce the time to rescue for unrecovered falls, the inclusion of technology to improve the efficacy of fall prevention interventions such as perturbation, digital training, exergaming or Virtual Reality/ Augmented Reality and finally the use of technology to manage of injurious fallers.

9.8 Improving Fall Risk Prediction with Technology

Technology can alleviate burden by automating and standardizing some of the quantifications. Computerized posturography and accelerometry have been used in fall risk assessment as well. These risk assessments provide objective quantifications of various mobility features. However, cost of these devices can inhibit clinicians from acquiring the necessary equipment and the need for specific training on using these devices is another limiting factor. Recent work has delved into using consumer-available devices for assessing fall risk. Smartphones, tablets, and gaming systems have been shown to be comparable to laboratory equipment for quantifying body movement. Many of these devices have not only been used in the clinic and laboratory spaces but can also be used in community settings. For example, Kinesis Balance is a smartphone app that allows older adults to have their balance assessed in an unsupervised setting [21]. Wii Fit boards have also been successful in quantifying balance to give general fall risk assessments, as well as Xbox's Kinect motion tracking system [22]. All of these types of technology allow for more access to healthcare, as these devices are more widely available and cheaper than standard laboratory equipment. These devices have also been optimally designed for layman use and do not require lots of speciality training. Again, several groups have developed apps for balance assessments (Kinesis Balance, iSway, Senior Sway, etc.) [21, 23, 24]. Furthermore, some groups have developed machine learning algorithms to predict falls and those at risk of falling [25–29]. The successfulness of these algorithms could go a long way to identify who is in most need of preventative or interventional treatment.

9.9 Technological Approaches to Fall Detection and Managing Falls

Advancement in technology specifically sensor networks, internet of things, and human-computer interaction are being regarded as effective approaches to fall detection and management. The earliest form of emergency alert systems, also called *Manual alert systems*, date back to the 1970s. Wilhelm Hormann introduced the German 'Hausnotruf' system and American International Telephone Company introduced the 'Emergency Dialer' (Popular Science 1975). These allowed individuals to contact caretaker or call centre for assistance in case of emergency. With rapid rise in the ageing population, and a pandemic situation such as COVID-19 may result in limited access to in-person healthcare facilities. Remote health monitoring will eventually gain popularity for rapid diagnosis, early detection of disability, and increased healthcare accessibility to underserved communities. *Technology for automated fall detection* looks promising and is the focus of this section.

Technology for fall detection can be divided into two categories—exosensors and wearables. *Exosensors* are set in the environment and may include visual sensors such as RGB and infrared cameras, as well as ambient sensors that are based on feedback from environment due to falling, for example, pressurized floors, microphones, ultrasonic sensors, etc. Feasibility studies with smart carpets and smart floors using pressure-sensing tiboelectric nanogenerators have been conducted for in-home use [30, 31]. The smart carpets are shown to exhibit an excellent electrical response to trigger, such as pressure sensitivity of 0.07 kPa^{-1} in the region from 0.8 to 11.8 kPa, fast response time of less than 28 ms and has an ability of precisely judging the falling action [31], and these systems are shown to achieve a classification accuracy of 96% in identifying actual falls [30]. Some of the key advantages are low cost, sending alarm without involving personal privacy, easy installation, and notable accuracy, making the proposed system potentially useful for homes and hospitals. Challenges for managing interference signal from cell and contact and for building higher fault tolerance remain [31]. Exosensors can also be incorporated in assistive-robot-based systems, as proposed in a recent study [32]. The assistive robot autonomously patrols an indoor environment, and when it detects falls, it activates an alarm. The system was designed to recognize lying-poses in single images. The robustness of the method has been tested using Fallen Person Dataset, which is publicly available dataset with eight different scenarios, various person heights, more than one person in an image, and several lying-position perspectives.

Before experiencing a fall, an individual's body can exhibit a range of physiological changes such as heart rate variability, change in breathing rate, body balance and orientation. *Wearables* comprising of sensors like accelerometers, gyroscopes, electrocardiography, electromyography, etc. can be leveraged to record these bodily variations and assist with fall detection. The key flow for building a fall detection system consists of selecting sensors, embedding them in suitable device (wearable as well as non-wearable installed in the environment), gathering and dynamically monitoring signals, and finally assisting with fall detection (Fig. 9.2).

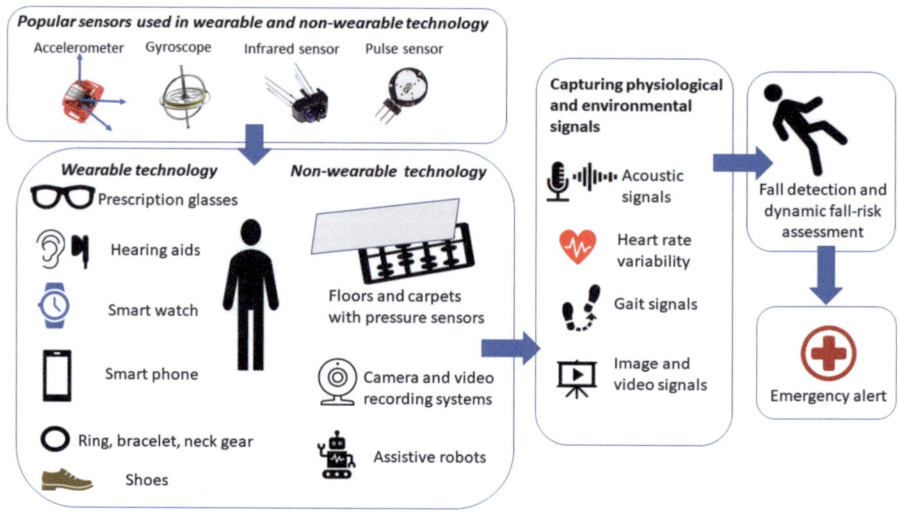

Fig. 9.2 Fall detection and dynamic risk monitoring systems using wearable technology consisting of sensors that can be placed on individuals and exosensors installed in the environment. The process involves embedding sensors into devices or objects, dynamically monitor the signal, and via algorithms detect falls, perform dynamic fall-risk assessments, and finally generate emergency alert

Some of the other questions in the field include—How many sensors are required? What is the best body location to install the sensor? What type of sensors are best suited for usage in the real-world? In a thorough investigation by Cleland and colleagues [33], it was found that although data from all locations provided similar levels of accuracy, the hip was the best single location to record data for activity detection providing better accuracy than the other investigated locations. Increasing the number of sensing locations from one to two or more statistically increased the accuracy of classification. There was no significant difference in accuracy when using two or more sensors. It was noted, however, that the difference in activity detection using single or multiple accelerometers may be more when trying to detect finer grain activities. For differentiating transitional activities, such as sitting (from standing) and lying down (also from standing), which are those most similar to falls, the most suitable positions have turned out to be the waist, chest, and knee [34]. In fall detection the waist accelerometer proved to have almost same performances as the chest accelerometer [35].

Wearable sensors based on *threshold values* have been proposed to distinguish near-falls from normal range of acceleration range, gait parameters, and other activities [36–38]. One of the milestone fall detection algorithms [38] was able to detect all fall events at least 70 msec before the impact, with the threshold adapted to each individual subject. Based on real-world fall recordings using body-worn sensors, a five-phase fall model has been proposed which includes the stages: pre-fall phase, falling phase, impact phase, resting phase, and recovery phase [39]. A preimpact fall detection study, utilizing *pattern recognition approaches* obtained an average lead time (i.e. the time between the fall detection and the collision) of 280 ± 10 ms with the experimental data that had 6 types of falls and 14 types of physical activity [40]. Another system predicts a fall event (300–700 msec) before occurring. Fall incidence will trigger an alarming notice to the appropriate healthcare providers via the Internet [41].

Literature shows that fusing the signals of different sensors could result in higher accuracy and lower false alarms, while improving the robustness of such systems [42]. More public datasets (Table 9.1) are now available for understanding fall-related signals and developing better detection solutions.

Machine learning and deep learning approaches based on existing multimodal datasets that utilize a combination of accelerometer and camera sensors have shown high accuracies in fall event detection of the order of 95% [52–54]. Using existing datasets such as UMAFall and SisFall with machine learning algorithms, a comprehensive study found that the multi-class approach to identify the phases of a fall showed promising results with an accuracy close to 99% [55]. It has been observed that ensemble learning algorithms perform better than lazy or eager learning models. Furthermore, a high sampling rate usually produces better results than a lower one. These neural network-based propositions may show high accuracies, however, very often lack transparency and interpretability. More investigation is warranted. Context-aware systems considering individual underlying conditions, surrounding environments, light exposure, and real-life complexities are needed to develop practical solutions.

The future of wearable technology to advance health outcomes such as fall detection appears to be promising. Fall detection from smartphones has been reviewed [56]. Built-in fall detection multiple sensor-based mechanisms can be installed in daily objects, gadgets, or tools that an individual uses. Pilot studies have been conducted to test the capability of fall detection using hearing aids [57], walking aids [58], prescription glasses [59], and other eyewear [60]. Watches are popular in step count monitoring but had been proposed for fall detection as early as the 2000s [61]. A proposed belt system also appears to be promising, since waist is an acceptable location for accuracy in terms of activity monitoring. This system records steps and falls [62]. Smart shoe-, chest bands-, and smart shirt-based systems have also been in development that make use of body temperature, ECG, and respiratory functionalities [63]. Although these systems may sound modern, we should also keep in mind if the system is too complicated, it may suffer from technology adherence issues from the users [64]. In the digital age, we should avoid adding to the cognitive load of the stakeholders involved. Moreover, making affordable technology is another aspect.

The fall detection problem may appear straightforward but is rather complex in *real-world settings*. For example, a system using accelerometer, magnetometer, gyroscopes, along with GPS and audio feedback capabilities recorded 83 of 84 false alarms, i.e. the system detecting a fall when it was not [65]. The authors

Table 9.1 Selected recent public datasets to develop understanding of fall mechanism, building fall detection algorithms using classical, machine learning and deep learning methods

Public dataset	Subject demographics	Fall samples	Types of sensors	Other Activities of Daily Living (ADL)	Reported performance for fall detection	Reported challenges
SisFall [43]	$N = 38$ (23 between 19 and 30 years, 15 between 60 and 75 years) 19 M, 19 F	15 types of falls (1798 falls)	Accelerometer, gyroscope	19 types of ADL (2706 ADLs)	84% accuracy with best feature, fails in every 7 of 10 ADLs	Young people simulate falls and ADL with more acceleration than that expected with elderly people.
UMAFall [44]	$N = 17$ (between 18 and 55, mean age 26.9 ± 10.2 years) 10 M, 7 F	3 types of falls (209 falls)	Accelerometer, gyroscope, magnetometer	8 types of ADLs (322 total ADLs)	Dataset description with some statistics-related visualizations	To detect falls, combined use of two sensors placed on the wrist and waist was proposed to characterize the mobility of the human body.
MobiFall [45]	$N = 24$ (between 22 and 47 years old) 17 M, 7 F	4 types of falls	Accelerometer, gyroscope	12 types of ADLs	The best performance of 99% achieved by the manually selected feature set. Entropy measure was found to be single best predictor	The performance could be a result of the relative low number of subjects in each split. Dataset extension with more subjects and activities as next steps to account for any ambiguity.
UR Fall [46]	$N = 5$ (above 26 years old) 5 M	3 types of falls (210 images)	Accelerometer, Kinect cameras	5 ADLs (402 images)	99% accuracy	A limitation of the Kinect sensor is that sunlight interferes with the pattern-projecting laser, so the proposed fall detection system is most suitable for indoor use only.
tFall [47]	$N = 10$ (between 20 to 42 years old, 31.3 ± 8.6 years) 7 M, 3F	8 types of falls (503 falls recorded)	Accelerometer in smartphone, placed in pocket	Under real-life conditions (on average about 800 ADL records per subject were collected)	90% specificity	A restricted set of falls simulated by young and middle-age people, all of them healthy subjects.

DLR [48]	$N = 20$ (between 23 and 58 years) 14 M, 6 F	One type of fall	Accelerometer, gyroscope, magnetometer, barometer	15 types of ADLs	75% for falling	Walking up and downstairs and falling were sometimes confused. It is also suggested to extend the algorithm to recognize sensor posture, such as "pocket-based", "handheld" and "swinging".
KFall x([49])	$N = 32$ (24.9 ± 3.7 years) 32 M	15 types of falls	Accelerometer, gyroscope, magnetometer	21 types of ADLs	99% specificity and sensitivity using deep learning	The dataset only contains simulated falls from young male adults due to safety concerns and practical convenience. Additionally, it does not include normal ADLs from older subjects
FARSEEING [18]	$N = 2000$ contributed physical activity data, 76 ± 12.6 years, mean age of 94 fallers	208 real-world fall events	Accelerometer, 58% additionally include gyroscope and magnetometer	24 h of physical activity monitored	Dataset description only	Underreporting might occur, especially in populations with cognitive impairment.
CMDFall [50]	$N = 50$ (21–40 years old) 30 M, 20 F	8 types of falls (400 falls)	Accelerometer, Kinect sensors	12 ADLs (600 normal activities)	Fusion of modalities resulted in 98% F1 score	Depth of field is quite noisy, and the skeleton is unreliable due to the complex and various human poses. Acceleration cannot distinguish a fall from many other fall-like activities.
FallAllD [51]	$N = 15$	35 types of falls	Accelerometer, gyroscope, magnetometer, barometer	44 types of ADL	93% accuracy	More challenges with wrist-worn sensors due to complicated movements, compared to waist-worn sensors.

found that largest percentage of these false alarms (42.2%) were during normal device use. Another 16.9% of false alarms occurred when the participant dropped the device. Device misuse and putting down the device each constituted 10.8% of false alarms. Finally, 19.3% of false alarms occurred for unknown reasons, perhaps it was almost a fall which the individual was able to correct. Sensitivity and specificity are both critical aspects to building a reliable fall-detection system. Distinguishing sitting (specially sitting on the ground), standing, and lying from each other remains challenging [66, 67]. A technology system may depend on age range and whether falls are to be detected indoors, in hospital settings, or in community settings. Infrared and Kinect sensors cannot be used in sunlight and are preferred for indoor usage; thus, they won't be useful in outdoor settings. Video-based monitoring is great at visualizing human body movement however they have privacy and security considerations if used inside homes. Furthermore, these cameras' sensor-based fall detection is computationally expensive; they need cloud-based approaches for faster processing and data storage. Response time is critical in falling situations. Accelerometers are sensitive to movement, so their location on the body becomes crucial in distinguishing falls from other movements and body transitions between activities of daily living. Thus, each sensor will have an advantage and limitation. Demographics of individuals based on which fall detection systems are being built are also critical. For example, many of the subjects in the fall datasets (Table 9.1) are young individuals, with falls simulated in laboratory conditions. For improving accuracy and sensitivity of fall detection, more data may not necessarily be better for supervised learning approach, emphasis instead should be on diverse data in terms of types of activity of daily life (ADL), studying the characteristics of falls that are false-positive, and those going undetected.

9.10 Digital Mobility Parameters for Monitoring

Monitoring of gait speed and walking endurance are popular in laboratory assessment of mobility function [68, 69]. Physical function and life-space have popularly been self-reported in past research. Self-report is quick however is prone to recall bias and may be influenced by individual perceptions. Over the last two decades, accelerometer-based wearable devices have become popular in objective monitoring of physical activity and overall mobility in daily life. These are lightweight, compact, and cheap devices. Activity volume can be quantified as step-count, transitions between postures, and number of activity bouts. Activity intensity can be quantified as light, moderate, and vigorous depending on energy spent. Besides, recent interest has been in daily-life measures for gait variability such as cadence and entropy (Table 9.2). Association of physical function, cognitive capabilities, psychosocial health, and environmental-related factors with digital mobility measures from accelerometer sensors have been detailed [70]. An Australia-based randomized controlled trial found that daily feedback to patients and therapists using an accelerometer increased walking times during rehabilitation admissions [71]. In regard to falls, there is no consensus on if volume, quality, or both aspects of mobility are important considerations to reduce fall risk. For example, fall history was not associated with volume-based accelerometry measures, such as steps per day but instead was associated with quality of walking [72, 73]. This contrasts with studies that showed non-recurrent fallers (less than two falls) took more steps per day than recurrent fallers [74, 75] and that fall risk was reduced in those walking greater than 5000 steps per day (volume measure) [76]. Among other mobility markers, spatio-temporal measures from Global Positioning System are also becoming popular [77]. A general flowchart for extracting mobility measures in daily-life is given in Fig. 9.3. Overall, wearable technology-enabled interventions can assist in delaying mobility-related disability and improving participation of older adults in the community.

Table 9.2 Accelerometer-based parameters to assist digital mobility monitoring (Table adapted from [70]). Accelerometer measures can be classified under the umbrella categories of Volume, Intensity, and Gait Quality. Specific measures can be extracted and put to these categories

Volume	Intensity	Gait Quality
Step count Walking bouts count Daily activity counts Up-down transitions High-low activity transitions	Minutes spent, Metabolic equivalents (METs), and accumulation of the following: – Light physical activity. – Moderate physical activity. – Vigorous physical activity.	Step variability Cadence Complexity Entropy Acceleration range

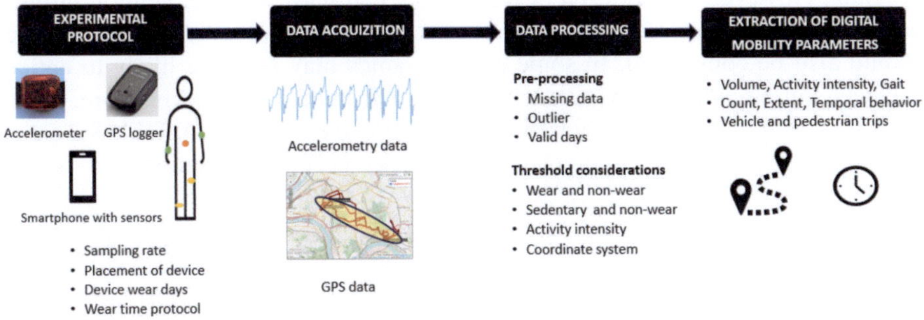

Fig. 9.3 A flowchart depicting extraction of digital mobility parameters from sensors and various considerations in the process, modified from Fig. 9.1 of [70]

9.11 Interventions to Reduce the Risk of Falling Based on Technology

Many interventions utilizing technology have been developed, in the hopes that the interventions are more appealing, easier to follow, and can be done more independently. All these factors would help increase adherence to the interventions and reduce fall risk more consistently. The table shows some examples such as StandingTall [78], Nymbl [79], and KOKU (keep on keep up) [80]. These programs have shown that they can reduce fall risk or incident rate of falls. Interventions that require facilitation also show improvement in fall risk. V-Time [81] and treadmill perturbation [82] are promising in their reduction of falls. However, availability of such interventions would be limited and requires significant equipment and staff training.

Exergames have also shown to be promising, often using Nintendo Wii or Xbox Kinect to allow for visual feedback as well as fun and engaging platforms for individuals to interact with. A review found that exergame-based interventions did improve physical or cognitive function in older adults but whether exergames were superior to standard physical therapy interventions remains to be seen [22]. Using commercially available systems makes these interventions more accessible as they are more widely available, cheaper, and do not require extensive training to use. Exoskeleton systems have also been developed, more specifically for individuals with neurological conditions that have led to gait deficits such as stroke, Parkinson's disease, or multiple sclerosis. The Lokomat has shown promising results for improving gait function in these groups but there is conflicting evidence as to whether the exoskeleton is better than traditional mobility interventions [83].

Higher rates of adherence have been shown in both supervised and unsupervised settings for technology-based versus traditional interventions [84]. The increased adherence is most often due to increased enjoyment of the exercise program. However, the addition of technology can make the intervention intimidating or confusing to older adults who are its intended audience. Societal nuance should also be considered. In some places, games may be more likely to entice subjects, but elsewhere they may repel subjects instead. Like in Singapore, game exercise was found to be less helpful than traditional exercise [85]. Table 9.3 summarizes ongoing as well as completed technology-based intervention studies.

Table 9.3 Technology-based intervention studies (ongoing as well as completed)

Technological interventions	Intervention/technology description	Intervention environment	Success of intervention Implication on fall prevention
Standing Tall [78]	Phone app that delivers personalized instruction for balance exercises. Subjects completed two hours of standing tall per week in addition to health education for 2 years.	Free-living, unsupervised Adherence:40% adherence over first 6 months, 30% adherence over 24 months	Significantly reduced rate of falls and injurious falls over 2 years by 16% and 20% respectively ($p = 0.027$, $p = 0.031$)
Nymbl [79]	Phone app developed to follow the guidelines set by the STEADI (Stop Elderly Accidents, Deaths, and Injuries) best practices protocol [86]. The app requires the subject to undergo an assessment and then provides personalized exercises based on the subject's performance for 6 min every day. Subjects used the app for 3 or 6 weeks.	Laboratory-based for balance assessments then free-living setting and unsupervised for app usage Adherence: 95% ± 24% for 3 weeks (21 days), 90% ± 26% for 6 weeks (42 days)	Improvements seen after 3 weeks in tandem stance AP sway (-3.2 mm; $p < 0,00$), ML sway (-1.3 mm; $p = 0.01$), and sway area (-682.7; $p = 0.001$); one legged stance AP sway (-1.5 mm; $p = 0.02$), and feet together stance sway area (-128.7mm^2; $p = 0.01$).
KOKU [80]	Gamified strength and balance tablet-based app guided by Otago Exercise Program [87] accompanied by health education, home safety test, gait training, and a medication review. Subjects had follow-up visits at 6 and 12 weeks.	In-home setting supervised for initial 4 weeks and encouraged via telephone check-ins the next 2 weeks to continue intervention independently Adherence: 61% still used app at least once per week at 6 week follow up	Improvements in exercise efficacy ($p = 0.014$), exercise frequency ($p = 0.018$), sleep quality ($p = 0.003$), and self-rated physical health ($p = 0.048$), and reductions in disability ($p = 0.027$) and sleep medication use ($p = 0.016$).
V-Time [81]	Combines treadmill training and VR to target physical and cognitive aspects of walking, real-time foot movement projected to subject and the simulated environment included obstacles, multiple pathways, and distractions. Subjects did training for 45 min 3 times per week for 6 weeks.	Laboratory-based	Fall rate significantly reduced for subjects who did treadmill and VR (11.9 compared to 6.00 falls per 6 months, $p < 0.0001$)

(continued)

Table 9.3 (continued)

Technological interventions	Intervention/technology description	Intervention environment	Success of intervention Implication on fall prevention
Treadmill Perturbations [82]	Dual-belt treadmill walking with anterior-posterior perturbations administered by abruptly changing belt speed or adjusting platform beneath treadmill*. 2 visits one week apart.	Laboratory-based	No group differences were found between the subjects that were given perturbation training versus regular treadmill walking. Perturbation recovery was significantly improved for both groups for AP and ML perturbations ($p < 0.001$ for both).
Vibrating insoles [88]	Provided subsensory vibrations to soles of the feet to improve sensation, balance, and gait. Subjects attended 3 6-h study sessions on separate days over the course of 2 weeks.	Laboratory-based, supervised	Significantly improved TUG, decreased area of postural sway, and reduced temporal gait variability ($p < 0.01$ for all)
Wii Fit exergame [89]	Used a Wii fit balance board for subjects to use to play a range of games that target different static and dynamic components of balance of varying difficulty. Subjects completed 10 training sessions of at least 30 min over the course of 5 weeks.	Laboratory-based, supervised	Significantly improved BBS (45.93 increased 50.10; $p < 0.001$) and ABC scores (62.25 increased to 72.25; $p < 0.001$). COP displacement and dynamic balance performance also improved with the experimental group significantly better than the control group ($p < 0.001$ for both tests).
Xbox Kinect exergame [90]	Exergames involved picking up apples, tight-rope walking, and balloon popping. Subjects played the exergames 24 total times with a frequency of one to three times per week.	Laboratory-based, supervised	Decreased double standing time ($P = 0.03$), minimum foot clearance ($P = 0.04$), BBS scores ($P < 0.01$), CS-30 scores ($P < 0.01$), and FRT scores ($P < 0.01$) significantly improved in the intervention group compared with values in the control group.

Table 9.3 (continued)

Technological interventions	Intervention/technology description	Intervention environment	Success of intervention Implication on fall prevention
Lokomat exeoskeleton [83]	Static, robotic exoskeleton device integrated into a treadmill with a bodyweight support system and monitor that provides feedback. Used to help individuals regain walking ability. Subjects are often recovering from stroke or have Parkinson's disease or multiple sclerosis.	Laboratory-based, supervised,	Review finds Lokomat does improve mobility, but it is unclear if better than standard therapy

9.12   Future Perspectives

The consumer electronics sector of industry is driving the developments at a breathtaking speed. This leads to novel situations where many research projects are in a defence situation or try to validate industrial approaches that have been developed by start-up companies or established players. Data on the accuracy, false positive and false negative and other test measurement properties are often lacking for industrial products. Thousands of Apps on exercise intervention are available, and many claim to improve balance and strength. The evidence from randomized controlled trials is non-existent for most of them. That leaves patients and clinicians in a dilemma.

The world's leading experts on falls concluded in their recent paper on the state-of-the-art that they all see a huge potential in using technology for fall detection and fall risk assessment but rated the evidence as preliminary and incomplete (Montero-Odasso 2022). Likewise, this group recognizes the need and opportunities to use web-based and mobile applications for exercise programs addressing fall prevention. For the time being, the evidence base for this is insufficient. A further aspect that was identified is the use of actigraphy to monitor patients and older citizens if they reach sufficient levels of physical activities and how certain clinical interventions influence these physical activity levels. Most clinicians also acknowledge that personal emergency response systems such as fall detectors are required for a reduction of long-lying periods and avoid potentially life-threatening situations. If older persons panic or lose their consciousness only technology will compensate these events.

The clinical uptake of digital mobility measures will occur, but the timing is not clear. The adoption of technology as part of the clinical routines has been slow. There are some early adopting pioneers that embrace sensor-derived data and encourage their patients to use technology. The recent release of the iOS 18 platform surprisingly offers a mobile mobility lab profiling patients on their levels of dynamic balance. This push and others need to be accompanied with rigorous and independent cross-validation. Intuitive use of technology by older adults is key.

The usability and user experience should be in the centre of future developments. Co-design approaches need to be started in the embryonic phase of most projects. This has been a deficit in the development of many fall alarm systems when relatives and clinicians pushed hard for older persons to use the technology, but the actual adherence was limited. The digital exercise programs should not be considered as a substitute for personal contact but rather as an augmenting approach or sometimes as a bridging intervention, e.g. after discharge before a regular training program or physiotherapy is started. It is unlikely that habit formation will be sufficient to use these approaches for more than 2–3 months.

Technology assisting risk profiling in order to tailor and personalize prevention is great, but it will take time for healthcare professionals to understand the relevance of digital mobility biomarkers beyond gait volume, cadence and pace. There is also a need for better visualization of data that are face valid, informative and comprehensible for patients and healthcare professionals.

References

1. Lamb SE, Jørstad-Stein EC, Hauer K, Becker C. Development of a common outcome data set for fall injury prevention trials: the prevention of falls network Europe consensus. J Am Geriatr Soc. 2005;53(9):1618–22. https://doi.org/10.1111/J.1532-5415.2005.53455.X.
2. Schwenk M, Lauenroth A, Stock C, Moreno RR, Oster P, McHugh G, Todd C, Hauer K. Definitions and methods of measuring and reporting on injurious falls in randomised controlled fall prevention trials: a systematic review. BMC Med Res Methodol. 2012;12 https://doi.org/10.1186/1471-2288-12-50.
3. Kempen GIJM, Yardley L, Van Haastregt JCM, Zijlstra GAR, Beyer N, Hauer K, Todd C. The short FES-I: a shortened version of the falls efficacy scale-international to assess fear of falling. Age Ageing. 2008;37(1):45–50. https://doi.org/10.1093/AGEING/AFM157.
4. Rapp K, Freiberger E, Todd C, Klenk J, Becker C, Denkinger M, Scheidt-Nave C, Fuchs J. Fall incidence in Germany: results of two population-based studies, and comparison of retrospective and prospective falls data collection methods. BMC Geriatr. 2014;14(1) https://doi.org/10.1186/1471-2318-14-105.
5. Campbell AJ, Robertson MC. Implementation of multifactorial interventions for fall and fracture prevention. Age Ageing. 2006;35(SUPPL.2):ii60. https://doi.org/10.1093/AGEING/AFL089.
6. Deandrea S, Lucenteforte E, Bravi F, Foschi R, La Vecchia C, Negri E. Risk factors for falls in community-dwelling older people: a systematic review and meta-analysis. Epidemiology. 2010;21(5):658–68. https://doi.org/10.1097/EDE.0B013E3181E89905.
7. Ballinger C, Brooks, C. An overview of best practice for falls prevention from an occupational therapy perspective Foundation 2 An overview of best practice for falls prevention from an occupational therapy perspective. 2013. www.balancetraining.org.uk/fallsAdvice/findPath.
8. Clemson L, Fitzgerald MH, Heard R. Content validity of an assessment tool to identify home fall hazards: the Westmead home safety. Assessment. 2016;62(4):171–9. https://doi.org/10.1177/030802269906200407.
9. CDC. Clinical resources | STEADI–older adult fall prevention | CDC Injury Center. 2016a. https://www.cdc.gov/steadi/materials.html

10. Drootin M. Summary of the updated American Geriatrics Society/British geriatrics society clinical practice guideline for prevention of falls in older persons. J Am Geriatr Soc. 2011;59(1):148–57. https://doi.org/10.1111/J.1532-5415.2010.03234.X.
11. NICE. 1 Recommendations | Falls in older people: assessing risk and prevention | Guidance | NICE. 2013. https://www.nice.org.uk/guidance/cg161/chapter/1-recommendations#preventing-falls-in-older-people-2
12. CDC. POCKET GUIDE preventing falls in older patients. 2016b. www.cdc.gov/steadi.
13. British Columbia. Fall prevention - province of British Columbia. 2016. https://www2.gov.bc.ca/gov/content/family-social-supports/seniors/health-safety/disease-and-injury-care-and-prevention/fall-prevention.
14. AGS/BGS. Prevention of falls in older persons. AGS/BGS Clinical Practice Guideline; 2016.
15. Close JCT, Lord SR. Fall assessment in older people. BMJ. 2011;343(7823) https://doi.org/10.1136/BMJ.D5153.
16. CDC. Assessment Timed Up & Go (TUG). 2017. www.cdc.gov/steadi
17. ProFouND. Prevention of falls network for dissemination | ProFouND Project | Fact Sheet | CIP | CORDIS | European Commission. 2016. https://cordis.europa.eu/project/id/325087
18. Klenk J, Schwickert L, Palmerini L, Mellone S, Bourke A, Ihlen EAF, Kerse N, Hauer K, Pijnappels M, Synofzik M, Srulijes K, Maetzler W, Helbostad JL, Zijlstra W, Aminian K, Todd C, Chiari L, Becker C, for the FARSEEING Consortium, et al. The FARSEEING real-world fall repository: a large-scale collaborative database to collect and share sensor signals from real-world falls. Eur Rev Aging Phys Act. 2016;13(1):1–7. https://doi.org/10.1186/S11556-016-0168-9/FIGURES/3.
19. Lord SR, Sherrington C, Menz HB. Falls in older people: risk factors and strategies for prevention. Cambridge University Press; 1999.
20. Neuroscience Research Australia. FallScreen© risk of falls calculator for rehabilitation. Occupational Therapy NeuRA Research. 2016; https://www.neura.edu.au/research-clinic/fbrg/
21. Greene BR, McManus K, Ader LGM, Caulfield B. Unsupervised assessment of balance and falls risk using a smartphone and machine learning. Sensors. 2021;21(14):4770. https://doi.org/10.3390/S21144770.
22. Choi SD, Guo L, Kang D, Xiong S. Exergame technology and interactive interventions for elderly fall prevention: a systematic literature review. Appl Ergon. 2017;65:570–81. https://doi.org/10.1016/J.APERGO.2016.10.013.
23. Mancini M, Salarian A, Carlson-Kuhta P, Zampieri C, King L, Chiari L, Horak FB. ISway: a sensitive, valid and reliable measure of postural control. J Neuro Engg Rehabil. 2012;9(1):59. https://doi.org/10.1186/1743-0003-9-59.
24. Pergolotti M, Deal AM, Bryant AL, Bennett AV, Farley E, Covington K, Lucas K, Williams GR. Senior sway: using a Mobile application to measure fall risk. J Geriatr Phys Ther. 2019;42(3):E101–7. https://doi.org/10.1519/JPT.0000000000000223.
25. Gillain S, Boutaayamou M, Schwartz C, Brüls O, Bruyère O, Croisier JL, Salmon E, Reginster JY, Garraux G, Petermans J. Using supervised learning machine algorithm to identify future fallers based on gait patterns: a two-year longitudinal study. Exp Gerontol. 2019;127:110730. https://doi.org/10.1016/J.EXGER.2019.110730.
26. Hu Y, Bishnoi A, Kaur R, Sowers R, Hernandez ME. Exploration of machine learning to identify community dwelling older adults with balance dysfunction using short duration accelerometer data. In: Proceedings of the Annual International Conference of the IEEE engineering in medicine and biology society, EMBS, vol. 2020; 2020. p. 812–5. https://doi.org/10.1109/EMBC44109.2020.9175871.
27. O'Sullivan M, Blake C, Cunningham C, Boyle G, Finucane C. Correlation of accelerometry with clinical balance tests in older fallers and non-fallers. Age Ageing. 2009;38(3):308–13. https://doi.org/10.1093/ageing/afp009.
28. Rivolta MW, Aktaruzzaman M, Rizzo G, Lafortuna CL, Ferrarin M, Bovi G, Bonardi DR, Caspani A, Sassi R. Evaluation of the Tinetti score and fall risk assessment via accelerometry-based movement analysis. Artif Intell Med. 2019;95:38–47. https://doi.org/10.1016/j.artmed.2018.08.005.

29. Shahzad A, Ko S, Lee S, Lee JA, Kim K. Quantitative assessment of balance impairment for fall-risk estimation using wearable Triaxial accelerometer. IEEE Sensors J. 2017;17(20):6743–51. https://doi.org/10.1109/JSEN.2017.2749446.
30. Jeon SB, Nho YH, Park SJ, Kim WG, Tcho IW, Kim D, Kwon DS, Choi YK. Self-powered fall detection system using pressure sensing triboelectric nanogenerators. Nano Energy. 2017;41:139–47. https://doi.org/10.1016/J.NANOEN.2017.09.028.
31. Yu A, Wang W, Li Z, Liu X, Zhang Y, Zhai J. Large-scale smart carpet for self-powered fall detection. Adv Material Technol. 2020;5(2):1900978. https://doi.org/10.1002/ADMT.201900978.
32. Maldonado-Bascón S, Iglesias-Iglesias C, Martín-Martín P, Lafuente-Arroyo S. Fallen people detection capabilities using assistive robot. Electronics. 2019;8:915. https://doi.org/10.3390/ELECTRONICS8090915.
33. Cleland I, Kikhia B, Nugent C, Boytsov A, Hallberg J, Synnes K, McClean S, Finlay D. Optimal placement of accelerometers for the detection of everyday activities. Sensors (Basel, Switzerland). 2013;13(7):9183–200. https://doi.org/10.3390/S130709183.
34. Atallah L, Lo B, King R, Yang GZ. Sensor positioning for activity recognition using wearable accelerometers. IEEE Transactions on Biomedical Circuits and Systems. 2011;5(4):320–9. https://doi.org/10.1109/TBCAS.2011.2160540.
35. Gjoreski H, Luštrek M, Gams M. Accelerometer placement for posture recognition and fall detection. In: Proceedings−2011 7th International Conference on intelligent environments, IE; 2011. p. 47–54. https://doi.org/10.1109/IE.2011.11.
36. Kostopoulos P, Kyritsis AI, Deriaz M, Konstantas D. F2D: a location aware fall detection system tested with real data from daily life of elderly people. Procedia Comp Sci. 2016;98:212–9. https://doi.org/10.1016/J.PROCS.2016.09.035.
37. Weiss A, Shimkin I, Giladi N, Hausdorff JM. Automated detection of near falls: algorithm development and preliminary results. BMC Res Notes. 2010;3:62. https://doi.org/10.1186/1756-0500-3-62.
38. Wu G, Xue S. Portable preimpact fall detector with inertial sensors. IEEE Trans Neural Syst Rehabil Eng. 2008;16(2):178–83. https://doi.org/10.1109/TNSRE.2007.916282.
39. Becker C, Schwickert L, Mellone S, Bagalà F, Chiari L, Helbostad JL, Zijlstra W, Aminian K, Bourke A, Todd C, Bandinelli S, Kerse N, Klenk J. Proposal for a multiphase fall model based on real-world fall recordings with body-fixed sensors. Zeitschrift Fur Gerontologie Und Geriatrie. 2012;45(8):707–15. https://doi.org/10.1007/S00391-012-0403-6.
40. Jung H, Koo B, Kim J, Kim T, Nam Y, Kim Y. Enhanced algorithm for the detection of Preimpact fall for wearable airbags. Sensors. 2020;20:1277. https://doi.org/10.3390/S20051277.
41. Saadeh W, Butt SA, Altaf MA, Bin. A patient-specific single sensor iot-based wearable fall prediction and detection system. IEEE Trans Neural Syst Rehabil Eng. 2019;27(5):995–1003. https://doi.org/10.1109/TNSRE.2019.2911602.
42. Wang X, Ellul J, Azzopardi G. Elderly fall detection systems: a literature survey. Front Robotics AI. 2020;7:71. https://doi.org/10.3389/FROBT.2020.00071/BIBTEX.
43. Sucerquia A, López JD, Vargas-Bonilla JF. SisFall: a fall and movement dataset. Sensors. 2017;17:198. https://doi.org/10.3390/S17010198.
44. Casilari E, Santoyo-Ramón JA, Cano-García JM. UMAFall: a multisensor dataset for the research on automatic fall detection. Procedia Comp Sci. 2017;110:32–9. https://doi.org/10.1016/J.PROCS.2017.06.110.
45. Vavoulas G, Pediaditis M, Tsiknakis M. The MobiFall dataset: fall detection and classification with a smartphone. Int J Monitor Surv Technol Res. 2014;2(1):44–56. https://doi.org/10.4018/ijmstr.2014010103.
46. Kwolek B, Kepski M. Human fall detection on embedded platform using depth maps and wireless accelerometer. Comput Methods Prog Biomed. 2014;117(3):489–501. https://doi.org/10.1016/J.CMPB.2014.09.005.
47. Medrano C, Igual R, Plaza I, Castro M. Detecting falls as novelties in acceleration patterns acquired with smartphones. PLoS One. 2014;9(4):e94811. https://doi.org/10.1371/JOURNAL.PONE.0094811.

48. Frank K, Diaz EM, Robertson P, Sánchez FJF. Bayesian recognition of safety relevant motion activities with inertial sensors and barometer. In: Record–IEEE PLANS, Position Location and Navigation Symposium; 2014. p. 174–84. https://doi.org/10.1109/PLANS.2014.6851373.
49. Yu X, Jang J, Xiong S. A large-scale open motion dataset (KFall) and benchmark algorithms for detecting pre-impact fall of the elderly using wearable inertial sensors. Front Aging Neurosci. 2021;13:399. https://doi.org/10.3389/FNAGI.2021.692865/BIBTEX.
50. Tran TH, Le TL, Pham DT, Hoang VN, Khong VM, Tran QT, Nguyen TS, Pham C. A multi-modal multi-view dataset for human fall analysis and preliminary investigation on modality. In: Proceedings–International Conference on pattern recognition, 2018-august; 2018. p. 1947–52. https://doi.org/10.1109/ICPR.2018.8546308.
51. Saleh M, Abbas M, Le Jeannes RB. FallAllD: an open dataset of human falls and activities of daily living for classical and deep learning applications. IEEE Sensors J. 2021;21(2):1849–58. https://doi.org/10.1109/JSEN.2020.3018335.
52. Galvão YM, Ferreira J, Albuquerque VA, Barros P, Fernandes BJT. A multimodal approach using deep learning for fall detection. Expert Syst Appl. 2021;168:114226. https://doi.org/10.1016/J.ESWA.2020.114226.
53. Garg S, Panigrahi BK, Joshi D. An accelerometer based fall detection system using deep neural network. In: 2019 IEEE 5th International Conference for convergence in technology, I2CT; 2019. https://doi.org/10.1109/I2CT45611.2019.9033556.
54. Santos GL, Endo PT, de Monteiro KHC, Rocha, da ES, Silva I, Lynn T. Accelerometer-based human fall detection using convolutional neural networks. Sensors. 2019;19:1644. https://doi.org/10.3390/S19071644.
55. Zurbuchen N, Wilde A, Bruegger P. A machine learning multi-class approach for fall detection systems based on wearable sensors with a study on sampling rates selection. Sensors (Basel, Switzerland). 2021;21(3):1–23. https://doi.org/10.3390/S21030938.
56. Islam MM, Neom NH, Imtiaz MS, Nooruddin S, Islam MR, Islam MR. A review on fall detection systems using data from smartphone sensors. Ingenierie Des Systemes d'Information. 2019;24(6):569–76. https://doi.org/10.18280/ISI.240602.
57. Rahme M, Folkeard P, Scollie S. Evaluating the accuracy of step tracking and fall detection in the Starkey Livio artificial intelligence hearing aids: a pilot study. Am J Audiol. 2020;30(1):182–9. https://doi.org/10.1044/2020_AJA-20-00105.
58. Taghvaei S, Jahanandish MH, Kosuge K. Autoregressive-moving-average hidden Markov model for vision-based fall prediction-an application for walker robot. Assist Technol. 2017;29(1):19–27. https://doi.org/10.1080/10400435.2016.1174178.
59. Chen OTC, Kuo CJ. Self-adaptive fall-detection apparatus embedded in glasses. In: Annual International Conference of the IEEE engineering in medicine and biology society. IEEE engineering in medicine and biology society. Annual International Conference, vol. 2014; 2014. p. 4623–6. https://doi.org/10.1109/EMBC.2014.6944654.
60. Lin CL, Chiu WC, Chu TC, Ho YH, Chen FH, Hsu CC, Hsieh PH, Chen CH, Lin CC, Sung PS, Chen PT. Innovative head-mounted system based on inertial sensors and magnetometer for detecting falling movements. Sensors. 2020;20(20):5774. https://doi.org/10.3390/S20205774.
61. Degen T, Jaeckel H, Rufer M, Wyss S. SPEEDY: a fall detector in a wrist watch. In: Proceedings–International Symposium on Wearable Computers, ISWC; 2003. p. 184–9. https://doi.org/10.1109/ISWC.2003.1241410.
62. Liu B, Wang D, Li S, Nie X, Xu S, Jiao B, Duan X, Huang A. Design and implementation of an intelligent belt system using accelerometer. In: Annual International Conference of the IEEE engineering in medicine and biology society. IEEE engineering in medicine and biology society. Annual International Conference, vol. 2015; 2015. p. 2043–6. https://doi.org/10.1109/EMBC.2015.7318788.
63. Costa SEP, Rodrigues JJPC, Silva BMC, Isento JN, Corchado JM. Integration of wearable solutions in AAL environments with mobility support. J Med Syst. 2015;39(12):184. https://doi.org/10.1007/S10916-015-0342-Z.

64. Wilson J, Heinsch M, Betts D, Booth D, Kay-Lambkin F. Barriers and facilitators to the use of e-health by older adults: a scoping review. BMC Public Health. 2021;21(1):1–12. https://doi.org/10.1186/S12889-021-11623-W/TABLES/2.

65. Chaudhuri S, Oudejans D, Thompson HJ, Demiris G. Real world accuracy and use of a wearable fall detection device by older adults. J Am Geriatr Soc. 2015;63(11):2415. https://doi.org/10.1111/JGS.13804.

66. Bourke AK, Ihlen EAF, Van De Ven P, Nelson J, Helbostad JL. Video analysis validation of a real-time physical activity detection algorithm based on a single waist mounted tri-axial accelerometer sensor. In: Proceedings of the Annual International Conference of the IEEE engineering in medicine and biology society. EMBS; 2016. p. 4881–4. https://doi.org/10.1109/EMBC.2016.7591821.

67. Jatesiktat P, Ang WT. An elderly fall detection using a wrist-worn accelerometer and barometer. In: Proceedings of the Annual International Conference of the IEEE Engineering in Medicine and Biology Society, EMBS; 2017. p. 125–30. https://doi.org/10.1109/EMBC.2017.8036778.

68. Studenski S, Perera S, Patel K, Rosano C, Faulkner K, Inzitari M, Brach J, Chandler J, Cawthon P, Connor EB, Nevitt M, Visser M, Kritchevsky S, Badinelli S, Harris T, Newman AB, Cauley J, Ferrucci L, Guralnik J. Gait speed and survival in older adults. JAMA. 2011;305(1):50–8. https://doi.org/10.1001/JAMA.2010.1923.

69. Van Swearingen JM, Perera S, Brach JS, Cham R, Rosano C, Studenski SA. A randomized trial of two forms of therapeutic activity to improve walking: effect on the energy cost of walking. J Gerontol A Biol Sci Med Sci. 2009;64(11):1190–8. https://doi.org/10.1093/GERONA/GLP098.

70. Suri A, VanSwearingen J, Dunlap P, Redfern MS, Rosso AL, Sejdić E. Facilitators and barriers to real-life mobility in community-dwelling older adults: a narrative review of accelerometry- and global positioning system-based studies. Aging Clin Exp Res. 2022;2022:1–14. https://doi.org/10.1007/S40520-022-02096-X.

71. Peel NM, Paul SK, Cameron ID, Crotty M, Kurrle SE, Gray LC. Promoting activity in geriatric rehabilitation: a randomized controlled trial of Accelerometry. PLoS One. 2016;11(8):e0160906. https://doi.org/10.1371/JOURNAL.PONE.0160906.

72. Ihlen EAF, Weiss A, Bourke A, Helbostad JL, Hausdorff JM. The complexity of daily life walking in older adult community-dwelling fallers and non-fallers. J Biomech. 2016;49(9):1420–8. https://doi.org/10.1016/J.JBIOMECH.2016.02.055.

73. Weiss A, Brozgol M, Dorfman M, Herman T, Shema S, Giladi N, Hausdorff JM. Does the evaluation of gait quality during daily life provide insight into fall risk? A novel approach using 3-day accelerometer recordings. Neurorehabil Neural Repair. 2013;27(8):742–52. https://doi.org/10.1177/1545968313491004.

74. Jefferis BJ, Iliffe S, Kendrick D, Kerse N, Trost S, Lennon LT, Ash S, Sartini C, Morris RW, Wannamethee SG, Whincup PH. How are falls and fear of falling associated with objectively measured physical activity in a cohort of community-dwelling older men? BMC Geriatr. 2014;14(1) https://doi.org/10.1186/1471-2318-14-114.

75. Jefferis BJ, Merom D, Sartini C, Wannamethee SG, Ash S, Lennon LT, Iliffe S, Kendrick D, Whincup PH. Physical activity and falls in older men: the critical role of mobility limitations. Med Sci Sports Exerc. 2015;47(10):2119–28. https://doi.org/10.1249/MSS.0000000000000635.

76. Aranyavalai T, Jalayondeja C, Jalayondeja W, Pichaiyongwongdee S, Kaewkungwal J, Laskin JJ. Association between walking 5000 step/ day and fall incidence over six months in urban community-dwelling older people. BMC Geriatr. 2020;20(1):1–11. https://doi.org/10.1186/S12877-020-01582-Z/FIGURES/2.

77. Fillekes MP, Kim EK, Trumpf R, Zijlstra W, Giannouli E, Weibel R. Assessing older adults' daily mobility: a comparison of GPS-derived and self-reported mobility indicators. Sensors. 2019;19(20) https://doi.org/10.3390/S19204551.

78. Delbaere K, Valenzuela T, Lord SR, Clemson L, Zijlstra GAR, Close JCT, Lung T, Woodbury A, Chow J, McInerney G, Miles L, Toson B, Briggs N, Van Schooten KS. E-health StandingTall

balance exercise for fall prevention in older people: results of a two year randomised controlled trial. BMJ. 2021;373 https://doi.org/10.1136/BMJ.N740.

79. Papi E, Chiou S-Y, Mcgregor AH. Feasibility and acceptability study on the use of a smartphone application to facilitate balance training in the ageing population; n.d. https://doi.org/10.1136/bmjopen-2020-039054.

80. Choi NG, Stanmore E, Caamano J, Vences K, Gell NM. A feasibility study of multicomponent fall prevention for homebound older adults facilitated by lay coaches and using a tablet-based, gamified exercise application. J Appl Gerontol. 2021;40(11):1483–91. https://doi.org/10.1177/0733464821991024.

81. Mirelman A, Rochester L, Maidan I, Del Din S, Alcock L, Nieuwhof F, Rikkert MO, Bloem BR, Pelosin E, Avanzino L, Abbruzzese G, Dockx K, Bekkers E, Giladi N, Nieuwboer A, Hausdorff JM. Addition of a non-immersive virtual reality component to treadmill training to reduce fall risk in older adults (V-TIME): a randomised controlled trial. Lancet. 2016;388(10050):1170–82. https://doi.org/10.1016/S0140-6736(16)31325-3.

82. Rieger MM, Papegaaij S, Pijnappels M, Steenbrink F, van Dieën JH. Transfer and retention effects of gait training with anterior-posterior perturbations to postural responses after medio-lateral gait perturbations in older adults. Clin Biomech. 2020;75:104988. https://doi.org/10.1016/J.CLINBIOMECH.2020.104988.

83. Calabrò RS, Cacciola A, Bertè F, Manuli A, Leo A, Bramanti A, Naro A, Milardi D, Bramanti P. Robotic gait rehabilitation and substitution devices in neurological disorders: where are we now? Neurol Sci. 2016;37(4):503–14. https://doi.org/10.1007/S10072-016-2474-4/FIGURES/2.

84. Valenzuela T, Razee H, Schoene D, Lord SR, Delbaere K. An interactive home-based cognitive-motor step training program to reduce fall risk in older adults: Qualitative descriptive study of older adults' experiences and requirements. JMIR Aging. 2018;1(2):e11975. https://doi.org/10.2196/11975.

85. Wu Z, Li J, Theng YL. Examining the influencing factors of exercise intention among older adults: a controlled study between Exergame and traditional exercise. Cyberpsychol Behav Soc Netw. 2015;18(9):521–7. https://doi.org/10.1089/CYBER.2015.0065/ASSET/IMAGES/LARGE/FIGURE2.JPEG.

86. Stevens JA, Phelan EA. Development of STEADI: a fall prevention resource for health care providers. Health Promot Pract. 2013;14(5):706–14. https://doi.org/10.1177/1524839912463576.

87. Shubert TE, Smith ML, Jiang L, Ory MG. Disseminating the Otago exercise program in the United States: perceived and actual physical performance improvements from participants. J Appl Gerontol. 2018;37(1):79–98. https://doi.org/10.1177/0733464816675422.

88. Lipsitz LA, Lough M, Niemi J, Travison T, Howlett H, Manor B. A shoe insole delivering subsensory vibratory noise improves balance and gait in healthy elderly people. Arch Phys Med Rehabil. 2015;96(3):432–9. https://doi.org/10.1016/J.APMR.2014.10.004.

89. Whyatt C, Merriman NA, Young WR, Newell FN, Craig C. A Wii bit of fun: a novel platform to deliver effective balance training to older adults. Games for Health J. 2015;4(6):423–33. https://doi.org/10.1089/G4H.2015.0006/ASSET/IMAGES/LARGE/FIGURE8.JPEG.

90. Sato K, Kuroki K, Saiki S, Nagatomi R. Improving walking, muscle strength, and balance in the elderly with an exergame using Kinect: a randomized controlled trial. Games Health J. 2015;4(3):161–7. https://doi.org/10.1089/G4H.2014.0057/ASSET/IMAGES/LARGE/FIGURE2.JPEG.

Part III

Older People and Technologies

Robots in Geriatric Care: A Future with No Return?

10

Lorenzo De Michieli, Alexey Petrushin, Matteo Bustreo, Alessio Del Bue, and Giacinto Barresi

10.1 Introduction

Robots' role in healthcare is steadily rising and older adults constitute a demographic group that can greatly benefit from these gerontechnologies [1, 2]. Ubiquitously and timely, smart mechatronic systems can provide seniors with personalized responses to their needs, caused by mild-to-severe impairments due to health or pathological senescence, during the execution of clinical exercises or activities of daily living (ADLs). This chapter will present such opportunities for elderly care in the next sections.

Section 10.2 discusses robots as tools for motor recovery and aid. Section 10.3 describes mechatronic assistive agents with social, service, and telepresence functions. Section 10.4 introduces distributed robotics, based on Internet of Things (IoT) and Artificial Intelligence (AI) technologies for monitoring and personalized care. Finally, Section 10.5 summarizes these examples of senior-centered robotics.

10.2 Robotic Systems for Motor Rehabilitation and Assistance

Different medical conditions (e.g., diabetic neuropathy) and accidents (e.g., falls) generate motor and postural deficits in older adults. Long-term care must manage these issues according to their musculoskeletal, neurophysiological, perceptual, and cognitive-behavioral causes and their impact on elderly daily life. Indeed, heterogeneous reasons can lead to a loss of motor autonomy, like degenerative processes of

L. De Michieli (✉) · A. Petrushin · G. Barresi
Rehab Technologies Lab, Istituto Italiano di Tecnologia, Genoa, Italy
e-mail: lorenzo.demichieli@iit.it

M. Bustreo · A. Del Bue
Pattern Analysis and Computer Vision (PAVIS), Istituto Italiano di Tecnologia, Genoa, Italy

© The Author(s), under exclusive license to Springer Nature Switzerland AG 2023
A. Pilotto, W. Maetzler (eds.), *Gerontechnology. A Clinical Perspective*, Practical Issues in Geriatrics, https://doi.org/10.1007/978-3-031-32246-4_10

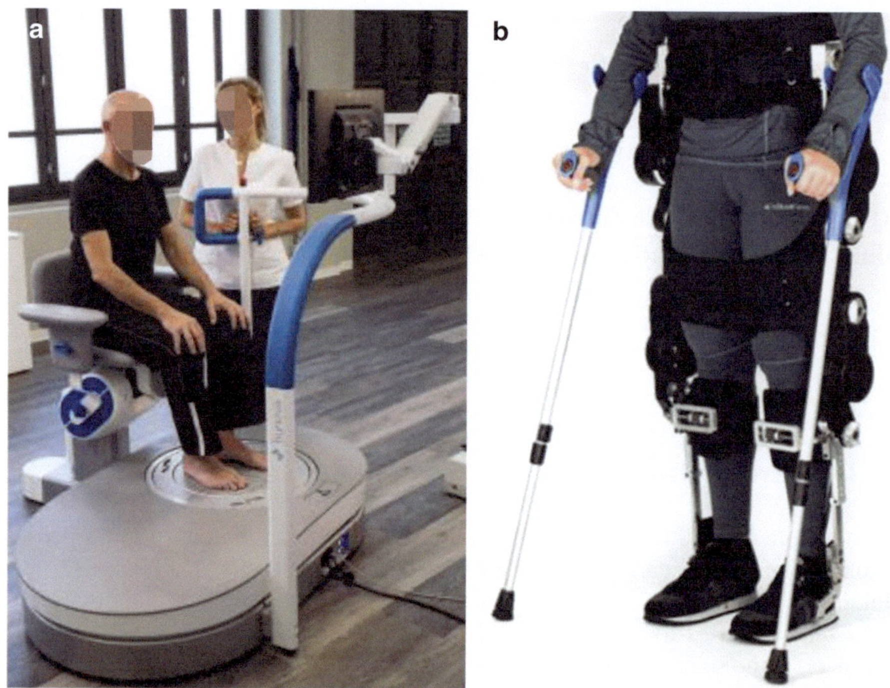

Fig. 10.1 (**a**) a patient on hunova (courtesy of Movendo Technology, https://www.movendo.technology) (**b**) the TWIN exoskeleton for lower limbs (credits: Rehab Technologies Lab, Istituto Italiano di Tecnologia, https://rehab.iit.it/twin)

dementia, inappropriate or late interventions after events like strokes, or even a lack of motivation in performing physical activity [3–8].

This section will show how robotic devices offer smart responses to such needs of recovery and assistance of elderly motor skills (Fig. 10.1). In fact, intelligent mechatronic systems can act as tools for physiotherapy or neurorehabilitation. They can also constitute assistive solutions to counter deficits in dexterous object manipulation, maintaining the posture, and walking steadily.

Most rehabilitation robots implement modalities based on passive training (robot-driven, position control strategy) and active training (patient-driven). Among these, active assistive training modalities can especially help the users to move their impaired limbs according to the strategies of physical and occupational therapy. The approach of assistance-as-needed is especially useful to reduce the risk for the patient to rely exclusively on the robot during the exercises. Each control modality can be enhanced by synergies with other devices, as in the case of neurotechnologies like brain-computer interfaces. According to [9], these robotic systems can work as "neuro-gerontechnologies" when they stimulate the nervous system according to biosignals or to neural principles of plasticity. In this way, they effectively promote the older patients' recovery or exploit their residual abilities (detectable according to biosignals and gaze motions) to assist their capability to interact with the world.

Rehabilitation robots mainly belong to two categories: end-effectors (designed to mechanically constrain, guide, and alter the motion of the distal part of a limb) and exoskeletons (wearable robots). Different exemplary solutions in these classes are described in reviews like [10]. The clinician can select the most appropriate type of robotic system for a certain patient according to the severity and the features of their impairments. For instance, an exoskeleton could be more impactful for people with low residual motor capabilities, and end-effectors can effectively deliver forces and perturbations during the exercises of patients who can more actively perform actions during the re-training.

Furthermore, robotic devices can also provide clinicians with reliable quantitative assessments of sensory, motor, and cognitive skills and of therapeutic outcome of the patients, even in terms of biomarkers [11]. These examples are not specifically based on elderly cases, but they must be considered as the background for developing novel rehabilitative gerontechnologies.

An example of end-effector for the upper limb is the Wristbot of Rewing (https://www.rewing.it) [12, 13], and an example of lower-limb end-effector is hunova of Movendo Technology (Fig. 10.1a) [14].

Both these solutions are devised for being empowered by the engaging design of exergames (video games that promote exercising), especially effective in motivating older adults to perform physical activity [15].

Alongside the opportunity of integrating robotic and virtual rehabilitation solutions [16], these systems propose groundbreaking AI solutions to monitor the individual conditions and predict their upcoming changes, even the risk of fall (as in the case of the Silver Index based on data collection during hunova sessions) [17, 18]. Through this type of machine learning-powered approaches [19], it is possible to adapt the treatments to the individual needs alongside the daily care interventions according to a precision medicine perspective.

Unlike end-effectors, exoskeletons are worn by the user. They anthropomorphically align with the mechanical joints of the human body, physically interacting with them to modify their motion. They can assist the posture or guide a movement, completing its execution or correcting its trajectory. Consequently, they can work as both rehabilitative and assistive devices, as highlighted in [20] about upper limb exoskeletons like Spexo [21]. This also is the case of lower limb exoskeletons [22] like TWIN (Fig. 10.1b), designed as a user-friendly wearable robot for rehabilitation and assistance of lower limbs motion for people with severe conditions like spinal cord injury (SCI) [23]. Exosuits are another type of wearable robots, typically lightweight and soft (thus ideal for daily use) systems for assistance of upper [24] and lower [25] limbs with mild deficits.

Considering typical motor assistive robots (in both clinical and domestic contexts), we need to highlight that they can encompass a wide range of solutions. Among these: robotic wheelchairs [26] and robotic arms [27], robotic hand tools (e.g., tremor-countering spoons for people with Parkinson's Disease) [28], and bionic prostheses (especially artificial lower limbs in case of older people who lost a foot because of diabetes) [29].

However, introducing a robotic device in the everyday life can be especially challenging in terms of acceptance, as it happens for exoskeletons [30]: user-centered design practices must be adopted to prevent elderly's frustration and embarrassment in using such devices (avoiding their abandonment) [31].

Interestingly, certain motor assistive robots tend to solve the problem of acceptance through the introduction of agent-like features (with a head, possibly limbs too), as in the case of Kompai robot, a multi-purpose artificial assistant that can function as a walking aid too [32]. Another example is human-lifting RIBA II [33], providing the mobilization of the patient from and off the bed or the chair, working as a help for nurses according to multiple patterns of physical human-robot interaction.

Going beyond the definition of a clinical robotic tool for elderly care through morphologies and functionalities, these devices lead us to introduce the topic of the next section: assistive robotic agents.

10.3 Assistive Robotic Agents

Heterogeneous progressive impairments occurring in healthy and pathological senescence definitely alter the capability of the older person to autonomously perform ADLs alongside typical patterns of communicative, social, and affective functioning, especially in cases of isolation and loneliness. These situations may easily worsen the difficulties of seniors, generating obstacles to sustain their physical and psychological wellness. Consequently, older people lose important daily routines and social connections: without being part of such processes and networks, they will start losing practical—especially communicative and relational—skills and healthy mood (facilitating the clinical emergence of apathy and depression). These issues became especially clear for the isolation exacerbated by the social distancing and the lockdown periods enforced as restrictions during the COVID-19 pandemic [34–38].

Within this context, assistive robotic agents—apparently characterized as "artificial individuals" with a certain degree of autonomous behavior—can work as companions and helpers that share the same daily living setting of the elder people, helping them to perform ADLs, to self-care, and to be involved in cognitively, emotionally, and socially stimulating interactions. As a special case in this domain, telepresence robots can help older people to establish social connections and experiences with people located away from them, including the caregivers.

10.3.1 Robotic Companions and Helpers

Seniors can establish different degrees of physical and social interactions with assistive robotic agents. Most reviews [39–43] on this field show how human-robot interactions can contribute to counter social isolation and help to live a safer and more independent life through functions like bringing goods, monitoring health conditions and habits, alerting patients to perform physical exercises or to ingest medicaments at expected times, mitigating stress and improving mood, stimulating mental functions. These properties are advantageous even in severe cases of dementia.

Overall, care robots can be designed to be affective companions [44, 45] for providing social and cognitive stimulations (sometime with therapeutic goals in cases of depression or anxiety) or they can be exclusively dedicated to services like cleaning or shopping in order to support a positive aging "in place" [46, 47]. However, even the latter can become part of social dynamics [48] thanks to the role they occupy as agents in the everyday routine of people. A well-known example of animal-like robotic companion based on minimal actuation, totally dedicated to expressive functions, is Paro, a seal "pup" designed to provide emotional and social support for people with dementia (Fig. 10.2a). As an exemplary evidence of its impact, a study suggests that making elderly interact with Paro improves social interactions and reduces the use of painkillers [49].

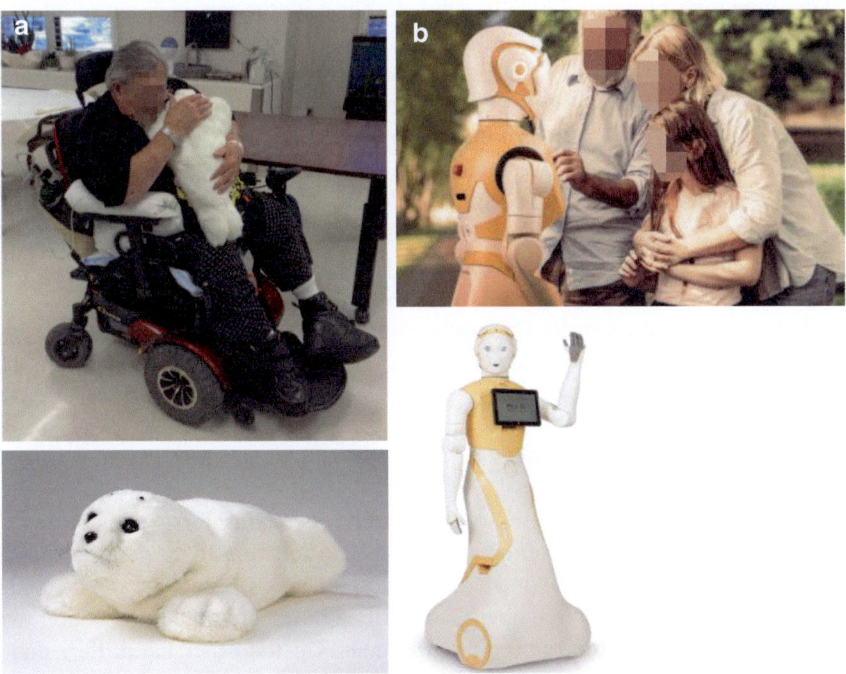

Fig. 10.2 (a) the robotic seal Paro (www.parorobots.com). Picture by Takanori Shibata published in the article "PARO as a Biofeedback Medical Device for Mental Health in the COVID-19 Era", CC BY 4.0 (b) ARI the Social Robot by PAL Robotics (https://pal-robotics.com/robots/ari/)

Beyond a morphology designed for establishing affective dynamics, other solutions can be even more effective to engage and help older adults in a wider set of applications. This is the case of humanoid robots [50] like Nadine, which is used in [51] to demonstrate how this agent made recreational activities more promptly available for elder people in a nursing home. The goal of the authors was to demonstrate how a humanoid robot can address the emotional needs of the elderly, reducing the workload for caretakers during leisure activities.

The success of this solution can be attributed to the facilitated interaction based on the humanoid shape alongside the agent's capability to read gestures and facial expressions of humans for providing feedback accordingly. The seniors appeared happier, more focused on the entertainment activities, and less prone to turn to the clinical staff with their requests. In addition, literature offers numerous cases of robotic companions and helpers with partially humanoid features enabling, for example, bipedal locomotion. Robots like Pepper [52] and ARI [53] (Fig. 10.2b) can exploit their arms for communication (even for guiding physical exercises of older people) and for offering physical support, while their wheels-based mobility can be considered a sufficient compromise in order to reach a proper technology readiness level and, consequently, to release such aids in real settings of daily living.

The academic and industrial communities cooperate with patients and clinicians in order to understand how to improve the engaging features of these robots alongside their functions in ADLs. Facing topics like technology acceptance and rejection [54] requires long-term ecologically valid studies with the involvement of all stakeholders—in particular the users in their daily living settings. Taking account of cohort-effects and, overall, cultural differences will be a critical factor for investigating the assistive robots user experience and for refining the "social competence" of these artificial agents in their context [55], making them able to adapt to user's conditions (e.g., data about state and change of mood) [56].

User research will guide the design and development of novel solutions that can empower the existing robotic platforms even through virtual and augmented solutions to enhance their expressive impact [57].

Interestingly, a certain category of assistive robots can have companionship features even if they are controlled by someone: this is the case of telepresence robots that bring social contacts to the older adults, as discussed in the next subsection.

10.3.2 Telepresence Robots

Telepresence robots (TRs) are remote-controlled mechatronic systems capable of providing a perception of presence in a real-world location that operator does not physically inhabit [58]. On the one hand, this type of assistive robots can be considered as a special case of service devices described in the previous sub-section when they are operated from the remote environment. On the other hand, they can be perceived as social companions when they serve as means for non-physical presence of the remote operator in the daily life of older person. Considering this dual peculiarity, and according to our perspective, they constitute their own category.

Fig. 10.3 Example of telepresence robot: (**a**) Texai by Willow Garage (willowgarage.com), CC BY 2.0 (**b**) UBBO Maker by AXYN Robotique (http://gostai.com)

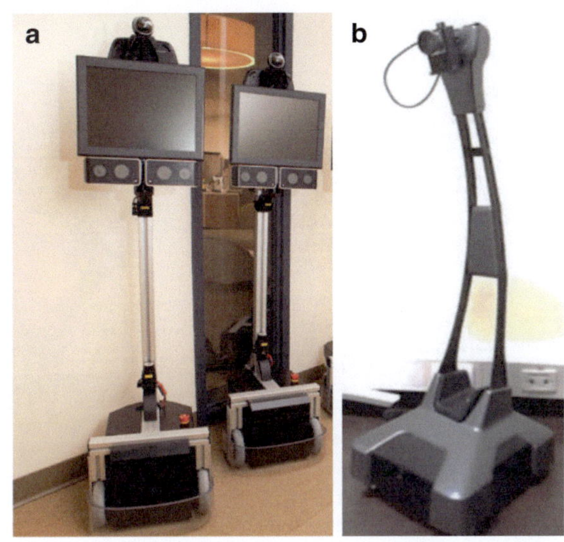

TRs come in different shapes and sizes but generally consist of a wheeled platform with a mounted screen, video camera, microphone, and speakers. Some of the TRs on the market have reached an advanced stage of development. They are capable of autonomous navigation throughout environment, docking, adjusting height, and inclination of the screen, acquiring physiological data of the user and environmental parameters (Fig. 10.3). Giraff [59], Double (Double Robotics®) [60], and AMY-M2 (AMY-Robotics®) [61] are examples of TRs used in healthcare domain.

Telepresence systems can support older people in two ways. In certain cases, the robot is placed in the remote environment and controlled by older adult (to interact with family, for instance). Alternatively, the robot is found in the local environment and controlled by a remote user (e.g., a relative, a caregiver), which can navigate in the local environment and communicate with older adult through the implemented robot functionalities.

When used in the first modality TR can provide a highly realistic sensation of existence in the remote environment for the older person and be particularly beneficial for people with physical disabilities and long-term patients.

Escolano et al. [62] demonstrated how patients with amyotrophic lateral sclerosis (ALS, often occurring in the sixth decade of life) can control a TR through brain-computer interface (BCI) and independently explore space otherwise inaccessible to them. People with[1] severe motor disabilities can control TRs using only their eyes by means of gaze tracking system [63]. TRs can provide mobility-impaired people with the possibility to participate actively in visits of museums and archeological sites that cannot offer them a dedicated infrastructure for visits in person [64].

---

[1] https://www.axyn.fr/

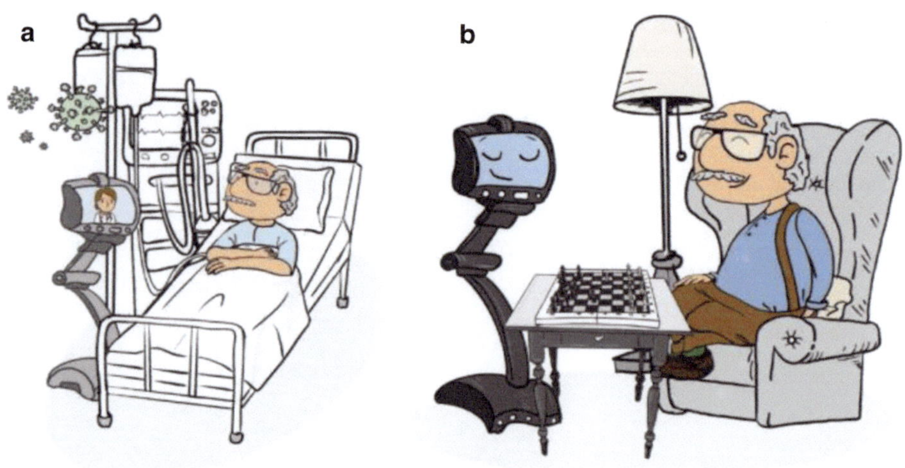

Fig. 10.4 (**a**) Telepresence application in which a doctor can assess a COVID-19 patient. In this application, TR works as a surrogate of the doctor eliminating a need for protective equipment and making the medical visit much safer. (**b**) TR facilitates successful aging through creation of a social interaction and providing assistance in activities of daily living

When used in the second modality TRs enable medical personal to practice real-time telemedicine, provide assistance in certain activities of daily living and increase the social participation of older people through video calls.

Usage of telepresence for healthcare services can help the medical personal to work more efficiently and much safer through respecting physical distancing (Fig. 10.4a). With the beginning of the COVID-19 pandemic, the number of TRs deployed in the hospitals significantly increased. TRs are used for ward rounds that doctors can do even when they are at home or under quarantine themselves, triage and registration in emergency department, virtual family member visits without exposing them to the virus [65], disinfecting clinical rooms with ultraviolet radiation [66], logistic support [67] as well as meals and medication delivery [68].

TRs enable quicker care delivery and access to the best care possible even in rural areas where there is not enough medical personal. Vespa et al. [69] demonstrated that a TR can help to assist neurologic patients faster and with a cost-benefit. Newman et al. [70] used a TR to connect a pharmacist with the patients discharged from a rural community hospital. During the interview, the pharmacist reviewed the discharge prescription list and identified that in 8 out of 9 cases the patient had at least one unintentional discharge medication discrepancy. TRs robots not only "teleport" a doctor to the patient but they can also do automatic translation to overcome the language barrier if needed [71]. When equipped with sensors the TRs can measure user's bio signals for purposes of monitoring, diagnosing, and improving user experience.

Stricker et al. [72] compared different approaches to measure cardiac pulse from video stream of the face acquired by a camera installed on a mobile platform. Authors demonstrated that pulse rate can be estimated under ambient illumination even when subject is moving. Some TRs can communicate or directly equipped with diagnostic instruments, for instance, RP-VITA telepresence robot [73] has a built-in electronic stethoscope.

As discussed above, aging is often associated with higher risks of social isolation and loneliness as well as the loss of independence and self-autonomy. The restrictions during the COVID-19 outbreaks further lowered the quantity and quality of contacts of older adults and negatively affected their physiological well-being [74]. Through bridging physical distance, TRs can mitigate these problems facilitate social interactions and improve emotional health of older people (Fig. 10.4b).

In addition, some TRs are capable of helping to maintain independent mobility and decrease risk of falls in older adults. For example, Astro robot [75] is equipped with a hand bar and can assist person while they are walking, standing up, and sitting down [66]. Thus, they can also provide the users with motor assistive features as the systems in the previous section.

Currently available TRs have proven their usefulness; however, in order to become ubiquitous in geriatric care and older adults' assistance they should overcome existing barriers. Some of the implementations were found to have such limitations as: too expensive [76, 77], poor economics [78], privacy concerns [77–79], audio problems [77, 79], insufficient control [79], and low video quality [77].

However, the studies investigating the user experience indicate that TRs are generally accepted [80, 81]. Koceski et al. [81] evaluated perceived usefulness and perceived ease of use of various TR functionalities (navigation, vital signal measurements, manipulator function, reminder, video conference). The results showed a high-level acceptance of the TR technology by both older people and by professional caregivers.

Nevertheless, most telepresence systems on the market are not specifically designed for older adults. Additional user-centered design requirements should be implemented and evaluations performed to close the gap between the existing functionality and the needs and expectations of older people.

The range of interaction of the existing telepresence systems can be further enhanced with haptic feedback and the ability to physically manipulate the remote environment, alongside alternative and augmentative modalities of control. This is particularly important for improving telepresence accessibility for people with severe motor impairments as the ones of Locked-In Syndrome (LIS, which typically occurs in ALS), requiring novel interaction concepts based on cognitive ergonomics and neuroergonomics [82]. Interpretation of the working environment, measuring of person's emotional state, and their behavioral traits can improve the user experience and make TR operation more effective. This information can be acquired and integrated with the TR by a distributed multi-sensor system that is capable of providing continuous monitoring of the environment.

This section quickly introduced robotic agents for elderly care, dedicating special space to telepresence devices. However, we must consider these agents as part of a wider ecosystem serving and caring for older adults, as the next section will depict.

10.4 Ambient Intelligence and Distributed Robotics

Live data collection and analysis are fundamental steps to properly assist older adults according to their fragilities. Meaningful information can be exploited to deploy a smart environment system that adjusts to individual needs. Such a setting should be equipped with technologies designed for sensing, monitoring, interpreting, and managing a physical system (including people): summing up, it would appear like a "distributed robot". Key components of such a robotic ecosystem are a set of sensors, artificial intelligence (AI) solutions, and mechatronic devices—including assistive and, possibly, rehabilitative robots—that work synergistically as the parts of a robotic environment. Such an advance is based on a background in ubiquitous robotics [83] to coordinate different devices. However, any current framework needs to be updated to the most recent advances in connected care in order to provide the most appropriate services to elder people, moving towards healthcare 4.0 and 5.0 [84–87].

More than other population groups, the elderly might benefit from the development of an assistive technology solution that is continually available, personalized, affordable, and non-invasive, which can monitor persons' health and behavior during routine daily activities. Such an assistive technology can only be achieved in living environments, where people spend most of their time. Bringing automatic assistive technologies in the form of distributed robotics inside people's houses can make the habitation a safer and less solitary place, reducing the requirement of regular assistance provided by the family or by the healthcare system.

Furthermore, we must consider the burden of chronic conditions. Worldwide, elderly chronic diseases are among the most common and costly health issues and they are the main cause of death, accounting for 60% of all death [88]. The early symptoms of the chronic diseases emerge gradually, therefore they are hard to observe with periodic scheduled screening tests, which, most of the times, are not personalized but based on the average population risk of disease [89].

Nevertheless, since early detection of chronic diseases can significantly reduce their impact and debilitative effects in the population, it is critical to observe their symptoms as early as possible [88]. The integration of the modern advances in the field of computation and electronics can give huge support for the definition of a health system that can effectively manage the rapid rising of the population age with minimal workforce, making use of IoT-powered environments [90].

These solutions bring the potential of multiple, ubiquitous devices to serve people with fragilities in their own daily living setting, including TRs acting as integrated parts of the whole system, when needed. Next subsections will introduce the technologies and the perspectives on such a breakthrough in elderly care.

10.4.1 Multi-Sensor Environments

Homes of older individuals and hospitals can be equipped with distributed and pervasive sensors capable of sensing the surrounding environment in real time, sharing collected information with interested parties (e.g., other robotic systems, older adults, family members, caregivers), and storing sensor data in the cloud that are then used to design accurate models, monitor current health conditions, and predict future insights. Such multi-sensor solutions are enabled by the Internet of Things (IoT) technologies. The application of multi-sensor IoT systems in the medical fields, especially in geriatric care [91], introduces new approaches in care with shift from a centralized healthcare system towards pervasive model based on preventive and personalized therapies.

A number of devices can be of service for an IoT-based healthcare system: (i) ambient sensors that serve to collect environmental data—including people's conditions and activities—and, accordingly, intervene through domotic systems; (ii) implantable and wearable devices that are mostly used to measure a person's state and vital signals and provide feedback (Fig. 10.5a).

Environmental and wearable sensors can make well-being, health monitoring, and healthcare support accessible anywhere, anytime, and by anyone, without the need of moving to any external location. Meanwhile, domotic and wearable systems can provide feedback solutions (e.g., domotic adaptation of indoor temperature, alarms) and personal robots like R1 [92] (Fig. 10.5b) with valuable information for safe and personalized interventions.

Multi-sensor environments still constitute a new concept and they are mostly limited to small-scale pilot studies. However, they have already been successfully used for mitigating and managing issues like: risk of fall, heart rate monitoring,

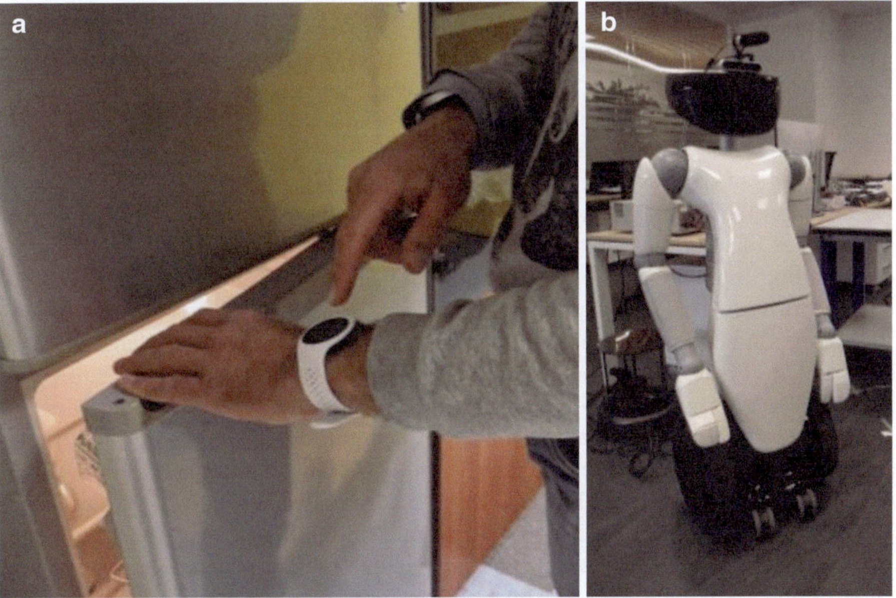

Fig. 10.5 Examples of interconnected systems. (**a**) a wearable device (Empatica wristband, http:// empatica.com). (**b**) R1 an assistive robotic agent (R1 of iCub Facility at IIT)

cancer treatment, depression recovery, Parkinson's Disease, asthma monitoring, and risk of exposure to contagious diseases.

Currently [91], the typical implementation of the multi-sensor IoT technology in healthcare is accompanied by various challenges. Intelligent environments are complex systems that can include a number of types of employed sensors, communication protocols, and data processing algorithms. The lack of the reference standard in the industry makes data aggregation a challenging task and slows down the adoption ratio. Another barrier for a broad adoption of these systems is related to security and privacy concerns and processing of personal health data. Whenever it is possible, IoT sensors should follow principles of privacy-by-design. In particular, when they have sufficient computational power, they should be provided with algorithms for anonymizing, elaborating, and interpreting the acquired data on the edge, before sending them to the cloud for further analysis. Sophisticated AI algorithms are necessary to process collected information, particularly when dealing with continuous arrays of data gathered from multiple sensors. These algorithms play a crucial role in interpreting big data and providing valuable support in making health-related decisions. Certainly, the iterative and participatory design of IoT-based systems for geriatric care should involve older adults' needs in large-scale studies.

These aspects must be considered when IoT also embrace robots in its connected care applications, unveiling further perspectives in elderly care: the home itself will literally command intelligent embodied agents to help older adults in need according to the live collection and processing of information on them, as next sub-section will discuss.

10.4.2 The EDITH Setup

Considering the issues described in the previous subsection—from the need of IoT for health monitoring and diagnostics into everyday life [93] to the management of large amount of data, avoiding network congestion and countering privacy issues— we envision the development of innovative solutions that exploit the most recent capabilities of intelligent and interactive technologies. For instance, a multi-layer computation pipeline should be taken into consideration for granting higher standards of privacy. A first computational level should take place as soon as possible, in the robotic acquiring device itself when it is possible: the human interpretable collected raw data should be converted to compact and informative features by either using hand-crafted or data-driven AI approaches [91]. Following processing stages can combine different data sources for highlighting the emergence of data patterns that are relevant from a diagnostic point of view, by using either supervised or unsupervised algorithms. Finally, an application layer can collect the organized and interpreted data, manage the data transmission and reception with the health clinic, encrypt and store the data, provide feedback and proactively support the elder in his/her daily activities. This is just a sample of the solutions that are converging into the EDITH (Embodied Distributed Intelligent Technologies for Health) Setup of IIT (Fig. 10.6).

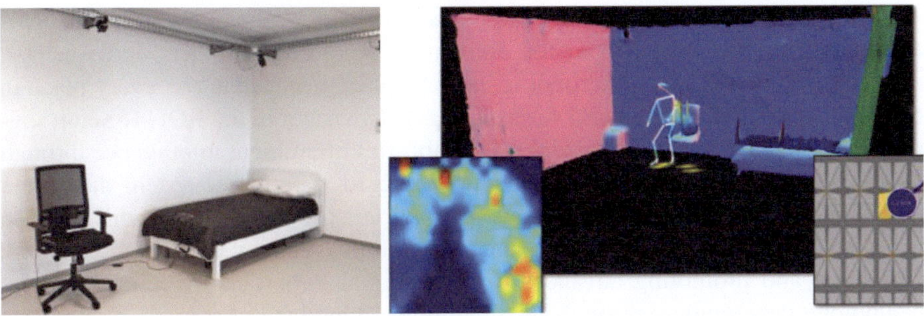

Fig. 10.6. A portion of the IoT sensors installed to implement the EDITH Setup (left) and the pre-processed data collected by the cameras and the sensors of seat and floor (right)

The EDITH Setup consists of a sensorized living environment where the furniture has been equipped with a series of sensing technology for monitoring the elderly health status during their daily routine activities. The EDITH Setup is also equipped with an R1 humanoid assistive robot, to support the elders in their daily activities and to reduce isolation, constituting a promising solution to implement the principles of Active Ageing [94] in Ambient Assisted Living [95] frameworks. Smart cameras and robot's eyes frame the monitored rooms and extract the body joints of the persons, immediately discarding any visual information about the people in the scene. Pressure sensors are installed in the seats and under the mattress, while the floor is sensorized for monitoring person changes of positions.

A thermal camera collects information about the person and the environment temperature. Force sensing resistors are placed in the door handles for monitoring the strength of the persons. Infrared sensors are used for quantifying the time spent by each person in different areas of the rooms and the bathroom. In case the persons wear smartwatches or wristbands, they can be interfaced with the Setup and share their data. The robot and the IoT sensors collect the data and stream them to a LAN where a centralized AI-powered computational unit encrypts, merges, and stores the collected information. By using AI, the EDITH Setup can aggregate the data to understand individual's health both at baseline and during disease [B] [89]: by learning the behavioral patterns of the monitored person, when sudden changes in their habits appear it rises flags or alarms. Particular focus has been dedicated to the study of elderly balance (i.e., irregularities in the gait, sudden changes in the walking speed, irregular dynamics during standing and seating, falls) and in the study of the sleep disorders. The centralized computing system takes care of communicating the analyzed data with the caregivers and notifying the emergency services. When treatment has been prescribed, the centralized computing system can remind the elder to take the appropriate medicaments at the right time using Bluetooth speakers. Moreover, the EDITH Setup proactively gives suggestions against sedentary lifestyles and bad food habits.

Managing the complexity of elder people problems (and the issues of any person with difficulties) in their own daily living environment requires an effort of holistic understanding that only a distributed machine can proficiently perform. This approach gets inspiration from the domain of ubiquitous robotics and we must observe that, in this case, the robot is in every place because it "is" every place in that context. The presence of R1 humanoid assistive robot in the EDITH Setup suggests how this approach can extend the capabilities of ambient intelligence through its distributed embodiment with a human-centered robotic ecosystem that could include even rehabilitation robots designed for home use. Furthermore, this solution is devised as the node of a network connecting clinical centers and laboratories too, sustaining and promoting advances in translational geriatric research and gerontechnology development through an "ubiquitous living lab".

10.5 Conclusions

Among gerontechnologies, care robots already constitute important opportunities to help older adults.

Indeed, rehabilitation robots can offer solutions for the functional recovery of older adults, and exoskeletons can work as wearable assistive devices for supporting elderly mobility. These and other rehabilitative and assistive tools are the most typical examples of robots for elderly care in clinical centers, even if they will certainly become home solutions in the future.

However, homes are already starting to be inhabited by assistive robotic agents that can execute specific services to empower the individual autonomy. Moreover, robotic agents can be designed as helpers and companions, also caring for the mental conditions of a person through an experience of social interactions as opportunities for cognitive and affective stimulations. Furthermore, their applications in telepresence can spatially and socially extend the daily experience of older people. Indeed, TRs enable long-term patients and people with limited mobility to connect with outside world and extend relational capability beyond their surroundings (e.g., visiting museums and archeological sites, interacting with friends and relatives). Furthermore, TRs allow caregivers to reach more patients in a timely and safe manner from virtually any place thereby providing access to the best care possible. When navigated by family members TRs provide the best social connection when in-person social interaction is not possible.

After considering elderly care robots as tools and agents, we can also see them as environments themselves. Indeed, technologies like IoT—connecting multiple sensors and actuated systems, including assistive robots—can enable distributed robotic systems, based on the embodiment of ambient intelligence. Such a concept requires advanced AI-powered devices, spread around the daily living setting for collecting and analyzing data and for providing the inhabitants with personalized care.

We presented an example of such a distributed robotic ecosystem: the EDITH Setup at IIT. As all connected care solutions, this Setup highlights the need of an intensive and extensive level of data collection that can create issues related to privacy violation. Indeed, the pervasive and almost invisible presence of environmental and wearable sensors and feedback sources in the daily life of an individual must be appropriately assessed in terms of users' dignity and privacy. Older people-centered design can also overcome these issues alongside the users' distrust towards innovations, and, consequently, improving the technology acceptance and, consequently, the quality of elderly life. This scenario is just a sample to pave the way toward a robot-assisted positive aging.

References

1. Sale P. Gerontechnology, domotics, and robotics. In: Rehabilitation medicine for elderly patients. Springer; 2018. p. 161–9.
2. Osaka K, Tanioka T, Tanioka R, Kai Y, Locsin RC. Effectiveness of care robots, and the intermediaries' role between and among care robots and older adults. In: 2020 IEEE/SICE International Symposium on System Integration (SII). IEEE; 2020. p. 611–6.
3. Bianchi AB, Antunes MD, Santos NQ, Bulla HA, Silva ES, Marques AP, Bertolini SMMG. Posture and balance in elderly who practice and who do not practice physical activities. J Phys Educ. 2020;31
4. Curreri C, Trevisan C, Carrer P, Facchini S, Giantin V, Maggi S, Noale M, De Rui M, Perissinotto E, Zambon S. Difficulties with fine motor skills and cognitive impairment in an elderly population: the progetto Veneto anziani. J Am Geriatr Soc. 2018;66(2):350–6.
5. Rand D. Proprioception deficits in chronic stroke—upper extremity function and daily living. PLoS One. 2018;13(3):e0195043.
6. Zhang Q, Lin Y, Liu X, Zhang L, Zhang Y, Zhao D, Lu Q, Jia J. Diabetic peripheral neuropathy affects pinch strength and hand dexterity in elderly patients. Neural Plast. 2021;2021:1.
7. Park H-J, Lee N-G, Kang T-W. Fall-related cognition, motor function, functional ability, and depression measures in older adults with dementia. NeuroRehabilitation. 2020;47(4):487–94.
8. Cai Y, Leveille SG, Hausdorff JM, Bean JF, Manor B, McLean RR, You T. Chronic musculoskeletal pain and foot reaction time in older adults. J Pain. 2021;22(1):76–85.
9. Barresi G, Zenzeri J, Tessadori J, Laffranchi M, Semprini M, De Michieli L. Neuro-Gerontechnologies: applications and opportunities. In: Scataglini S, Imbesi S, Marques G, editors. Internet of things for human-centered design: application to elderly healthcare. Springer; n.d.
10. Molteni F, Gasperini G, Cannaviello G, Guanziroli E. Exoskeleton and end-effector robots for upper and lower limbs rehabilitation: narrative review. PM&R. 2018;10(9):S174–88.
11. Garro F, Chiappalone M, Buccelli S, De Michieli L, Semprini M. Neuromechanical biomarkers for robotic neurorehabilitation. Front Neurorobot. 2021;15
12. Iandolo R, Marini F, Semprini M, Laffranchi M, Mugnosso M, Cherif A, De Michieli L, Chiappalone M, Zenzeri J. Perspectives and challenges in robotic neurorehabilitation. Appl Sci. 2019;9(15):3183.
13. Masia L, Casadio M, Giannoni P, Sandini G, Morasso P. Performance adaptive training control strategy for recovering wrist movements in stroke patients: a preliminary, feasibility study. J Neuroeng Rehabil. 2009;6(1):1–11.
14. Saglia JA, De Luca A, Squeri V, Ciaccia L, Sanfilippo C, Ungaro S, De Michieli L. Design and development of a novel core, balance and lower limb rehabilitation robot: hunova®. In: 2019 IEEE 16th International Conference on Rehabilitation Robotics (ICORR). IEEE; 2019. p. 417–22.
15. Godfrey SB, Barresi G. Video games for positive aging: playfully engaging older adults. In: Scataglini S, Imbesi S, Marques G, editors. Internet of things for human-centered design: application to elderly healthcare. Springer; n.d.
16. Baur K, Schättin A, de Bruin ED, Riener R, Duarte JE, Wolf P. Trends in robot-assisted and virtual reality-assisted neuromuscular therapy: a systematic review of health-related multiplayer games. J Neuroeng Rehabil. 2018;15(1):1–19.

17. Veerubhotla A, Ehrenberg N, Ibironke O, Pilkar R. Objective evaluation of risk of falls in individuals with chronic stroke: feasibility study. Arch Phys Med Rehabil. 2021;102(10):e101.
18. Cella A, De Luca A, Squeri V, Parodi S, Puntoni M, Vallone F, Giorgeschi A, Garofalo V, Zigoura E, Senesi B. Robotic balance assessment in community-dwelling older people with different grades of impairment of physical performance. Aging Clin Exp Res. 2020;32(3):491–503.
19. Ai Q, Liu Z, Meng W, Liu Q, Xie SQ. Machine learning in robot assisted upper limb rehabilitation: a focused review. In: IEEE Transactions on Cognitive and Developmental Systems; 2021.
20. Kapsalyamov A, Hussain S, Jamwal PK. State-of-the-art assistive powered upper limb exoskeletons for elderly. IEEE Access. 2020;8:178991–9001.
21. Latt WT, Luu TP, Kuah C. Tech AW towards an upper-limb exoskeleton system for assistance in activities of daily living (ADLs). In: Proceedings of the International Convention on Rehabilitation Engineering & Assistive Technology; 2014. p. 1–4.
22. Kapsalyamov A, Jamwal PK, Hussain S, Ghayesh MH. State of the art lower limb robotic exoskeletons for elderly assistance. IEEE Access. 2019;7:95075–86.
23. Laffranchi M, D'Angella S, Vassallo C, Piezzo C, Canepa M, De Giuseppe S, Di Salvo M, Succi A, Cappa S, Cerruti G. User-Centered Design and Development of the Modular TWIN Lower Limb Exoskeleton. Front Neurorobot. 2021;15:15.
24. Xiloyannis M, Chiaradia D, Frisoli A, Masia L. Physiological and kinematic effects of a soft exosuit on arm movements. J Neuroeng Rehabil. 2019;16(1):1–15.
25. Di Natali C, Poliero T, Sposito M, Graf E, Bauer C, Pauli C, Bottenberg E, De Eyto A, O'Sullivan L, Hidalgo AF. Design and evaluation of a soft assistive lower limb exoskeleton. Robotica. 2019;37(12):2014–34.
26. Sivakanthan S, Candiotti JL, Sundaram AS, Duvall JA, Sergeant JJG, Cooper R, Satpute S, Turner RL, Cooper RA. Mini-review: robotic wheelchair taxonomy and readiness. Neurosci Lett. 2022;136482:136482.
27. Phalaprom S, Jitngernmadan P. iFeedingBot: a vision-based feeding robotic arm prototype based on open source solution. In: International conference on computers helping people with special needs. Springer; 2020. p. 446–52.
28. Nazrin A, Abdulla R, San LY. A low cost stabilizing spoon for people with parkinson's disease. J Appl Technol Innov. 2021;5(3):32.
29. Prylińska M, Husejko J, Kwiatkowska K, Wycech A, Kujaciński M, Rymarska O, Sarnowska J, Rogala D, Jarosz K, Nieciecka A. Care for an elderly person after lower limb amputation. J Edu Health Sport. 2019;9(8):886–94.
30. Shore L, de Eyto A, O'Sullivan L. Technology acceptance and perceptions of robotic assistive devices by older adults–implications for exoskeleton design. In: Disability and rehabilitation: assistive technology; 2020. p. 1–9.
31. Sposito M, Poliero T, Di Natali C, Semprini M, Barresi G, Laffranchi M, Caldwell D, De Michieli L, Ortiz J. Exoskeletons in elderly healthcare. In: Scataglini S, Imbesi S, Marques G, editors. Internet of things for human-centered design: application to elderly healthcare. Springer; n.d.
32. Caleb-Solly P, Dogramadzi S, Huijnen CA, Heuvel H. Exploiting ability for human adaptation to facilitate improved human-robot interaction and acceptance. Inf Soc. 2018;34(3):153–65.
33. Ding M, Ikeura R, Mori Y, Mukai T, Hosoe S. Measurement of human body stiffness for lifting-up motion generation using nursing-care assistant robot—RIBA. In: SENSORS, 2013 IEEE. IEEE; 2013. p. 1–4.
34. Ford AB, Haug MR, Stange KC, Gaines AD, Noelker LS, Jones PK. Sustained personal autonomy: a measure of successful aging. J Aging Health. 2000;12(4):470–89.
35. Van der Weele GM, Gussekloo J, De Waal MW, De Craen AJ, Van der Mast RC. Co-occurrence of depression and anxiety in elderly subjects aged 90 years and its relationship with functional status, quality of life and mortality. Int J Geriatr Psychiatry. 2009;24(6):595–601.
36. Plagg B, Engl A, Piccoliori G, Eisendle K. Prolonged social isolation of the elderly during COVID-19: between benefit and damage. Arch Gerontol Geriatr. 2020;89:104086.

37. Bassuk SS, Glass TA, Berkman LF. Social disengagement and incident cognitive decline in community-dwelling elderly persons. Ann Intern Med. 1999;131(3):165–73.
38. Seeman TE, Lusignolo TM, Albert M, Berkman L. Social relationships, social support, and patterns of cognitive aging in healthy, high-functioning older adults: MacArthur studies of successful aging. Health Psychol. 2001;20(4):243.
39. Márquez-Sáncheza S, Mora-Simonb S, Herrera-Santosa J, Roncerod AO, Corchadoa JM. Intelligent dolls and robots for the treatment of elderly people with dementia. Adv Distrib Comput Art Intell J. 2020;9(1):99–112.
40. Abdi J, Al-Hindawi A, Ng T, Vizcaychipi MP. Scoping review on the use of socially assistive robot technology in elderly care. BMJ Open. 2018;8(2):e018815.
41. Thunberg S, Rönnqvist L, Ziemke T. Do robot pets decrease agitation in dementia patients? In: International Conference on Social Robotics. Springer; 2020. p. 616–27.
42. Sharma A, Rathi Y, Patni V, Sinha DKA. Systematic review of assistance robots for elderly care. In: 2021 International Conference on Communication information and Computing Technology (ICCICT). IEEE; 2021. p. 1–6.
43. Cooper S, Di Fava A, Villacañas Ó, Silva T, Fernandez-Carbajales V, Unzueta L, Serras M, Marchionni L, Ferro F. Social robotic application to support active and healthy ageing. In: 2021 30th IEEE International Conference on Robot & Human Interactive Communication (RO-MAN). IEEE; 2021. p. 1074–80.
44. Schellin H, Oberley T, Patterson K, Kim B, Haring KS, Tossell CC, Phillips E, de Visser EJ. Man's new best friend? Strengthening human-robot dog bonding by enhancing the dog-likeness of Sony's Aibo. In: 2020 Systems and Information Engineering Design Symposium (SIEDS). IEEE; 2020. p. 1–6.
45. Ihamäki P, Heljakka K. Robot pets as "serious toys"-activating social and emotional experiences of elderly people. Inf Syst Front. 2021:1–15.
46. Mois G, Beer JM. Robotics to support aging in place. In: Living with robots. Elsevier; 2020. p. 49–74.
47. Bajones M, Fischinger D, Weiss A, Puente PDL, Wolf D, Vincze M, Körtner T, Weninger M, Papoutsakis K, Michel D. Results of field trials with a mobile service robot for older adults in 16 private households. ACM Transactions on Human-Robot Interaction (THRI). 2019;9(2):1–27.
48. Forlizzi J. How robotic products become social products: an ethnographic study of cleaning in the home. In: 2007 2nd ACM/IEEE International Conference on Human-Robot Interaction (HRI). IEEE; 2007. p. 129–36.
49. Pu L, Moyle W, Jones C, Todorovic M. The effect of using PARO for people living with dementia and chronic pain: a pilot randomized controlled trial. J Am Med Dir Assoc. 2020;21(8):1079–85.
50. Tanioka T. Nursing and rehabilitative care of the elderly using humanoid robots. J Med Investig. 2019;66(1.2):19–23.
51. Mishra N, Tulsulkar G, Li H, Thalmann NM, Er LH, Ping LM, Khoong CS. Does elderly enjoy playing bingo with a robot? A case study with the humanoid robot nadine. In: Computer graphics international conference. Springer; 2021. p. 491–503.
52. Schrum M, Park CH, Howard A. Humanoid therapy robot for encouraging exercise in dementia patients. In: 2019 14th ACM/IEEE International Conference on Human-Robot Interaction (HRI). IEEE; 2019. p. 564–5.
53. Cooper S, Di Fava A, Vivas C, Marchionni L, Ferro FARI. The social assistive robot and companion. In: 2020 29th IEEE International Conference on Robot and Human Interactive Communication (RO-MAN). IEEE; 2020. p. 745–51.
54. Weiss A, Hannibal G. What makes people accept or reject companion robots? A research agenda. In: Proceedings of the 11th Pervasive Technologies Related to Assistive Environments Conference; 2018. p. 397–404.
55. Tuyen NTV, Jeong S, Chong NY. Emotional bodily expressions for culturally competent robots through long term human-robot interaction. In: 2018 IEEE/RSJ International Conference on Intelligent Robots and Systems (IROS). IEEE; 2018. p. 2008–13.

56. Giakoumis D, Peleka G, Vasileiadis M, Kostavelis I, Tzovaras D. Service robot behaviour adaptation based on user mood, towards better personalized support of MCI patients at home. In: Smart assisted living. Springer; 2020. p. 209–26.
57. Groechel T, Shi Z, Pakkar R, Matarić MJ. Using socially expressive mixed reality arms for enhancing low-expressivity robots. In: 2019 28th IEEE International Conference on Robot and Human Interactive Communication (RO-MAN). IEEE; 2019. p. 1–8.
58. Draper JV, Kaber DB, Usher JM. Telepresence. Hum Factors. 1998;40(3):354–75.
59. Kerr D, Serrano JA, Ray P. The role of a disruptive digital technology for home-based healthcare of the elderly: telepresence robot. Digital Med. 2018;4(4):173.
60. Double Robotics–Telepresence Robot. https://www.doublerobotics.com/.
61. AMY Service Robots. www.amyrobotics.com.
62. Escolano C, Murguialday AR, Matuz T, Birbaumer N, Minguez JA. Telepresence robotic system operated with a P300-based brain-computer interface: initial tests with ALS patients. In: 2010 Annual International Conference of the IEEE Engineering in Medicine and Biology. IEEE; 2010. p. 4476–80.
63. Hansen JP, Alapetite A, Thomsen M, Wang Z, Minakata K, Zhang G. Head and gaze control of a telepresence robot with an HMD. In: Proceedings of the 2018 ACM Symposium on eye tracking research & applications; 2018. p. 1–3.
64. Ng MK, Primatesta S, Giuliano L, Lupetti ML, Russo LO, Farulla GA, Indaco M, Rosa S, Germak C, Bona BA. Cloud robotics system for telepresence enabling mobility impaired people to enjoy the whole museum experience. In: 2015 10th International Conference on Design & Technology of Integrated Systems in Nanoscale Era (DTIS). IEEE; 2015. p. 1–6.
65. Aymerich-Franch L, Ferrer I. Socially assistive robots' deployment in healthcare settings: a global perspective. arXiv preprint arXiv:211007404; 2021.
66. UVD Robots. Blue Ocean robotics. https://uvd.blue-ocean-robotics.com/robots.
67. Diligent Robotics. "Moxi hospital robot". https://www.diligentrobots.com/moxi.
68. Beam Pro telepresence robot. Blue Ocean Robotics. https://gobe.blue-ocean-robotics.com/beam-to-gobe.
69. Vespa PM, Miller C, Hu X, Nenov V, Buxey F, Martin NA. Intensive care unit robotic telepresence facilitates rapid physician response to unstable patients and decreased cost in neurointensive care. Surg Neurol. 2007;67(4):331–7.
70. Newman P, Dhaliwall S, Bains S, Polyakova O, McDonald K. Patient satisfaction with a pharmacist-led best possible medication discharge plan via tele-robot in a remote and rural community hospital. Can J Rural Med. 2021;26(4):151.
71. Hai NDX, Nam LHT, Thinh NT. Remote healthcare for the elderly, patients by tele-presence robot. In: 2019 International Conference on System Science and Engineering (ICSSE). IEEE; 2019. p. 506–10.
72. Stricker R, Müller S, Gross H-M. Non-contact video-based pulse rate measurement on a mobile service robot. In: The 23rd IEEE International Symposium on Robot and Human Interactive Communication. IEEE; 2014. p. 1056–62.
73. InTouch Health. https://intouchhealth.com/telehealth-devices/intouch-vita/.
74. Kasar KS, Karaman E. Life in lockdown: social isolation, loneliness and quality of life in the elderly during the COVİD-19 pandemic: a scoping review. Geriatric Nursing; 2021.
75. Cavallo F, Aquilano M, Bonaccorsi M, Limosani R, Manzi A, Carrozza MC, Dario P. On the design, development and experimentation of the ASTRO assistive robot integrated in smart environments. In: 2013 IEEE international conference on robotics and automation. IEEE; 2013. p. 4310–5.
76. Vermeersch P, Sampsel DD, Kleman C. Acceptability and usability of a telepresence robot for geriatric primary care: a pilot. Geriatr Nurs. 2015;36(3):234–8.
77. Moyle W, Jones C, Cooke M, O'Dwyer S, Sung B, Drummond S. Connecting the person with dementia and family: a feasibility study of a telepresence robot. BMC Geriatr. 2014;14(1):1–11.
78. Niemelä M, Melkas H. Robots as social and physical assistants in elderly care. In: Toivonen M, Saari E, editors. Human-centered digitalization and services. Singapore: Springer; 2019. p. 177–97. https://doi.org/10.1007/978-981-13-7725-9_10.

79. Niemelä M, Van Aerschot L, Tammela A, Aaltonen I, Lammi H. Towards ethical guidelines of using telepresence robots in residential care. Int J Soc Robot. 2021;13(3):431–9.
80. Korblet V. The acceptance of mobile telepresence robots by elderly people. University of Twente; 2019.
81. Koceski S, Koceska N. Evaluation of an assistive telepresence robot for elderly healthcare. J Med Syst. 2016;40(5):121.
82. Petrushin A, Tessadori J, Barresi G, Mattos LS. Effect of a click-like feedback on motor imagery in EEG-BCI and eye-tracking hybrid control for telepresence. In: 2018 IEEE/ASME International Conference on Advanced Intelligent Mechatronics (AIM). IEEE; 2018. p. 628–33.
83. Shiomi M, Kamei K, Kondo T, Miyashita T, Hagita N. Robotic service coordination for elderly people and caregivers with ubiquitous network robot platform. In: 2013 IEEE Workshop on Advanced Robotics and its Social Impacts. IEEE; 2013. p. 57–62.
84. Abou Allaban A, Wang M, Padır T. A systematic review of robotics research in support of in-home care for older adults. Information. 2020;11(2):75.
85. Bonaccorsi M, Fiorini L, Cavallo F, Saffiotti A, Dario P. A cloud robotics solution to improve social assistive robots for active and healthy aging. Int J Soc Robot. 2016;8(3):393–408.
86. Mbunge E, Muchemwa B, Batani J. Sensors and healthcare 5.0: transformative shift in virtual care through emerging digital health technologies. Global Health J. 2021;5(4):169–77.
87. Li J, Carayon P. Health care 4.0: a vision for smart and connected health care. IISE Trans Health Sys Engg. 2021;11(3):171–80.
88. Almarashdeh I, Alsmadi M, Hanafy T, Albahussain A, Altuwaijri N, Almaimoni H, Asiry F, Alowaid S, Alshabanah M, Alrajhi D. Real-time elderly healthcare monitoring expert system using wireless sensor network. Int J Appl Engg Res. 2018;13(10):7541–50.
89. Gambhir SS, Ge TJ, Vermesh O, Spitler R, Gold GE. Continuous health monitoring: an opportunity for precision health. Sci Transl Med. 2021;13(597):eabe5383.
90. Majumder S, Aghayi E, Noferesti M, Memarzadeh-Tehran H, Mondal T, Pang Z, Deen MJ. Smart homes for elderly healthcare—recent advances and research challenges. Sensors. 2017;17(11):2496.
91. Petrushin A, Freddolini M, Barresi G, Bustreo M, Laffranchi M, Del Bue A, De Michieli L. IoT-powered monitoring Systems for Geriatric Healthcare: overview. In: Scataglini S, Imbesi S, Marques G, editors. Internet of things for human-centered design: application to elderly healthcare. Springer; n.d.
92. Parmiggiani A, Fiorio L, Scalzo A, Sureshbabu AV, Randazzo M, Maggiali M, Pattacini U, Lehmann H, Tikhanoff V, Domenichelli D. The design and validation of the r1 personal humanoid. In: 2017 IEEE/RSJ international conference on intelligent robots and systems (IROS). IEEE; 2017. p. 674–80.
93. Gambhir SS, Ge TJ, Vermesh O, Spitler R. Toward achieving precision health. Sci Transl Med. 2018;10(430):eaao3612.
94. Organization WH. Active ageing: a policy framework. World Health Organization; 2002.
95. Marques G. Ambient assisted living and internet of things. Harnessing the internet of everything (IoE) for accelerated innovation opportunities; 2019. p. 100–15.

Education and Training in Gerontechnology

Slawomir Tobis

11.1 Human Aging and Its Impact on Attitudes to Technology

European societies have been aging rapidly. According to WHO data, the percentage of people 60+ in the oldest countries in the world was approx. 20% in 1980 and approx. 30% in 2017, and following pre-pandemic forecasts, it will be approx. 40% in 2050 [1]. Even if unforeseen events modify these prognoses (e.g., COVID-19 has shortened life expectancy in the vast majority of European countries), a clear upward trend in the number and percentage of older people is still observed. At the same time, a gap in care arises as low birth rates lead to fewer people at work and gradually increase the old-age dependency ratio, which expresses the relative size of the older part of the population compared with the working-age population [2].

Since most of the older people live independently in their own homes where they want to remain as long as possible (to retain the surroundings they are familiar with and maintain their relationships with friends and their family), the essential question is what actions can be taken to enable them to stay at home. At the opposite pole, for people living in institutions, with restricted independence, entirely different activities are needed to improve their quality of life. Consequently, it is imperative to propose differentiated and targeted means and methods of care with the aim to satisfy the needs of its recipients. Care optimization means personalized care delivery, tailored to each subject [3], and taking into account support for the caregivers of older people (both formal and informal), in the face of their decreasing availability in the system—so that the care burden does not lead to frustration and burnout. Moreover, the implementation of new solutions should be cost-effective. Therefore, it appears that the above problems are difficult to solve without using modern

S. Tobis (✉)
Department of Occupational Therapy, Poznan University of Medical Sciences, Poznan, Poland
e-mail: stobis@ump.edu.pl

technologies. While the ideas of assistive technologies in all their possible aspects precede the present day, they lead, for example, to the image of socially assistive robots replacing humans in care. It is, however, a picture of the future as research in this field is not yet advanced enough to enable drawing such meaningful conclusions. Additionally, many questions remain unanswered, including particularly ethical questions as well as those related to education for the (unavoidable) new technological solutions.

When thinking of the design and implementation of new technologies for older subjects, it is vital to relate to the actual needs and preferences of end-users rather than technological advances (support for health and independence in daily functioning, safety, physical, social and cognitive activity, education, and entertainment).

11.1.1 Attitudes to Technology Along the Aging Trajectory

In the context of technologies, questions about the preparedness of older people for their use are particularly important. In a study performed by our team on a group of over 800 people of different ages ($n = 843$), only 66.5% declared that technologies were for them easy to use [4]. Notably, older participants were significantly less likely to report ease of use of technology than the rest (50.4% vs. 76.3%. $p = 0.00000$), which clearly signals educational needs in this group.

Golant et al. observed three main factors related to coping with technologies by older subjects: perceived efficaciousness, perceived usability, and perceived collateral damages. The likelihood of technology adoption is the higher, the better these factors are rated by prospective users [5]. Furthermore, according to a study by De Regge at el., to foster technology acceptance, trust in and attitude toward gerontechnologies must be strengthened. Additionally, family members' knowledge and beliefs in technology are the main factors contributing to the actual use of gerontechnologies by older persons. Also, the families' trust in technologies and provision of access to gerontechnologies positively influence the attitudes and usage intentions of their older relatives [6]. All these factors need to be taken into account when educational strategies are created.

11.2 Education in or for Gerontechnology: Target Groups and Starting Points

Increasing the interest of older people in the use of modern technologies requires the implementation of education focused on demonstrating the possibilities of technologies and their positive impact on everyday functioning. Moreover, it should be kept in mind that, in terms of the need for education for modern technologies, older people, as in many other respects, constitute a heterogeneous group, regardless of their education level (Fig. 11.1). Some of them can be considered enthusiasts of modern technologies, interested in, among others, new products entering the market. On the other extreme, there are skeptical individuals who believe that modern

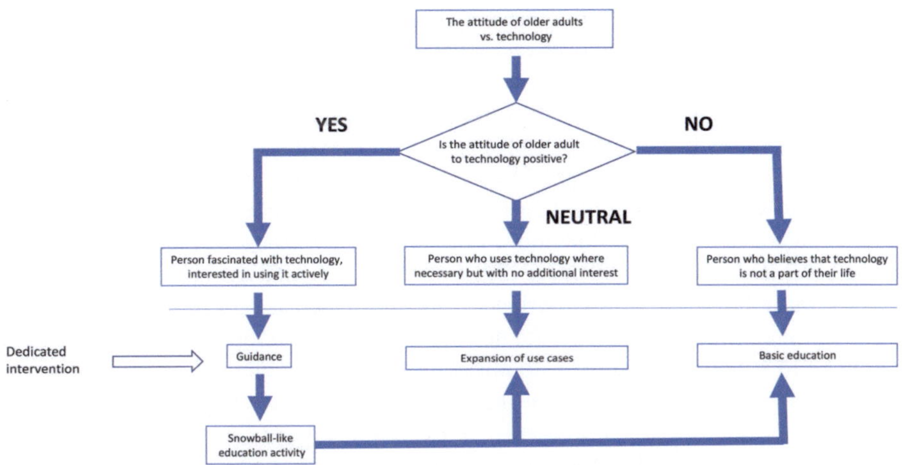

Fig. 11.1 Groups of older adults, their educational needs and possibilities of intervention

technologies are for young people, have nothing to do with them, and they can do without "these devices." Between these two extremes, there are persons, more or less indifferent, who use technological solutions because they make life easier and therefore have a utilitarian attitude to technology. It is evident that all these groups require a different educational approach.

Education tailored specifically for older people is of particular importance as they recognize opportunities and limitations differently from their younger counterparts and, consequently, often differently from both formal and informal caregivers. As we showed in our study on the use of social robots in care, they thought that *The elderly are able to manage with the robot* almost twice as frequently, and more than twice that *The elderly want to increase their knowledge about the robots to be able to operate them* [4]. Additionally, Xie observed that older subjects preferred older trainers, who shared the same learning processes, to younger ones who were "impatient" due to not understanding the learning speed, style, and difficulties experienced by older pupils [7]. These results are in line with the study by Chen & Chan, who showed that older adults did not want to be educated by their children [8]. This observation is particularly important in light of the study on older adults conducted in the USA and Israel by Heart & Kalderon [9], who noticed that the majority of studied subjects identified their primary sources of support as children and other family members.

The education of older persons requires an understanding of the ways and motivations of their learning. In the abovementioned study by Chen & Chan, the participants did not feel comfortable using advanced technological devices because, in their opinion, too much mental effort was necessary to learn to use such devices [8]. The learning curve frequently involved taking classes, making detailed notes, continuously reviewing information, and practicing, which was perceived as tiring or stressful. It is thus crucial to pay attention not only to the pace of training but also to its themes, methods, and structure—by providing effective aids and adapting the classes and sessions to match the receptive capacities of the learners. Furthermore, as far as learning skills in technology are concerned, it is imperative to take specific personal and cultural characteristics into account [9] (e.g., Asian elders may have different attitudes from those of European ones—we observed considerable readiness to collaborate with younger educators and helpers during our studies in Poland).

It is also worth pointing out that European Commission noticed in its European Digital Agenda for Europe "the more Europeans know [robots], the more they like them" [10]. Indeed, while teaching older subjects, it is vital to use the kind of technology that allows them to experience success, which is—in turn—essential for developing confidence in their own abilities. A possible approach for this purpose might be to structure the courses to allow for the acquisition of skills and create an effective feedback mechanism during the educational activities [11]. The well-trained older adults can subsequently be expected to be successful in the roles of educators to their less-educated peers, possibly as a kind of educational snowball, as shown in Fig. 11.1.

11.3 Older Adults, Aged Care and Gerontechnology: Stakeholders

Undoubtedly, education for gerontechnology cannot be limited to older subjects since their needs in this regard are different from those of their younger counterparts. For example, a frequent obstacle for older adults to get acquainted with information and communication technology (ICT) devices was that family members could operate these devices for them [12, 13]. In this case, negative attitude of older persons to technological devices was related to lack of motivation (not making an effort because of being substituted by other stakeholders—the younger ones—which should be taken into account when planning educational activities). Moreover, older adults may not be aware of technologies they could benefit from [14]; hence, technology promoters are needed to deliver advice and provide information.

The education of all the stakeholders is thus necessary, who are active not only in the field of creating new technological solutions but also in that of disseminating and implementing them (Fig. 11.2). Improved awareness and training in available and effective technological interventions among older adults and healthcare providers, combined with sustainable funding, are likely to promote the adoption of gerontechnologies [15]. Involving clinicians and caregivers at the time of designing technological interventions is also recommended. This is in agreement with our observations during mutual education of future biomedical engineers (students of Poznan University of Technology, Poland) and occupational therapists (students of Poznan University of Medical Sciences, Poland) who both benefited from the concurrent involvement of the other party when analyzing the older patients' needs and problems, and solving them using various technological approaches [16].

A study by Mikus showed that many technologies that had been considered successful failed with older adults. This was not because older users were uninterested

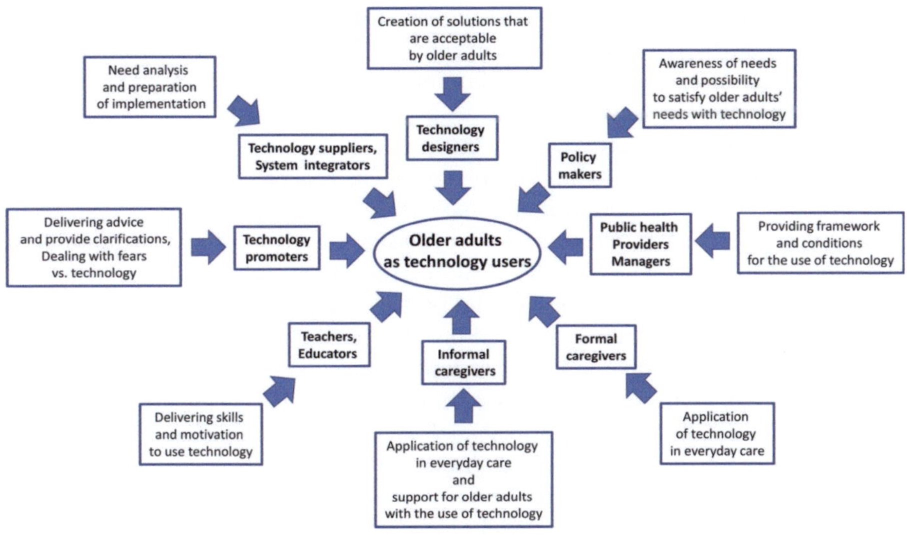

Fig. 11.2 Stakeholders and their roles in education for gerontechnologies

or incapable but rather because they tended to be left out of the design process of technologies [17]. D. Norman (an 83-year-old author of the industry bible *Design of Everyday Things* and a former Apple VP) even stated: "the world seems designed against the elderly" [18]. All the while, most technologies are designed for a younger user who is accustomed to using them—since they grow up surrounded by various technologies. Furthermore, the commonly applied top-down design methodology is not effective with older adults since it fails to engage users in the design process, which is typical for the bottom-up methodology [19]. Moreover, attention should be paid to the fact that there is a group of older persons with the education, ability, and desire to understand, use and procure technological devices. Their generational wealth and, consequently, buying potential should be observed when thinking about new products or solutions. Bearing all this in mind, technology designers clearly constitute a particular group of stakeholders who need to be educated in designing for the old. While improving "technology literacy" can help older users better inter-act with gerontechnologies, the issue of "aging literacy" (the understanding of the functioning of older people) must be properly addressed when considering the edu-cation of technologists. This education can involve exercises based on partnering with older persons to design new gerontechnologies. Such a preemptive approach can be applied for creating technologies that are both useful and capable of reducing barriers to use and is certainly more effective than intervening after the product has been placed on the market. Feedback loops are also a welcome addition to the design process, facilitating understanding and developing mutual trust between designers and users. Complying with the person-centered approach means here not only education, guidance, and close follow-up, but also co-design, involving the older participant in the development and evaluation of technology [20], which should additionally make their education easier and more effective. This is more important as the barriers to using gerontechnology are well established (including lack of interest, need for training and consumer assistance, and design problems); hence, more attention should be paid to tailoring technological solutions to the needs and preferences of prospective older users [21].

In a study consisting of mono-disciplinary focus groups (involving older adults, care professionals, managers within home care or social work organizations, technology designers and suppliers, and policymakers), each stakeholder group listed steps they considered necessary for a successful implementation of technologies. All groups agreed that technology should provide tangible profits to older persons; however, older adults uniquely pointed out that technologies providing too many benefits could make people lose their independence and make them dependent on technology [22]. Without taking this rudimentary rule into account, no effective activities for the acceptance of gerontechnologies by older people are imaginable. It is thus vital to create educational programs for various stakeholders to raise the awareness of the aging process and the needs of older persons for independence and aging in place. Furthermore, all stakeholders should join forces to work towards aging-friendly communities [23] with adequate educational support.

A special group of stakeholders, who are set to use gerontechnologies in practice, are caregivers, particularly the professional ones. A literature review provided by Zaman et al. showed that training could be a significant factor for the health professionals' eagerness to use or refer their clients or patients for using technologies at home [15]. Healthcare providers should, for example, signal the desire to get more available functions, such as voice demonstration or video chatting, for integrating [ICT] interventions into routine systems. Caregivers need education and practice on the use of modern technologies in care for older adults primarily—this applies to both inexperienced and experienced care professionals, but particularly for those who "have been working for a long time," which may be associated with doing the job routinely, without paying attention to new technologies. In a Danish study on a nationally representative group of nursing staff (employed in various healthcare institutions), the results indicated that the respondents who were confronted with the introduction of new technology in the last three years expressed a positive opinion on this introduction [24]. This conclusion also signals that semi-permanent educational support is necessary while using gerontechnology.

11.3.1 Barriers, Facilitators

It is generally believed that older and younger learners have different training performances. With older adults, apart from the importance of self-pacing (i.e., with the trainees defining the pace of learning), the Interest Bridge Model can be applied in learning how to use technology. This model states that, when the education of older adults is based on requests from interest, the trainees are generally likely to develop a more profound and longer-term engagement in technology and integrate technology into their everyday lives [25]. An observational and active learning method has also been shown as effective with older users of tablets [26]. Such approaches to education are crucial because findings indicate that less frequent use of technology and computers in the older age group potentially has severe social implications—persons with less technology use are more likely to become disadvantaged or excluded. Henceforth, predominantly the vulnerable social groups should obtain particular educational support in modern gerontechnologies due to their increased risk of social exclusion: lower socio-economic groups, minorities, the oldest-old, and those who are in general less educated [11].

According to Broady et al., stereotypes held by trainers and tutors who expect their pupils to learn more rapidly than they are able to, particularly so when new skills are not compatible with existing knowledge, constitute a barrier in the education of older adults [27]. This, in turn, makes them feel incapable of learning the particular topics and demotivated.

Further barriers have been signaled by Callahan et al., who performed an extensive analysis of the effects of three instructional methods (lecture, modeling, and active participation) and four instructional factors (materials, feedback, pacing, and group size) on the observed training performance of older learners. Their results suggest that all instructional methods and two instructional factors uniquely explain variance in observed training performance, whereas self-pacing, particularly combined with group size, explained the greatest proportion of the observed variance. As for the instructional methods, their selection should be considered according to the type of training and presented content [28].

Chen & Chang, who, using qualitative methodology, assessed barriers and facilitators for technology use defined by older subjects themselves, divided the former category into three groups: dispositional barriers (most common) and situational and technological barriers (which were less frequent) [8]. All these groups manifest barriers related to education. In first of them, understood as personal factors associated with the subject's attitude and self-perception as a technology user, these include lack of knowledge, difficulty or inability to learn, and not knowing how to use [technologies]. Among the situational barriers, that is, personal factors that are beyond the individual's control or are related to their life situation or environment, lack of assistance has been identified, and among the technological barriers—complexity of technologies or tasks. As for the facilitators, training, assistance, adaptive design, and encouragement have been pointed out. Also, excellent and trustworthy tutors can be viewed as facilitators, not only for educational activities but also for long-term technology use.

Based on the identified barriers and obstacles for education in gerontechnology, there is urgent need for discussion and action, since the majority of stakeholders appear not well prepared to deal with the older group. Systemic improvements aimed at common education for aging (at both pre- and postgraduate level) seem essential not only to improve intergenerational understanding but also to make the introduction of new technologies, along with education and training, more effective and smooth.

11.4   Educational Support of the Deployment of Assistive Technologies in Light of Own Studies

Our experiences show that students, when properly prepared for communication with older adults with mild cognitive impairment, are perfectly able to support them in using modern technologies if only they have sufficient motivation [29]. During the COVID-19 pandemic, our team organized and ran the Internet-Telephone Consultation Service for older adults. The participating students helped older persons get connected with the Internet, configure a communication service with video capability, and use this connectivity for medical consultations [30]. The students supported and supervised the first connections, which was important not only at the moment but also—as demonstrated by Peek et al.—for the stability of the use of technological devices in the future [31]. The experiences of young people, directly supporting older ones, were described as "valuable, truly intergenerational workshops."

Indeed, in our study on the possibilities of support for older adults with mild cognitive impairment by the TIAGo social robot, one of the participants who had the robot in her apartment for 10 weeks stated, "I was always afraid of everything, I was scared, and I do not like new things at all," but "the girls [from the technical staff] were here, (…) introduced, and thanks to that it was straightforward," and "I actually stopped being afraid of such new things." Importantly, the team members had been trained in gerontology and communication with older persons prior to their engagement in the study—it is thus evidently indispensable to train the trainers to understand old age. Tutors and helpers should give their trainees enough time to learn and provide step-by-step demonstrations. Our further study showed that students of Occupational therapy, who were engaged in care for older people, understood that if a social robot was to be implemented in this kind of care, the introduction of a robot in the life of an older person should be "gradual, allowing for gaining familiarity, increasing the number of available functions" [32]. Furthermore, the participants of our previously mentioned study with 843 subjects of different ages [4] expressed the belief that older adults would be better prepared to dealing with technology in the future than today—given that many older persons at present have no problems with, for example, smartphones and computers, they would easily manage to operate a robot. Others would require more education and assistance to get started—the process of introduction of technologies should be gradual, with broad availability of professional trainers. The implementation of any new technology should be sufficiently timed whilst educational activities around its introduction should be based on self-pacing. The involvement of training staff can diminish, in a flexible way, only when the users gain confidence in the robot's operation, depending on the degree of confidence obtained by the older persons.

11.5 Final Remarks

The following points should be observed when planning education and training in gerontechnology:

- Older adults have strongly varying attitudes to gerontechnology.
- Older adults have strongly varying knowledge and skills related to gerontechnologies.
- Educators need to provide appropriate structure, feedback, and timing of training activities, possibly based on self-pacing.
- Education should provide the opportunity to experience success and notice benefits for one's life activities, and should be based on requests from interests.
- Designing technological interventions should involve clinicians and caregivers, provide tangible benefits, and avoid unnecessary help to older adults.
- It is imperative to involve prospective users of gerontechnology in the design process, development, and evaluation of products and services, and educate the designers/developers for a successful collaboration.
- Educators should ascertain that new-to-obtain skills relate to existing knowledge and experience of trainees.
- Excellent and trustworthy tutors can be facilitators for education and use of technology.
- The implementation of gerontechnology should be appropriately timed and accompanied by competent helpers for as long as necessary.
- Semi-permanent educational support is needed while using gerontechnologies.

Education in gerontechnology is a complex issue. The process of learning by experience constitutes a good base for all educational activities related to gerontechnology, building on the well-proven concept of "experiential learning" developed by Kolb [33], which suggests that learning can be understood as transforming experiences into knowledge, skills, or attitudes. This applies not only to older individuals but also to all stakeholders engaged in any way in the creation, implementation, and use of gerontechnology. The education of individual stakeholders must comprise aging literacy and secure equity and diversity, especially in the context of vulnerable target groups.

References

1. United Nations, Economic Do, Social Affairs. World population prospects: the 2017 revision, key findings and advance tables. 2017.
2. Eurostat. Ageing Europe—statistics on population developments. 2020.
3. American Geriatrics Society Expert Panel on Person-Centered C. Person-centered care: a definition and essential elements. J Am Geriatr Soc. 2016;64(1):15–8.

4. Tobis S, Neumann-Podczaska A, Kropinska S, Suwalska A. UNRAQ—A questionnaire for the use of a social robot in care for older persons. A multi-stakeholder study and psychometric properties. Int J Environ Res Public Health. 2021;18(11):6157.

5. Golant SM. A theoretical model to explain the smart technology adoption behaviors of elder consumers (Elderadopt). J Aging Stud. 2017;42:56–73.

6. De Regge M, Van Baelen F, Beirao G, Den Ambtman A, De Pourcq K, Dias JC, et al. Personal and interpersonal drivers that contribute to the intention to use Gerontechnologies. Gerontology. 2020;66(2):176–86.

7. Xie B. Information technology education for older adults as a continuing peer-learning process: a Chinese case study. Educ Gerontol. 2007;33(5):429–50.

8. Chen K, Chan AH-S. Use or non-use of Gerontechnology—a qualitative study. Int J Environ Res Public Health. 2013;10(10):4645–66.

9. Heart T, Kalderon E. Older adults: are they ready to adopt health-related ICT? Int J Med Inform. 2013;82(11):e209–31.

10. Robots: the more Europeans know them, the more they like them: European Commission; 2015. Available from: https://digital-strategy.ec.europa.eu/en/news/robots-more-europeans-know-them-more-they-them.

11. Czaja SJ, Charness N, Fisk AD, Hertzog C, Nair SN, Rogers WA, et al. Factors predicting the use of technology: findings from the Center for Research and Education on aging and technology enhancement (CREATE). Psychol Aging. 2006;21(2):333–52.

12. Wildenbos GA, Peute L, Jaspers M. Aging barriers influencing mobile health usability for older adults: a literature based framework (MOLD-US). Int J Med Inform. 2018;114:66–75.

13. Harerimana B, Forchuk C, O'Regan T. The use of technology for mental healthcare delivery among older adults with depressive symptoms: a systematic literature review. Int J Ment Health Nurs. 2019;28(3):657–70.

14. Heinz M, Martin P, Margrett JA, Yearns M, Franke W, Yang HI, et al. Perceptions of technology among older adults. J Gerontol Nurs. 2013;39(1):42–51.

15. Zaman SB, Khan RK, Evans RG, Thrift AG, Maddison R, Islam SMS. Exploring barriers to and enablers of the adoption of information and communication technology for the care of older adults with chronic diseases: scoping review. JMIR Aging. 2022;5(1):e25251.

16. Tobis S, Cylkowska-Nowak M, Wieczorowski M. Occupational therapy and engineering in the battle for good aging–innovative teaching methods/Terapia zajęciowa i inżynieria w walce o dobrą starość–innowacyjne metody nauczania. Geriatria. 2017;11:253–8.

17. Mikus J. Designing with the digital divide to design technology for all. Australian Universal Design Conference; 2021.

18. Norman D. I wrote the book on user-friendly design. What I see today horrifies me. Fast Company. 2019.

19. Wang S, Bolling K, Mao W, Reichstadt J, Jeste D, Kim H-C, et al. Technology to support aging in place: older adults' perspectives. Healthcare. 2019;7(2):60.

20. Ollevier A, Aguiar G, Palomino M, Simpelaere IS. How can technology support ageing in place in healthy older adults? A systematic review. Public Health Rev. 2020;41(1):26.

21. Cohen-Mansfield J, Biddison J. The scope and future trends of Gerontechnology: consumers' opinions and literature survey. J Technol Hum Serv. 2008;25(3):1–19.

22. Peek ST, Wouters EJ, Luijkx KG, Vrijhoef HJ. What it takes to successfully implement technology for aging in place: focus groups with stakeholders. J Med Internet Res. 2016;18(5):e98.

23. Jeste DV, Blazer DG 2nd, Buckwalter KC, Cassidy KK, Fishman L, Gwyther LP, et al. Age-friendly communities initiative: public health approach to promoting successful aging. Am J Geriatr Psychiatry. 2016;24(12):1158–70.

24. de Veer AJ, Fleuren MA, Bekkema N, Francke AL. Successful implementation of new technologies in nursing care: a questionnaire survey of nurse-users. BMC Med Inform Decis Mak. 2011;11(1):67.

25. Beh J, Pedell S, Doubé W. Evaluation of interest-bridge model: older adults meditated learning of mobile technology. Proceedings of the 28th Australian Conference on Computer-Human

Interaction; Launceston, Tasmania, Australia: Association for Computing Machinery; 2016. p. 293–301.

26. Kim BJ, Ishikawa H, Liu L, Ohwa M, Sawada Y, Lim HY, et al. The effects of job autonomy and job satisfaction on burnout among careworkers in long-term care settings: policy and practice implications for Japan and South Korea. Educ Gerontol. 2018;44(5–6):289–300.

27. Broady T, Chan A, Caputi P. Comparison of older and younger adults' attitudes towards and abilities with computers: implications for training and learning. Br J Educ Technol. 2010;41(3):473–85.

28. Callahan JS, Kiker DS, Cross T. Does method matter? A meta-analysis of the effects of training method on older learner training performance. J Manag. 2003;29(5):663–80.

29. Tobis S, Wieczorowska-Tobis K, Neumann-Podczaska A. Internet-telephone consultation service for older persons. Ageing and COVID-19. Routledge; 2021. p. 274–84.

30. Neumann-Podczaska A, Seostianin M, Madejczyk K, Merks P, Religioni U, Tomczak Z, et al. An experimental education project for consultations of older adults during the pandemic and healthcare lockdown. Healthcare (Basel). 2021;9(4):425.

31. Peek STM, Luijkx KG, Vrijhoef HJM, Nieboer ME, Aarts S, van der Voort CS, et al. Understanding changes and stability in the long-term use of technologies by seniors who are aging in place: a dynamical framework. BMC Geriatr. 2019;19(1):236.

32. Tobis S, Cylkowska-Nowak M, Wieczorowska-Tobis K, Pawlaczyk M, Suwalska A. Occupational therapy students' perceptions of the role of robots in the care for older people living in the community. Occup Ther Int. 2017;2017:9592405.

33. Kolb D. Experiential learning experience as the source of learning and development. New Jersey: Prentice Hall; 1984.

Artificial Intelligence and the Medicine of the Future

12

Richard Woodman and Arduino Alexander Mangoni

12.1 Introduction

Artificial intelligence (AI), machine learning (ML) and Big Data are emerging as powerful tools of choice for solving complex problems in almost every domain of our lives. Within healthcare, the rapid adoption of Industry 4.0 technologies including interconnected wireless sensors and devices (the Internet of Things or IoT) as well as the continued expansion of electronic health records (EHRs) has resulted in unprecedented volumes of data. Together, the IoT, Smart mobile devices, EHRs and imaging data provide what can be viewed as the digital data foundation of a "Wisdom pyramid" for Healthcare 4.0 [1]. Lying above this knowledge base is a "digital" middle tier of digital knowledge representation consisting of the digitally captured medical ontologies and research publication databases such as PubMed. And at the pinnacle of the pyramid lies AI and ML which utilise both the digital data foundation base and digital knowledge representation to generate digital knowledge learning and prediction and includes ML, natural language processing and deep learning. In more common language and practical terms, this translates to informed and assisted decision-making for the end-user. Together these 3 pyramid tiers represent Healthcare 4.0, whose goal is to assist healthcare professionals in making accurate clinical decisions and to provide patients with more efficient personalised services. These goals are reflected via changes in the diagnosis, treatment [2] and monitoring [3] of patients together with effective resource management, and the alignment of the healthcare processes with the needs and complexity of modern medicine.

R. Woodman (✉)
Flinders Health and Medical Research Institute, Flinders University, Adelaide, Australia
e-mail: richard.woodman@flinders.edu.au

A. A. Mangoni
Department of Clinical Pharmacology, Division of Critical and Cardiac Care, Flinders Medical Centre and Flinders University Adelaide, Adelaide, Australia

Disease diagnosis, risk prediction, treatment setpoints, clinical decision support systems [4, 5], public health systems surveillance for disease outbreaks, surgical assistance, personalised healthcare service systems, drug discovery and repurposing, remote patient monitoring and healthcare staff and patient tracking systems [1] are just some of the major areas in which AI is advancing healthcare. Examples of successful projects include risk stratification and treatment decisions [6], triaging patients presenting to Emergency Departments [7], reducing the risk of falls [8, 9], delaying hospital readmission [10], cardiovascular risk prediction [11, 12], predicting the long-term prognosis of patients with frailty and disability [13] and mortality from COVID-19 [14]. The rapid rise of algorithm development within ML with ever more complex algorithms such as deep learning, neural networks and generative adversarial networks has been matched and assisted by the increasing availability of EHRs and other sources of Big Data, together with enhanced data access and transfer. Indeed, there appear to be almost unlimited opportunities to extract hidden insights from health and medical data leading to a transformation of modern healthcare.

In this chapter, we describe some of the backgrounds to AI and ML and provide examples of their application within medicine and healthcare with a special focus on the management of the older patient population. We also describe some of the theories behind ML and discuss some of the important challenges that remain for its use within healthcare.

12.1.1 What is Artificial Intelligence and Machine Learning?

Whilst the roots of AI and ML go back some 70 years, it is only more recently, with the expansion of computing power as well as the availability of Big Data that progress has made a quantum leap [15]. The terminology of AI began in 1950, when Alan Turing, the renowned Manchester University mathematician, developed his "Theory of computation" suggesting that a machine could simulate formal reasoning using a simple binary symbol approach. This insight is known as the Church–Turing thesis [16]. The term AI was not however formally conceptualised and named until 1956 and even today there is still no formal consensus on the definition of AI. Instead, the term is generally taken to refer to the ability of a machine to show "cognitive" capabilities, including the ability to learn, and perform inference and deduction [17].

ML is the sub-domain of AI in which mathematical and computational algorithms in software are used to predict patient outcomes and identify patterns, often in very large datasets. Arthur Samuel described ML as "The field of study that gives computers the ability to learn without being explicitly programmed". More recently, Tom Mitchell clarified that "A computer program is said to learn from experience E with respect to some class of tasks T and performance measure P, if its performance at tasks in T, as measured by P, improves with experience E" [18]. In this context, "learning" here simply refers to the reduction in error, and therefore improved accuracy, that comes with "training", rather than the more complex concept of human learning. Beyond these literal translations, the general aims of ML encompass prediction, pattern recognition and cluster formation [19].

Despite its long history, the development of AI over time has by no means been linear and unimpeded, having endured several so-called "AI-Winters" in its development, often a consequence of rate-limiting factors such as a lack of computational power, funding and the availability of specific data. Figure 12.1 describes an example timeline of ML, paying special attention to the landmark developments in medicine and healthcare. For example, the development of new types of algorithms (Neural Networks, Nearest Neighbours, Deep Learning) and new ML systems (CASNET, Dxplain, Deep Blue, IBM Watson, Pharmabot, Chatbot Mandy, Arterys).

12.1.2 Advantages of ML

Whilst other methods of prediction are also available, a major practical advantage offered by ML in comparison to, for example, standard regression-based methods, is their suitability to handle Big Data. This makes ML a natural fit for genomics, epigenetics and omics, as well as high-dimensional clinical lab data. Specifically, ML can deal with common issues that impede more traditional methods including those of high dimensionality, sparsity, multi-collinearity, interactions and insufficient computing power (Table 12.1). Indeed, many ML algorithms are implicitly designed to deal with these and other issues, which makes them especially suitable for accurate prediction in circumstances where hitherto unknown effect moderators or phenotypes exist, requiring the use of data-driven approaches [20]. An important additional virtue of ML is its focus on model validation. This includes the avoidance of developing over-fitting models during either training (resulting in high bias) or testing (resulting in high variance). The aim in doing so is to help ensure that the proposed models generalise well to future unseen datasets.

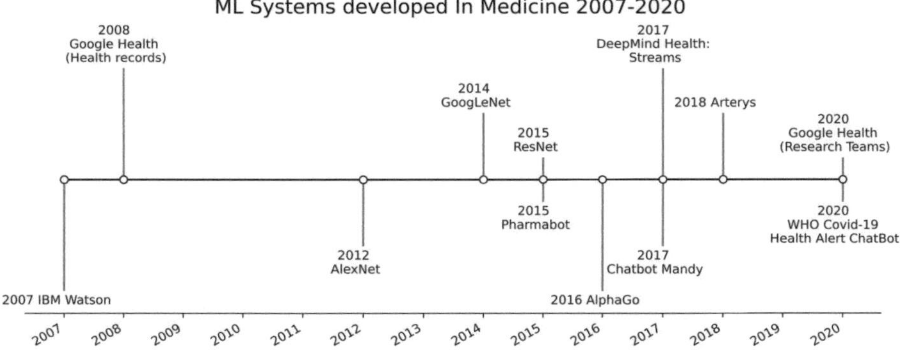

Fig. 12.1 An example timeline of machine learning in medicine and healthcare

Table 12.1 Examples of the advantages of the ML approach over more classical prediction methods

Advantage	Details
Handles large datasets	ML algorithms often perform better with large sets of data
Handles multi-collinearity	ML can include features (predictors) that are highly correlated
Feature extraction and data reduction	ML engineering techniques that help eliminate the problem of collinearity prior to training
Handles sparse data	ML can handle features with little variability within them, for example, data with mostly zeros
Handles high dimensionality	ML often performs better with more features (predictors)
Handles complex interactions	Many ML algorithms are implicitly designed to deal with complex interactions including those of second and third order
Good generalisation to new datasets	Strong attention paid to model validation by avoidance of over-fitting during training. The basic ML workflow helps ensure that the trained models also perform well in testing, validation and unseen datasets
Use of multiple algorithms	Common for ML to trial a range of different algorithms rather than just one, since different algorithms perform better with some types of data than others. This does not raise issues of multiple testing since the focus is on prediction and not inference
Different algorithmic sub-domains	The 3 major algorithmic subdomains: supervised, unsupervised and reinforcement learning allow flexibility in modelling
Model tuning	Adds an additional degree of flexibility to the models which does not exist with classical statistical models. The hyper-parameters can be tuned for better model fit during both training and validation (low bias and variance)
Learns over time with new data	The weights (hyperparameters) of the model are designed to be updated as new data is incorporated. Thus, the model rarely stays fixed like classical regression prediction models

12.1.3 Growth of AI and ML Research in Healthcare

The rapid rise in published articles on AI and ML research within healthcare including algorithm development and AI platforms (Fig. 12.2) reflects the involvement of ML research in the progress of healthcare within the last 50 years, and particularly the last decade. This includes diverse fields and applications such as the development of algorithms and AI platforms used in clinical decision support systems [5], patient monitoring [21–23], patient coaching [24], surgical assistance [25, 26], improvement in healthcare systems [27], prediction of in-hospital mortality, unplanned readmissions, and prolonged length of stay and final discharge diagnoses using EHRs [28].

Table 12.2 provides examples of some of the numerous clinical domains that have benefitted from an ML-based approach to prediction.

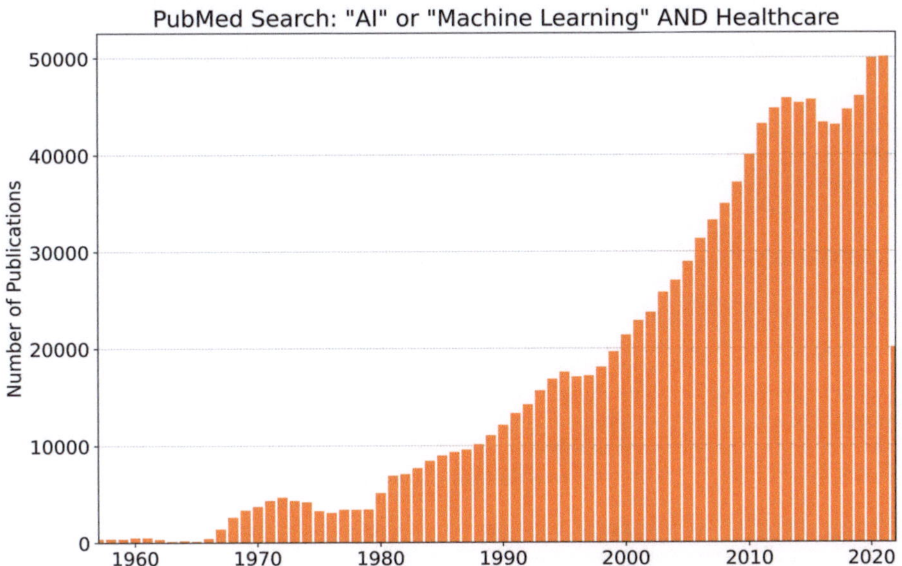

Fig. 12.2 The rise in research output related to AI and ML in healthcare since 1957 (PubMed)

Table 12.2 Examples of machine learning applications in medicine and healthcare

Area of medicine/ healthcare	Summary of findings
Orthotopic heart transplant [29]	Ensemble machine learning-based model to predict patient survival 1 year following orthotopic heart transplantation (OHT). Significantly outperformed established OHT algorithms.
Cardiac magnetic resonance (CMR) imaging [30]	Artery Inc.'s cardio AI deep learning (DL) algorithm became the first U.S. Food and Drug Administration–approved clinical cloud-based DL application in healthcare in 2017. It analyses CMR images in seconds with information such as cardiac ejection fraction. The application has since expanded to include liver and lung imaging, chest and musculoskeletal x-ray images, and non-contrast head CT images.
CMR imaging [31]	Provides reduced time required for image segmentation and analysis. An accurate and reproducible fully automated quantification of left and right ventricular mass and volume is now commercially available. Research areas currently include reduction of image acquisition and reconstruction time, improving spatial and temporal resolution, and analysis of perfusion and myocardial mapping.
Brain MRI analysis [32]	This is a review of deep learning for quantitative brain MRI image analysis architectures.
Melanoma and non-melanoma skin cancers [33]	Convolutional neural network (CNN) was used to identify nonmelanoma and melanoma skin cancers. CNN performance was comparable to expert dermatologists.
Cardiovascular risk prediction [34]	CNN improved prediction accuracy by 7.6% compared to the established algorithm defined by the American College of Cardiology guidelines
Alzheimer's disease [35]	Considerably improved prediction accuracy of Alzheimer's disease (81%) between people with and without AD, including the early form, mild cognitive impairment and is superior to standard hippocampal atrophy accuracy (26%) and cerebrospinal fluid beta-amyloid measure accuracy (62%).
Application of AI in surgery [26]	A review of recent successful and influential applications of AI in surgery including preoperative planning, intraoperative guidance, and surgical robots
Breast cancer [36]	Deep learning algorithm in detecting lymph node metastases in breast cancer
Retinopathy [37]	Higher accuracy for detecting retinopathy than manual detection systems
Colorectal polyps and adenomas [38]	An AI model named GI genius trained on endoscopic video differentiated diminutive adenomas from hyperplastic polyps with high accuracy (98% sensitivity for adenomas and 94% accuracy for polyps)
Colorectal neoplasia [39]	Meta-analysis of 5 RCTs. Deep learning systems with real-time computer-aided detection (CAD) for adenoma. Detection rate was higher in the CAD versus control (791/2163 [36.6%] vs 558/2191 [25.2%]; RR, 1.44(1.27–1.62)
Human resource planning in rural and remote areas [40]	Length of stay of healthcare workers in rural areas (less than 1 year, less than 2 years, less than 3 years, and more than 3 years). Three models achieved an average AUC of approximately 0.66 using only nationality, gender, profession and marital status as variables

(continued)

Table 12.2 (continued)

Area of medicine/ healthcare	Summary of findings
Mapping the probability of Zika epidemic outbreak at the global level [41]	High-risk areas for Zika transmission were identified. Prediction accuracy of 0.964–0.966 using backward propagation neural network (BPNN), gradient boosting machine (GBM) and random forest (RF). Used high-dimensional multidisciplinary covariate layers with comprehensive location data on recorded Zika virus infection in humans
Dengue severity in patients [42]	Used logistic regression, random forest, gradient boosting machine, support vector classifier and artificial neural network (ANN). The ANN accuracy was AUC = 0.8324. Provides potential to assist rapid prognosis during dengue outbreaks.

12.2   ML Methodology

Rather than being developed as a separate scientific field, the ML methodology either overlaps with or borrows from many other quantitative and mathematical fields. These include:

- Statistics (*Statistical Learning* is sometimes used as a synonym for ML).
- Mathematical optimisation (the minimisation of a loss function).
- Data mining and exploratory data analysis (unsupervised learning).
- Neural networks (which aim to mimic the working of the biological brain).
- Predictive analytics (often applied to Business but also Medicine).

Below we describe how these areas each contribute to ML methodology.

12.2.1 Statistics

Whilst the major focus of traditional statistical regression models within medicine is to draw inferences for a target population, the goals for ML are those of accurate prediction and pattern recognition. The latter is a particularly attractive strategy for improving management decisions in the older patient population, a group that is typically characterised by significant inter-individual variability in organ function, comorbidity burden, medication use, physical and cognitive function, social circumstances and life expectancy. Again, the data-driven ML approach borrows from whichever scientific field, including statistics, that helps achieve optimal prediction for the given task. The term statistical learning is sometimes used to describe the statistical approaches to ML prediction and includes well-established statistical regression and clustering techniques such as logistic regression and K-means clustering.

12.2.2 Mathematical Optimisation

ML prediction problems are formulated as minimisation of some loss function on a training set of examples. Mathematical optimisation is a systematic approach for optimising (minimising or maximising) the value of an objective function with respect to a set of constraints. It lies at the heart of many of the ML algorithms in which the objective function is the loss function, such as the discrepancy between the predictions of the model being trained and the actual events. For example, the prediction of a patient's vital status at 12 months after hospital discharge, which provides critical information regarding the appropriateness and cost-effectiveness of specific pharmacological and/or non-pharmacological treatments. Frameworks such as XGBoost, which uses extreme gradient "Boosting" in its algorithms, use mathematical optimisation to move across gradients in the solution space of the loss function and identify the local minima. Figure 12.3 shows a surface plot of a hypothetical complex surface function which is the solution space depicting all possible values. The local minima is the minimum gradient along the surface and is chosen as the solution. Mathematical optimisation is well-suited for both Big Data, and for finding the solution to otherwise intractable problems.

12.2.3 Data Mining

The major focus of data mining is that of identifying previously *unknown* properties or patterns within a set of data, for example, clusters of features that might be used to phenotype patients, or perhaps unknown relationships between features. This is also the aim of *Unsupervised* ML which might utilise clustering techniques either as the primary goal, or as a pre-processing step to help improve accuracy for a *Supervised* ML method. A key distinguishing feature between ML and data mining

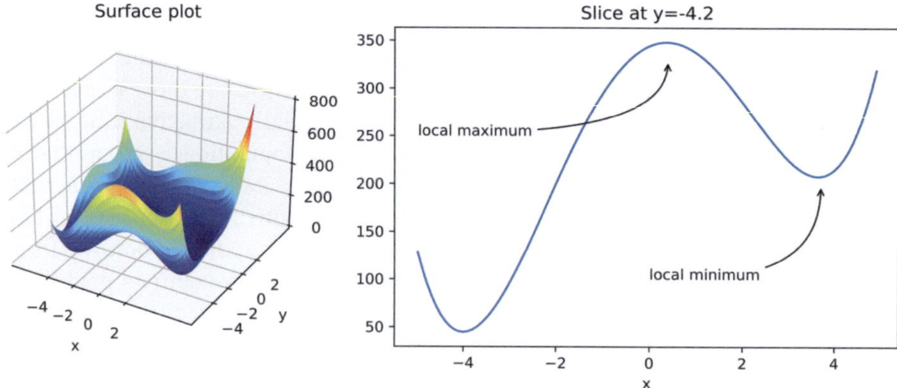

Fig. 12.3 Mathematical optimisation uses methods such as gradient descent to find the local minimum of complex surface functions. The surface gradients are calculated, and the algorithm moves slowly along the surface to the points with the minimum gradient to detect the local minima

however is on where the evaluation of their performance lies. For ML, the most common aim is to assess accuracy often with respect to *known* knowledge, e.g., accuracy compared to a gold standard. In comparison, since the key task for data mining is the discovery of previously *unknown* knowledge or clusters, evaluation is more focused on aspects such as the degree of cohesion and separation of points within the clusters.

12.2.4 Artificial Neural Networks and Deep Learning

Artificial neural networks (ANNs) are inspired by the ability of brains to learn complicated patterns in data. They work by modifying the weights for the (synaptic) connections between neurons [43], which then alters the transmission of signals between ANN layers. If the signals between layers in the ANN are sufficiently strong, they transverse between layers including the first (input) layer and the last (output layer). The nodes (artificial neurons) "learn" from the real value data provided as input, and the output predictions are based on a non-linear function of the input. As the learning process proceeds, the weights of both the neurons and the edges that connect them can either increase or decrease in strength. The term "deep Learning" refers to ANNs with multiple (hidden) layers of neurons in addition to the single input and output layers (Fig. 12.4). Given their ability to handle large amounts of data, many of the algorithms employed within medicine are now based on ANNs [44].

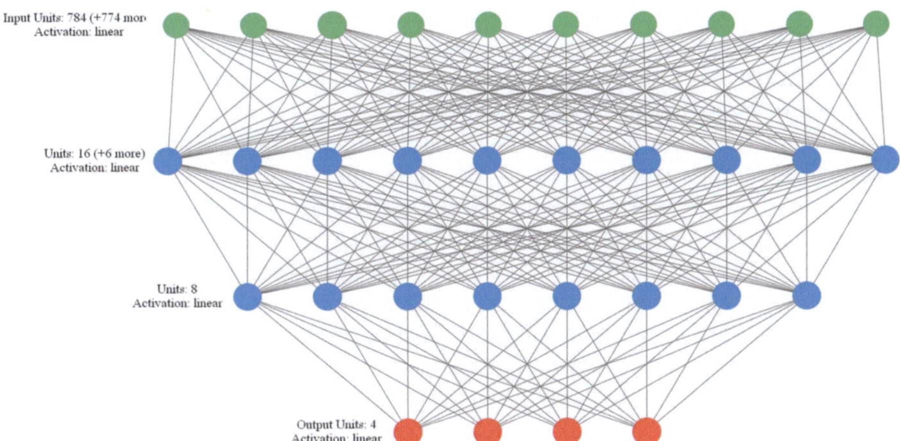

Fig. 12.4 Example of an artificial neural network (ANN). The ANN is an interconnected group of nodes, akin to the vast network of neurons in a brain. Here, each circular node represents an artificial neuron, and an edge between nodes represents a connection from the output of one artificial neuron to the input of another. Artificial neural networks (ANNs) with more than one hidden layer are often referred to as deep learning (DL) algorithms

12.2.5 Predictive Analytics

Predictive analytics is an umbrella term used for studies or domains that employ a blend of different forms of model-based and model-free analytics. For example, in a predictive study of Parkinson's disease, model-based approaches that were employed included generalised linear models (GLM), mixed effect modelling with repeated measurements (MMRM), change-based models and generalised estimating equations (GEE). In addition, the study utilised "model-free" predictive analytics including forecasting, classification and data mining using boosting algorithms, support vector machines (SVM), Naïve Bayes, decision trees, K-Nearest Neighbours and K-means classifiers [45].

12.3　The Machine Learning-Big Data Nexus

The rapid development of Healthcare 4.0 has been facilitated by a) increases in computing power, b) the availability of Big Data and c) significant improvements in AI algorithms including Deep Learning [1]. The increases in Big Data availability encompass increases in all of the 5 Vs of data: variety, volume, velocity, variability and veracity [46]. The digitisation of health data into EHRs, cloud-based storage, and the creation of vast datasets such as patient data from wearable devices has helped fast-track developments in ML in healthcare. Together with the increased volume of data and storage capacity, the ML healthcare environment has also developed because of computing power at low cost, and the resulting evolution in ML approaches to analyse complex high-dimensional datasets, that consists of structured, unstructured and heterogeneous (text, image, sensor) health data.

ML and Big Data have often been viewed as being the major components that define a spectrum of decision-making complexity from the involvement of a single human alone making a patient treatment decision, through statistical models with small- to medium-sized datasets, to ML algorithms combined with large, high-dimensional data [47]. The choice between approaches will often depend on the level of accepted interpretability as well as accuracy, with a trade-off between the use of large, complex datasets and more accurate algorithms with limited interpretability, to the smaller, simpler and more interpretable models such as linear or logistic regression. Thus, this trade-off between human specification of a predictive algorithm based on subject knowledge versus learning entirely from the data alone can be considered to be an ML spectrum [47] (Fig. 12.5). Consider, for example, the Framingham cardiovascular risk score, developed to predict 10-year mortality based on only eight predictors included in a standard binary logistic regression model [48]. Where do such clinical decision-support tools sit within the ML spectrum? The predictors were selected purposefully based on the available clinical knowledge of their effects at the time, rather than through any data-driven approach and might not therefore be considered as being a part of the ML spectrum. But the risk score

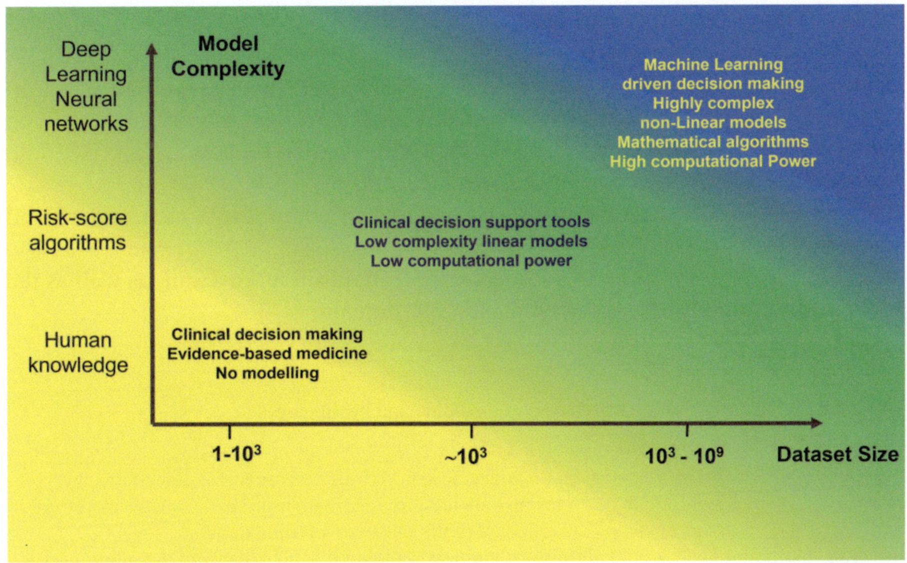

Fig. 12.5 The ML spectrum for clinical decision-making. At one end of the spectrum exists the sole clinician using evidence-based medicine with no modelling, and at the far end resides the highly complex "black-box" models that require vast computational power. Although the latter may be more accurate than either the clinician or a simple risk prediction model, they are also less transparent and interpretable. This trade-off is an important factor in considering the best approach for any treatment strategy

still required data on some 5300 patients to "learn" a risk prediction rule. As such, classical logistic regression can still be considered ML, although it likely has limited capacity for improved accuracy (and therefore learning) when provided with additional data.

In simplistic terms we can say that the more the ML algorithm depends on the raw data, and the less it depends on human input, the more it can be considered as ML. At the high end of the ML spectrum sit the deep learning (DL) algorithms and convolutional neural networks (CNN), involving multiple hidden layers and networks of artificial neurons that are expressly designed to teach themselves from the raw data and gradually reduce the prediction error with each successive iteration of the training cycle. Although first established as early as 2000, DL has gained rapid acceptance within the last 5 years as advances in computing power finally made their use feasible. For example, DL algorithms have now been deployed to detect diabetic retinopathy from retinal photographs at a sensitivity equal to or greater than that of ophthalmologists [49]. Whilst these high-complexity DL models cannot directly provide any intuitive interpretation, significant progress has been made recently, and many aspects of so-called "black-box" models are now interpretable with the proper tools [50].

12.4   The Taxonomy of ML

Many different branches of AI exist within industry in general as well as in healthcare. Within each of these branches there also exist various sub-branches. Based on the type of input and output data, ML algorithms can be broadly categorised into supervised, unsupervised or reinforcement learning.

Table 12.3 describes some of the various branches and sub-branches of AI and ML techniques [51].

Below we describe some of these AI and ML fields in more detail, as well as the specific algorithms employed within each sub-domain.

Table 12.3 The terminology of AI used in medicine and healthcare

Sub-field	Description
Machine learning	Pattern identification and analysis. Various mathematical algorithms that improve in accuracy as they are provided with more data and are therefore said to "learn" as reflected in the machine learning name.
Machine learning algorithms	The specific algorithms employed within machine learning including neural networks, random forests, support vector machines, gradient boosting, nearest-neighbours, naïve-bayes.
Supervised machine learning	Machine learning using algorithms that predict pre-defined outcomes such as vital status, disease status, blood pressure, etc. The training and test data are previously classified, that is, "labelled", by researchers and used to train an algorithm to predict the correct class (e.g. diseased/non-diseased).
Unsupervised machine learning	Machine learning using algorithms that identify "hidden" non-pre-specified clusters, or which identify patterns in the data. This may include statistical techniques such as latent class analysis, cluster analysis and hierarchical analysis.
Deep learning	An extension of neural networks. Multi-layer neural networks which enable machines to learn and make decisions. Includes convolutional neural networks (CNN) used in image processing, recurrent neural networks, deep belief networks and deep neural networks [52].
Natural language processing	The extraction of data from text as well as the ability to interpret and make decisions based on the extracted information. In healthcare the technique is widely employed to capture and make sense (semantic reasoning) of the large volumes of unstructured text stored in EHRs.
Analytical AI	Identifying, interpreting and communicating new insights, patterns and relationships or dependencies in data to assist in data-driven decision-making.
Functional AI	Exploring large quantities of data for patterns but executing actions rather than making recommendations. For example, robotics and IoT applications which take immediate actions.
Interactive AI	Enables efficient and interactive communication automation, such as chatbots, personal assistants. Employs various techniques such as machine learning, frequent pattern mining, reasoning, heuristic searches.
Textual AI	Textual analytics or natural language processing to provide text recognition, speech-to-text conversion, machine translation, answering questions.
Visual AI	Learning, classifying and sorting items, converting images and videos into insights. Often used in computer vision and augmented reality.

12.4.1 Supervised ML

In supervised ML, algorithms are trained on set of features that are used to predict an outcome. For example, a model might be trained to predict a cardiovascular event using data such as height, weight and smoking status. The true outcome in the datasets used for the purposes of training are known in advance, that is they have been "labelled" previously by researchers, but once successfully trained, can predict the outcomes for new data. The outcomes predicted can be either discrete (e.g. non-diseased/diseased) or continuous (e.g. quality-of-life (QOL) scores or required pain medication dose). Supervised ML models which predict discrete categories (or classes) are referred to as classification algorithms. Examples include predicting if a tumour is benign or malignant, or if a patient's comments regarding their care experience convey a positive or negative sentiment [53]. Supervised ML models which predict continuous values are referred to as regression algorithms, in comparison to statistics, where "regression" can refer to either binary outcomes (logistic regression) or continuous outcomes (linear regression). For some tasks, such as image recognition or language processing, the large number of features, consisting of pixels or words respectively, are typically pre-processed prior to using the chosen supervised ML algorithm, using a technique known as feature selection. This allows, for example, the selection of the identifiable characteristics from the dataset such as the colour of a pixel in an image or the number of times that a word appears in each text. The corresponding outcomes would be whether the image shows a malignant or benign tumour or whether transcribed interview responses indicate a positive or negative experience.

12.4.2 Examples of Supervised ML Algorithms

Some commonly used supervised techniques include decision trees, random forests, K-nearest neighbours (KNN), support vector machines (SVM) and logistic regression. The SVM is a discriminative classifier formally defined by a separating hyperplane. In other words, given labelled training data, the algorithm outputs an optimal hyperplane that is used to categorise new data.

The DT is the simplest tree-based supervised ML model. A tree structure is recursively created at a series of nodes, each of which represents a conditional statement (Yes or No) for the values of a given feature. The tree splits into branches/edges at each node and the end of the branch that does not split anymore is called the decision tree leaf. Importantly, trees can be combined using ensemble learning to yield far more accurate classifiers such as Random Forests (RF) and Boosted Trees. KNN is a supervised algorithm that classifies new data by using the most common value of its K neighbours, measured using a distance function. Logistic regression is a traditional statistical method for solving binary classification problems (problems with two class values). It predicts the probability of occurrence of an event by fitting data to a logistic function. Modifications of logistic regression include Ridge regression, LASSO (least absolute shrinkage selection operator) regression and Elastic net (a weighted combination of Ridge and LASSO). These algorithms all employ a penalty function (known as regularisation) that "shrinks" the coefficients of the basic logistic regression model towards zero to avoid overfitting. They therefore tend to perform better than standard logistic regression when applied to test and validation datasets. In LASSO, coefficients can be shrunk to zero, which thereby also allows the operator to employ it as a form of feature selection prior to training using a different algorithm.

Commonly, a suite of different supervised ML algorithms are employed together within the same study, with the final algorithm selected being the one that provides the best accuracy. For example, the diagnostic accuracy of logistic regression was assessed together with nine supervised ML algorithms: decision trees, random forests, extreme gradient boosting (XGBoost), support-vector machines, naive Bayes, K-nearest neighbours, ridge regression, logistic regression and neural networks to predict 12-month mortality in a group of older hospitalised patients. Prediction features included eight different geriatric assessment scoring domains together with laboratory values [54]. The XGBoost ML algorithm improved accuracy compared with logistic regression. Adding the laboratory data also improved accuracy.

12.4.3 Unsupervised ML

In contrast to supervised ML, where the objective is to predict an outcome, in unsupervised ML, the aim is to identify hidden patterns in the data from a given set of features. There is therefore no requirement for the training set to be pre-labelled and the techniques can be considered as exploratory, similar to data mining. Since the aim is to reduce many features into a far smaller number of groups based on the similarity of the features within the groups, these algorithms are often also referred to as clustering and dimension-reduction techniques. In medicine, they are extremely useful for "phenotyping" patients based on the similarity of their clinical features, symptoms and socio-demographics.

12.4.4 Examples of Unsupervised ML

Examples of unsupervised ML algorithms include principal components analysis, anomaly detection, fuzzy techniques, hierarchical clustering, agglomerative clustering, latent class analysis and K-means clustering. In healthcare, unsupervised ML is useful for assessing the heterogeneous efficacy and safety of interventions, treatments and care pathways in specific subgroups such as older patient populations [55]. One of the most popular methods, K-means clustering, partitions data into k clusters whereby each patient belongs to the cluster with the nearest mean. This technique produces exactly k different clusters with the maximum level of distinction between clusters. Since the best number of clusters k leading to the greatest separation (distance) is not known a priori, it must be computed from the data. Principal Component Analysis, or PCA, is a dimensionality-reduction method that can be used to reduce the dimensionality of high-dimensional data sets, that is, transforming a large set of features into a smaller set that still contains most of the information within the large set. Reducing the number of variables in this way inevitably reduces accuracy, but smaller data sets are easier to visualise and faster to analyse when the largely redundant features are removed. Latent class analysis and latent profile analysis are model-based methods of clustering which can be used to categorise or phenotype subjects into latent (hidden) classes based on a set of categorical (latent class) or continuous (latent profile) features, respectively [56]. Latent class analysis was used to categorise rheumatoid arthritis patients into five broad patterns (classes) of patterns (classes) of anti-inflammatory drug usage in rheumatoid arthritis patients [57]. Following classification into the five classes it was observed that reactive hyperaemia was relatively lower in the sulfasalazine or non-TNF inhibitors class users, suggesting these drugs may counteract the negative effects of RA on endothelial function. Similarly, LCA was used to characterise older hospital patients according to their type of drug usage resulting in three broad groups of patients (low overall drug use), high overall drug use with anticoagulants (class 2) and antiplatelet use (class 3) [58]. Mean serum sodium was significantly lower for patients in classes 2 and 3. Latent profile analysis was used to determine patterns of dietary fatty acids in a rheumatoid arthritis population which identified five broad groups of individuals [59]. Those with higher omega-3 fatty acid intake had significantly lower arterial stiffness than those in the other dietary patterns after accounting for numerous potential confounders.

12.4.5 Reinforcement Learning

Reinforcement learning (RL) involves a process of using trial and error to take one of several possible actions (initiation of patient treatment, optimal treatment dose, best medication combinations) that will maximise success or cumulative reward. RL was at the heart of the Alpha Go algorithm that learned to defeat the World Go champion in 2016 by four games to one. Its ability was such that it was eventually able to set up counter-intuitive strategies which led to winning moves [6]. RL makes decisions (actions) based on a set of derived rules and, rather than only looking for immediate success, aims to optimise the long-term rewards. The RL agent receives evaluative feedback about the performance of each of its actions that are performed at repeated steps, thereby improving by trial and error. Mathematically, this sequential decision-making process is called the Markov decision process (MDP) [17] and is defined by 4 major components: (1) a state that represents the environment at each time; (2) an action the agent takes at each time that influences the next state; (3) an estimated transition probability for reaching different subsequent states; and (4) a reward function which is the observed feedback given a state-action pair. The solution of the MDP is an optimal set of rules termed as the policy, which is analogous to a clinical protocol.

In the clinical setting, when the RL agent is well-trained, it is possible to pick the best action given the state of a patient and their specific set of clinical characteristics, giving the "policy" the edge over a standard clinical protocol. A policy might be a deep neural network (DNN) where for a given patient state, the DNN model estimates the highest probability of treatment success for a set of given treatments. Various RL algorithms have now been used to train policies including deep reinforcement learning [60, 61].

12.4.6 Examples of Reinforcement Learning

Outside of medicine, RL emerged as an effective tool to solve complicated control problems with large-scale, high-dimensional data including video games and board games. The ANN-based RL algorithm called AlphaGo that defeated the world Go champion in 2016 [62] was a significant moment in the field of AI because the average game of Go involves a possible 10^{170} possible different moves [63] meaning that for a computer to win, a rule-based approach was not possible. Instead, the algorithm learnt from its own mistakes. Recognising the huge potential for advancements in healthcare and other businesses using the same combination of RL and deep learning methods employed by AlphaGo, the technology giant Google, a subsidiary of Alphabet Inc. recently acquired the AlphaGo team of DeepMinds for a reported price of more than $500million with the aim of using the advantages offered by these transferable techniques [64]. Recently after the acquisition, DeepMind announced that their AI lab had developed an algorithm called AlphaFold that had determined the structure of 214 million proteins, including those in the human body, animals, plants, bacteria and other organisms. This represents a significant advance in biology that should accelerate the discovery of new drugs, as well as addressing problems such as sustainability and food insecurity [65].

Within medicine, RL has been applied within the critical care domain to optimise individual target laboratory values, medications, intervention timing, requests for lab tests and the optimal dosing of different drugs [66]. Within the elderly and frail population, deep RL was used to develop a strategy to explore the effect of ageing muscle on kinematics and muscle control before falls [67]. Multiple age-related factors were involved in the two steps taken prior to the fall, including overactivation of the hip extensors and inactivation of knee extensors, which led to a backward fall. An inactivated rectus femoris and right tibialis were the main actors of the forward fall.

12.5 The ML Workflow and Predictive Accuracy Evaluation

The process for training algorithms is very similar across the various ML algorithms available and analyses can therefore be characterised by a series of general workflow steps. Several important pre-processing steps take place prior to any analysis including splitting of the available data into either training/validation datasets using example, a 80/20 ratio, or if sufficient data exists, into training/validation/test sets in ratios such as a 60/20/20 split. Hyperparameters for each algorithm are selected in such a way as to help ensure that a similarly high levels of accuracy are attained in both the validation and test sets to that obtained for the training dataset. In other words, the final model should perform equally well with low bias (error in the training dataset) and low variance (error in the validation and test datasets). Other aspects of the data pre-processing workflow include data reduction and feature selection (to help reduce the number of highly correlated or redundant variables), the imputation of missing data with for example, the mean of the missing data, one-hot encoding (creating dummy variables) and the standardisation of continuous features, which might otherwise influence feature selection by virtue of having widely varying measurement units.

12.5.1 Accuracy Metrics

Many different measures of accuracy are available to assess the performance (accuracy) of ML algorithms and it is common for studies to utilise several accuracy metrics rather than relying on a single measure. For binary (classification) algorithms, the most common measures include:

Accuracy: The percentage of correct predictions.

Precision: Out of all subjects classified as positive, how many were truly positive? This is the same as Positive predictive value (PPV).

Recall: Out of the subjects that were truly positive, how many were classified as positive. This is the same as Sensitivity.

Specificity: Out of the subjects that were truly negative, how many were classified as negative.

F1 score: The harmonic mean of precision and recall. The harmonic mean tends towards the smaller of the 2 elements. Therefore, F1 is small if either precision or recall is small.

AUC: Area-under-the-curve is a common measure used within medical research when assessing diagnostic accuracy using statistical models such as logistic regression. Since it is well understood by clinicians and relevant in terms of diagnostic accuracy it is therefore often the metric of choice within medical research using ML. An AUC of 0.5 suggests no discrimination, 0.7 to 0.8 is considered acceptable, 0.8 to 0.9 is considered excellent and more than 0.9 is considered outstanding. AUC is calculated as the arithmetic mean of Sensitivity (Recall) and Specificity across all possible cut-points.

12.6 Challenges for AI and ML in Healthcare

12.6.1 Patient Confidentiality, Data Governance and Public Trust

Whilst innovations such as AI and ML offer exciting opportunities they can still falter without an adequate level of public trust and a consensus amongst all stakeholders around the role of data. To develop this trust, both the data custodians and the data analysts must be open and transparent about their real objectives, and the public needs reassurance that their data will be kept confidential when explicit consent is not required.

In 2016, DeepMind entered a collaboration with the Royal Free London NHS Foundation Trust to assist in the management of patients with acute kidney injury, a disease complication leading to a prolonged length of hospitalisation and an increased risk of morbidity and mortality. It was the first major health project for Deep Minds. After an investigation into the agreement following concerns over patient confidentiality, the UK Information Commissioner's Office declared that the Royal Free NHS Trust hospital had broken civil law when it transferred 5 years of health data for 1.6 million patients without their consent to DeepMind [68].

The business contract that the 2 companies entered into, and the data sharing arrangement, were ostensibly for the purpose of developing a mobile app for patients that would alert clinicians if there appeared imminent risk of acute kidney injury. But DeepMind was at that time a company renowned for expertise in AI rather than in software engineering and had no track record in either health research or technology. In addition, the mobile app was to be developed using an already defined standard risk scoring algorithm for AKI, rather than any new ML algorithm. Whilst UK Trusts are allowed to transfer data for direct care, they are not allowed to transfer it for testing purposes. In addition, the transferred data was identifiable and consisted of not just of those patients at risk of AKI, but of all the hospital's patients. Such an all-encompassing transfer would typically require that DeepMind maintains a "direct care" relationship with every patient in the Trust [69]. This example provides important lessons on the transfer of administrative datasets to large private companies looking to seek a head-start in innovative AI applications. It also highlights critical questions for policymakers, industry and individuals as healthcare moves forwards, as well as the existing insufficiencies of existing institutional and regulatory agencies in their governance of healthcare data.

Society already suffers from a "data trust deficit", and the DeepMind experience will not have helped [70]. Companies and healthcare institutions need to not only meet any legal requirements for data-sharing, but to also show themselves trustworthy. Data-sharing agreements should also specify clear limits and be proportionate to the task. In this case, developing a mobile app for AKI should not require the records of every admitted patient for multiple hospitals and over multiple years. The Nuffield Foundation in London has now established an independent convention on data ethics, and works with the British Academy, the Royal Society, the Royal Statistical Society and the Alan Turing Institute for data science, to bring society, policymakers, industry and researchers together to discuss the role of data in our society.

12.6.2 Other Ethical Considerations

Other ethical questions that also need to be addressed include the policing of privacy and consent given the continuous communication of data [70, 71], whether clinical decisions that are made based on an algorithm can be held accountable for health outcomes [72] and the ethical codes that "data scientists" work to [73]. From a legal perspective, AI algorithms are defined as decision-support tools making clinicians still morally and legally responsible for poor patient outcomes even if their decisions were influenced by AI-based systems. The National Health Service in the UK, for example, has recommended that stakeholders should work together to create a framework of AI explainability. This would require every organisation deploying an AI application within the NHS to explain clearly on their website the purpose of their AI application (including the health benefits compared to the current situation), what type of data is being used, how it is being used and how they are protecting individuals' anonymity [74].

12.6.3 Clinician and Patient Confidence

Whilst most clinicians today are also accepting of the idea that AI can lead to improvements in prediction accuracy and the automation of routine diagnostic tasks, a few remain sceptical of the ability of AI to assist and improve clinical decision-making [75]. In a recent survey, 108 of 118 clinicians (91%) said they would recommend the use of a SMART technology platform to their patients to address 5 chronic and disabling conditions prevalent in the older population (hearing loss, cardiovascular diseases, cognitive impairments, mental health problems and balance disorders). In addition, 20 of 24 (83%) of older adults expressed a desire to receive monthly reports on their health status via the same technology [76]. This and other similar data suggest that both clinicians and patients are in general strongly in favour of using smart technology that incorporates AI in the management of disease.

12.6.4 Transparency

As discussed earlier, as the higher end of the ML algorithm spectrum is reached and the algorithms become more complex and powerful, their solutions generally also become less transparent. This results in the potential for clinical decisions to be made that are increasingly reliant on predictions that may not be explainable. This trade-off between more accurate, yet less explainable algorithms and more interpretable, less accurate predictions derived from basic risk score models is what drives much of the "black-box" debate around the use of ML in healthcare. It is often cited as being a continuing frustration for clinicians since there is often no way to relate the predictions back to existing biological knowledge and traditional assumptions regarding the interpretation of specific signs and symptoms of disease [77]. This lack of transparency also leaves the data scientists with the task of convincing clinicians and stakeholders of the value of routinely using AI for decision-making within a high-risk clinical environment. This process might be easier if, rather than relying on a purely data-driven approach, an assurance could be offered that existing medical knowledge be incorporated into the models whenever possible to ensure that evidence-based clinical decisions are not dismissed. Others argue that the terms "transparency" and "interpretability" are themselves nebulous poorly defined terms. For example, if a heavy transformation of features is undertaken in order for a linear model to achieve at least comparable accuracy to a neural network, can the linear models still be considered as being more interpretable [78]?

For these reasons, AI practitioners are researching and implementing *explainable AI,* or XAI [16]. XAI techniques include partial dependency plots, Shapley Values and LIME analysis. For example, Shapely values are scores that represent the contribution of each individual's data points in determining the overall prediction for any given feature [79]. Thus, whether a given feature such as age reduces predicted risk in patients with positive outcomes but increases the predicted risk in those with negative outcomes can be presented graphically using SHAP values which display the relative impact of each feature for each patient [80] (Fig. 12.6).

12.6.5 Data Bias

There is now a growing recognition in AI for the use of transparency by data scientists in their algorithm development. For example, a well-recognised selection bias exists if the population used for the chosen development dataset is not representative of the target population to which the algorithms will eventually be applied. Such a bias may ultimately lead to worse accuracy and outcomes in socially disadvantaged groups that have not been included in the development data [81]. A population-specific level of knowledge of the training data used would assist healthcare regulators in assessing the algorithms potential for bias. Of course, a lack of external validity has been a longstanding and vexing issue in medicine, particularly in geriatric care. In fact, most of the randomised controlled clinical trials supporting the efficacy and safety of marketed drugs are typically conducted in younger and healthier cohorts using stringent inclusion and exclusion criteria. The use of AI applied to observational datasets of "real-life" older patient populations might significantly improve our knowledge regarding the use of medications in this complex group.

12.6.6 Integration of AI into Healthcare

If AI and ML are to achieve their goal of being generalisable between different geographic populations, a level of consistency in the captured data needs to be achieved between health networks in different jurisdictions, whose EHR systems deployed by individual healthcare networks can differ in a variety of ways. Differences in diagnostic coding, assignment to care type, definitions for patient admission, missing values, their respective potential for error, and recorded clinical and demographic features including disease history, medical notes, data from medical devices, physical examinations and laboratories, diagnostic images, gene expressions, clinical symptoms and medications are some of the many examples. Whilst

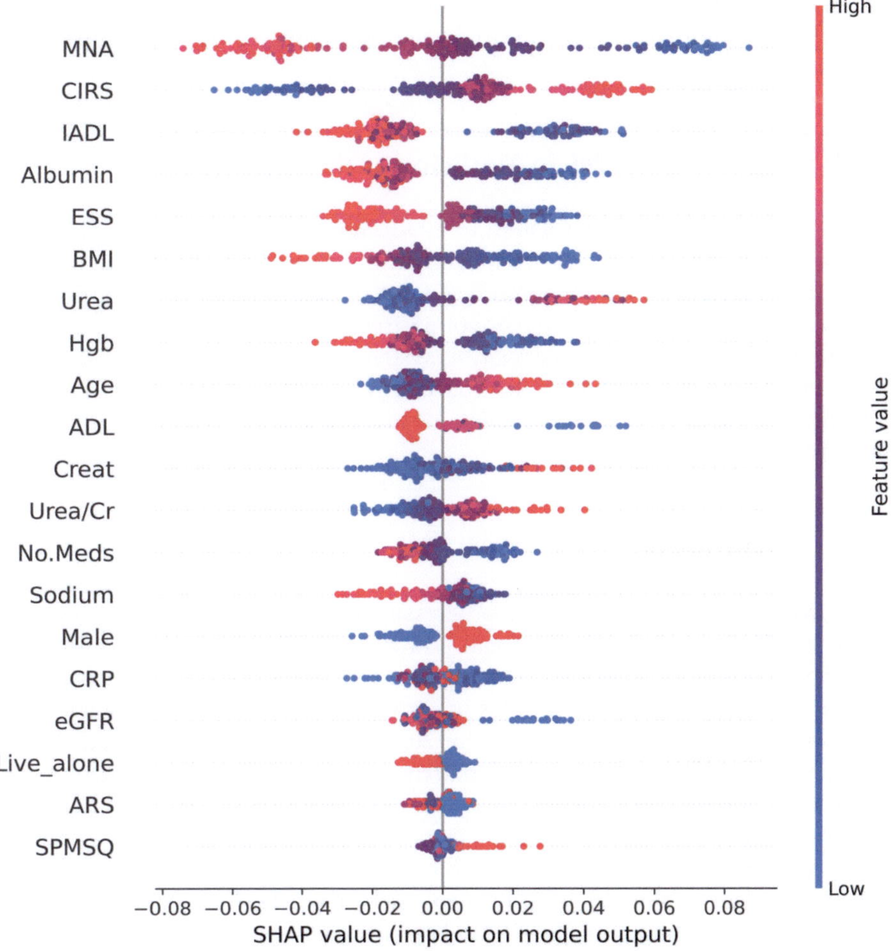

Fig. 12.6 Plot showing both the feature importance, the feature values (high or low) and the direction of the impact on the target variable (positive or negative SHAP values). Figure generated from data for [54]

such data is now commonly captured with electronic health records (EHRs), robust AI algorithms will be those that can reliably analyse integrated national and international EHR databases and similar observational data.

The Observational Health Data and Informatics project (OHDSI) [82] is an international network of researchers and observational health databases with a central coordinating centre housed at Columbia University and aimed at improving knowledge of health and disease via observational data. A similar initiative, the Transformational Data Collaboration (TDC) has begun in Australia [83]. Its aims include the mapping of administrative, hospital and primary care databases to support the common data model—the Observational Health Data Sciences and

Informatics (OHDSI), as well as a move to a standard-based model to ensure transparency of the information available to researchers within the various administrative datasets.

12.7   The Future of ML in Medicine and Healthcare

Beyond these current issues relating to ethics, regulation, bias, transparency and healthcare integration, a variety of longer-term challenges related to the development of the AI in healthcare are also beginning to be addressed. These include the adequacy of computing power, the use of unstructured health data, the requirement for decentralised data storage and analysis systems, the capacity to streamline workflows in algorithmic development, drug discovery and repurposing and optimal treatment via precision medicine. Solutions to these challenges will enable ML to progress to the next level.

12.7.1 Quantum ML

A common rate-limiting step in the progression of AI and ML has been the availability of the necessary computational power required to harness the ever more complex algorithms. Quantum computing is one advancement that has the potential to boost machine learning capabilities by virtue of simultaneous multi-state operations, enabling faster data processing. In 2019, Google's Sycamore quantum processor completed a specific task in 200 seconds, which was also estimated to take the world's current best supercomputer 10,000 years to complete [84]. Scientists have been working on quantum computers that operate at near zero degrees for many decades, driven by the promise of their vastly superior computing speed. At present, quantum computers are not yet commercially available and the application of Quantum computing in medicine and healthcare is therefore still a dream rather than a reality. But the hope is that quantum computing will enhance our access and use of Big Data which includes not just our best evidence knowledge, but also the massive volumes of continuously generated patient electronic data from the Internet of Things (IoT). State-of-the-art personalised medicine to determine best treatment for individual patients will likely require the analysis of mega-data from physiology, imaging, genomics, wearable technology, screening measures, EHRs, environmental data from sensors and more [85].

12.7.2 Federated Learning Approaches

Federated learning, also known as collaborative learning, is a machine learning technique that trains an algorithm across multiple decentralised networks, utilising datasets from each of the various networks, but without their physical exchange. This contrasts with other decentralised approaches that use only the local data but without combining results, and with centralised ML approaches where the separate local datasets are uploaded to a single server and analysed as a whole. Federated learning therefore combines input data from multiple sources which allows the creation of a robust collaborative, consensus machine learning model without the need to share patient data, which remains instead within the firewalls of the various institutions in which they reside. ML modelling of the local data is undertaken at each participating institution and the resulting parameters and gradients (but not data) are transferred to a central location for central model updating. The approach helps in addressing issues of data governance, privacy, security and access rights. Crucially, it also enables access to heterogeneous data, essential for training and rigorous validation to remove the potential for biased results arising from using more selective datasets. Models trained by FL achieve performance comparable to ones trained on both centrally hosted multiple datasets and single institution datasets [86]. Whilst originally developed for other technology domains, FL is now gaining support within healthcare.

12.7.3 Automated ML; End-to-End Model Development

The utilisation of ML within healthcare has the proven potential to improve health outcomes, cut healthcare costs and advance clinical research. However, most healthcare institutions do not currently deploy ML, in part due to the lack of ML expertise amongst healthcare professionals. The use of ML requires the ability to build an accurate model and then to integrate it within the clinical workflow. In order to make ML techniques easier to apply and to reduce the demand on data scientists, automated machine learning (AutoML) has emerged as a growing field that seeks to automatically select, compose and parametrise ML models, whilst still achieving optimal performance for the given dataset [87]. For example, Google's Cloud AutoML enables researchers and developers with limited ML expertise to train high-quality models specific to their needs [88]. The process of AutoML includes automated *data pre-processing* to improve data quality, transform and reduce dimensionality, *automated feature engineering* to create more adaptable features from the data, automated *feature extraction* for improved accuracy with smaller datasets, *automated feature selection* to retain only the most useful features, automated *algorithm selection* and *hyperparameter optimisation* to select the optimal algorithms and hyperparameters, and finally *model deployment and monitoring* of the model's performance via dashboards [89]. Future medical education undergraduate and postgraduate programmes are likely to increasingly incorporate AI and ML topics in their curriculum and an AutoML approach would likely improve acceptability for both students and faculty.

12.7.4 Natural Language Processing of EHRs

As much as 80% of the data in electronic health records (EHR) is believed to be stored in the form of unstructured, free-form text entries which cannot immediately be analysed by ML models [90]. To enable analysis, data sharing and eventual algorithm validation, they require conversion to a more standard format which can be achieved by applying Natural Language Processing (NLP). Recently, newer Neural Network and Deep Learning approaches to NLP have made considerable advances, outperforming traditional statistical and rule-based systems on a variety of tasks [90].

12.7.5 Drug Discovery

Drug development is time-consuming and costly. Average cost estimates for developing a new drug range from US$314 M to US$2.1billion, with a median of $985 million [91]. Using datasets with a drug compound's chemical structure, ML algorithms can predict the impact the drug compound could have on different cell lines and genes and detect possible side effects. ML can accelerate drug testing and speed at which drugs are brought to the market [92]. This is particularly important during public health emergencies, such as the ongoing COVID-19 pandemic, and was a major factor in facilitating the discovery of new treatments [93–95].

12.7.6 Precision Medicine Using Reinforcement Learning

The term "precision medicine" was termed synonymously with "personalised medicine" [96], which it eventually superseded based on the need to distinguish it from the personalised level of patient care that clinicians already provide [97]. Beyond the stratification of patients according to underlying conditions, signs and symptoms, precision medicine involves adding data such as biochemical, genetic and lifestyle information into the mix to assist in the decision-making process [96].

Examples include precision oncology that utilises molecular tumour profiling to look for features that predict the response to a particular therapy, or the likelihood of unacceptable side-effects. For example, the use of trastuzumab being provided only to HER-2-positive female breast cancer patients [98], and the phenotyping of patients with asthma and atopic eczema based on information including medical history and physical examination, lifestyle, laboratory tests, functional diagnostics, immunology and omics [96]. However, in practice, determining optimal treatments for complex patients with interacting comorbidities remains a considerable challenge. This is particularly true in the presence of additional patient characteristics such as frailty, which can itself interact both with co-existing disease states and with pharmacological treatment [99]. ML algorithms might offer the potential for enhanced decision-making beyond that witnessed so far with precision medicine.

Amongst the 3 major types of ML algorithms, reinforcement learning (RL) is at the forefront for progressing precision medicine. The large volumes of detailed EHRs with repeated measures make RL ideally suited to provide sequential optimal treatment recommendations and improve patient outcomes. Initially, RL was confined to the definition of the so-called dynamic treatment regimes (DTRs), which consist of multi-step clinical decision processes [100]. More recently, it has been successfully applied to multimorbidity management, HIV therapy, cancer treatment and management of anaemia in haemodialysis patients [61]. RL algorithms are also well aligned with the sequential decision-making process that occurs in ICUs and has consistently outperformed physicians in simulated studies including treatment strategies for sepsis, sedation dosage [66] and ventilator support for Covid-19 patients [101].

Nonetheless, challenges regarding RL system design, evaluation metrics and model choice exist. For example, whilst RL has been applied to more than 20 studies in the ICU to identify optimal treatment strategies, all applications relied on simulations and retrospective data. Further work is therefore required to prospectively validate RL in authentic clinical environments [66].

12.8   Conclusions

Our review of AI and ML in medicine has provided a brief history of ML with a special focus on its development within medicine and healthcare and the elderly patient. In the last decade, there has been a clear exponential increase in not only the volume of research that helps drive advancement in technology but also in the actual development of applications and their transformation of medicine and healthcare. Big Data arising from EHRs and electronic patient tracking systems combined with the development of self-learning algorithms for dynamic personalised medical treatment and decision-making suggests that ML in healthcare has arrived and is here to stay.

Evidence-based medicine dictates that medical treatment should be based on empirical evidence rather than either clinical experience alone, or at the other end of the spectrum, a purely data-driven Deep Learning algorithm. In this respect, algorithms that can also still incorporate clinical knowledge might offer more potential in moving forward. For example, clinical knowledge of the laboratory values that predict mortality was used when selecting from a wide variety of possible lab values to include within an RL model designed to determine optimal oxygen therapy for COVID-19 patients [101].

The rapid development in AI and ML suggests that the most likely next potential obstacle will be in maintaining a similar speed of progress in building the necessary structures for the governance of highly confidential patient data, as well as the regulations for safe and ethical use of AI. Without these, the support and trust of end-users including the clinical workforce and public might evaporate quickly and put any further progress on hold. However, assuming vigilance in these matters can be achieved, the tremendous gains offered by AI and ML towards better outcomes for patients, clinicians and healthcare systems suggest a bright and positive future ahead for AI in medicine.

References

1. Jayaraman PP, Forkan ARM, Morshed A, Haghighi PD, Kang Y-B. Healthcare 4.0: A review of frontiers in digital health. WIREs data mining and knowledge. Discovery. 2020;10(2):e1350.
2. Park SH, Do KH, Kim S, Park JH, Lim YS. What should medical students know about artificial intelligence in medicine? J Educ Eval Health Prof. 2019;16:18.
3. Topol EJ. High-performance medicine: the convergence of human and artificial intelligence. Nat Med. 2019;25(1):44–56.
4. Pappada SM. Machine learning in medicine: it has arrived, let's embrace it. J Card Surg. 2021;36:4121.
5. Garcia-Vidal C, Sanjuan G, Puerta-Alcalde P, Moreno-Garcia E, Soriano A. Artificial intelligence to support clinical decision-making processes. EBioMedicine. 2019;46:27–9.
6. Sutton RT, Pincock D, Baumgart DC, Sadowski DC, Fedorak RN, Kroeker KI. An overview of clinical decision support systems: benefits, risks, and strategies for success. NPJ Digit Med. 2020;3:17.
7. Hong S, Lee S, Lee J, Cha WC, Kim K. Prediction of cardiac arrest in the emergency department based on machine learning and sequential characteristics: model development and retrospective clinical validation study. JMIR Med Inform. 2020;8(8):e15932.
8. Dykes PC, Burns Z, Adelman J, Benneyan J, Bogaisky M, Carter E, et al. Evaluation of a patient-centered fall-prevention tool kit to reduce falls and injuries: A nonrandomized controlled trial. JAMA Netw Open. 2020;3(11):e2025889.
9. Li JJ, Jiang S, Zhu ML, Liu XH, Sun XH, Zhao SQ. Comparison of three frailty scales for prediction of adverse outcomes among older adults: A prospective cohort study. J Nutr Health Aging. 2021;25(4):419–24.
10. Giscombe SR, Baptiste DL, Koirala B, Asano R, Commodore-Mensah Y. The use of clinical decision support in reducing readmissions for patients with heart failure: a quasi-experimental study. Contemp Nurse. 2021;57(1–2):39–50.
11. Chiang J, Furler J, Boyle D, Clark M, Manski-Nankervis JA. Electronic clinical decision support tool for the evaluation of cardiovascular risk in general practice: A pilot study. Aust Fam Physician. 2017;46(10):764–8.
12. Shi X, He J, Lin M, Liu C, Yan B, Song H, et al. Comparative effectiveness of team-based care with a clinical decision support system versus team-based care alone on cardiovascular risk reduction among patients with diabetes: rationale and design of the D4C trial. Am Heart J. 2021;238:45–58.
13. McIsaac DI, Taljaard M, Bryson GL, Beaule PE, Gagne S, Hamilton G, et al. Frailty and long-term postoperative disability trajectories: a prospective multicentre cohort study. Br J Anaesth. 2020;125(5):704–11.
14. Maltese G, Corsonello A, Di Rosa M, Soraci L, Vitale C, Corica F, et al. Frailty and COVID-19: A systematic scoping review. J Clin Med. 2020;9(7)
15. Beam AL, Kohane IS. Translating artificial intelligence into clinical care. JAMA. 2016;316(22):2368–9.
16. Quest D, Upjohn D, Pool E, Menaker R, Hernandez J, Poole K. Demystifying AI in healthcare: historical perspectives and current considerations. Physician Leadership. 2021;8(1):59–66.
17. Greco M, Caruso PF, Cecconi M. Artificial intelligence in the intensive care unit. Semin Respir Crit Care Med. 2021;42(1):2–9.
18. Mitchell TM. Machine learning. McGraw-Hill; 1997.
19. Eloranta S, Boman M. Predictive models for clinical decision making: deep dives in practical machine learning. J Intern Med. 2022;292:278.
20. Engelhard MM, Navar AM, Pencina MJ. Incremental benefits of machine learning-when do we need a better mousetrap? JAMA Cardiol. 2021;6(6):621–3.
21. Alazzam MB, Mansour H, Alassery F, Almulihi A. Machine learning implementation of a diabetic patient monitoring system using interactive E-app. Comput Intell Neurosci. 2021;2021:5759184.

22. Tomasev N, Glorot X, Rae JW, Zielinski M, Askham H, Saraiva A, et al. A clinically applicable approach to continuous prediction of future acute kidney injury. Nature. 2019;572(7767):116–9.
23. Chan L, Vaid A, Nadkarni GN. Applications of machine learning methods in kidney disease: hope or hype? Curr Opin Nephrol Hypertens. 2020;29(3):319–26.
24. de Cock C, Milne-Ives M, van Velthoven MH, Alturkistani A, Lam C, Meinert E. Effectiveness of conversational agents (virtual assistants) in health care: protocol for a systematic review. JMIR Res Protoc. 2020;9(3):e16934.
25. Svoboda E. Your robot surgeon will see you now. Nature. 2019;573(7775):S110–S1.
26. Zhou XY, Guo Y, Shen M, Yang GZ. Application of artificial intelligence in surgery. Front Med. 2020;14(4):417–30.
27. Nasr M, Islam M, Shehata S, Karray F, Quintana Y. Smart healthcare in the age of AI: recent advances, challenges, and future prospects. 2021.
28. Rajkomar A, Oren E, Chen K, Dai AM, Hajaj N, Hardt M, et al. Scalable and accurate deep learning with electronic health records. NPJ Digit Med. 2018;1:18.
29. Ayers B, Sandholm T, Gosev I, Prasad S, Kilic A. Using machine learning to improve survival prediction after heart transplantation. J Card Surg. 2021;36(11):4113–20.
30. Crotti N. Startup Arterys wins FDA clearance for AI-assisted cardiac imaging system. 2017.
31. Leiner T, Rueckert D, Suinesiaputra A, Baessler B, Nezafat R, Isgum I, et al. Machine learning in cardiovascular magnetic resonance: basic concepts and applications. J Cardiovasc Magn Reson. 2019;21(1):61.
32. Akkus Z, Galimzianova A, Hoogi A, Rubin DL, Erickson BJ. Deep learning for brain MRI segmentation: state of the art and future directions. J Digit Imaging. 2017;30(4):449–59.
33. Esteva A, Kuprel B, Novoa RA, Ko J, Swetter SM, Blau HM, et al. Dermatologist-level classification of skin cancer with deep neural networks. Nature. 2017;542(7639):115–8.
34. Weng SF, Reps J, Kai J, Garibaldi JM, Qureshi N. Can machine-learning improve cardiovascular risk prediction using routine clinical data? PLoS One. 2017;12(4):e0174944.
35. Inglese M, Patel N, Linton-Reid K, Loreto F, Win Z, Perry RJ, et al. A predictive model using the mesoscopic architecture of the living brain to detect Alzheimer's disease. Commun Med (Lond). 2022;2:70.
36. Ehteshami Bejnordi B, Veta M, Johannes van Diest P, van Ginneken B, Karssemeijer N, Litjens G, et al. Diagnostic assessment of deep learning algorithms for detection of lymph node metastases in women with breast cancer. JAMA. 2017;318(22):2199–210.
37. Krause J, Gulshan V, Rahimy E, Karth P, Widner K, Corrado GS, et al. Grader variability and the importance of reference standards for evaluating machine learning models for diabetic retinopathy. Ophthalmology. 2018;125(8):1264–72.
38. Byrne MF, Chapados N, Soudan F, Oertel C, Linares Perez M, Kelly R, et al. Real-time differentiation of adenomatous and hyperplastic diminutive colorectal polyps during analysis of unaltered videos of standard colonoscopy using a deep learning model. Gut. 2019;68(1):94–100.
39. Hassan C, Spadaccini M, Iannone A, Maselli R, Jovani M, Chandrasekar VT, et al. Performance of artificial intelligence in colonoscopy for adenoma and polyp detection: a systematic review and meta-analysis. Gastrointest Endosc. 2021;93(1):77–85 e6.
40. Moyo S, Doan TN, Yun JA, Tshuma N. Application of machine learning models in predicting length of stay among healthcare workers in underserved communities in South Africa. Hum Resour Health. 2018;16(1):68.
41. Jiang D, Hao M, Ding F, Fu J, Li M. Mapping the transmission risk of Zika virus using machine learning models. Acta Trop. 2018;185:391–9.
42. Huang SW, Tsai HP, Hung SJ, Ko WC, Wang JR. Assessing the risk of dengue severity using demographic information and laboratory test results with machine learning. PLoS Negl Trop Dis. 2020;14(12):e0008960.
43. Hinton G. Deep learning-A technology with the potential to transform health care. JAMA. 2018;320(11):1101–2.

44. Kooi T, Litjens G, van Ginneken B, Gubern-Merida A, Sanchez CI, Mann R, et al. Large scale deep learning for computer aided detection of mammographic lesions. Med Image Anal. 2017;35:303–12.

45. Dinov ID, Heavner B, Tang M, Glusman G, Chard K, Darcy M, et al. Predictive big data analytics: A study of Parkinson's disease using large, complex, heterogeneous, incongruent, multi-Source and incomplete observations. PLoS One. 2016;11(8):e0157077.

46. Benke K, Benke G. Artificial intelligence and big data in public health. Int J Environ Res Public Health. 2018;15(12)

47. Beam AL, Kohane IS. Big data and machine learning in healthcare. JAMA. 2018;319(13):1317–8.

48. Doust JA, Bonner C, Bell KJL. Future directions in cardiovascular disease risk prediction. Aust J Gen Pract. 2020;49(8):488–94.

49. Gulshan V, Peng L, Coram M, Stumpe MC, Wu D, Narayanaswamy A, et al. Development and validation of a deep learning algorithm for detection of diabetic retinopathy in retinal fundus photographs. JAMA. 2016;316(22):2402–10.

50. Yones SA, Annett A, Stoll P, Diamanti K, Holmfeldt L, Barrenas CF, et al. Interpretable machine learning identifies paediatric systemic lupus erythematosus subtypes based on gene expression data. Sci Rep. 2022;12(1):7433.

51. Sarker IH. AI-based modeling: techniques, applications and research issues towards automation, intelligent and smart systems. SN Comput Sci. 2022;3(2):158.

52. Jiang F, Jiang Y, Zhi H, Dong Y, Li H, Ma S, et al. Artificial intelligence in healthcare: past, present and future. Stroke Vasc Neurol. 2017;2(4):230–43.

53. Alexander G, Bahja M, Butt GF. Automating large-scale health care service feedback analysis: sentiment analysis and topic modeling study. JMIR Med Inform. 2022;10(4):e29385.

54. Woodman RJ, Bryant K, Sorich MJ, Pilotto A, Mangoni AA. Use of multiprognostic index domain scores, clinical data, and machine learning to improve 12-month mortality risk prediction in older hospitalized patients: prospective cohort study. J Med Internet Res. 2021;23(6):e26139.

55. Kautzky A, Moller HJ, Dold M, Bartova L, Seemuller F, Laux G, et al. Combining machine learning algorithms for prediction of antidepressant treatment response. Acta Psychiatr Scand. 2021;143(1):36–49.

56. Mangoni AA, Woodman RJ. The potential value of person-centred statistical methods in ageing research. Age Ageing. 2019;48(6):783–4.

57. Mangoni AA, Woodman RJ, Piga M, Cauli A, Fedele AL, Gremese E, et al. Patterns of anti-inflammatory and Immunomodulating drug usage and microvascular endothelial function in rheumatoid arthritis. Front Cardiovasc Med. 2021;8:681327.

58. Woodman RJ, Wood KM, Kunnel A, Dedigama M, Pegoli MA, Soiza RL, et al. Patterns of drug use and serum sodium concentrations in older hospitalized patients: A latent class analysis approach. Drugs Real World Outcomes. 2016;3(4):383–91.

59. Woodman RJ, Baghdadi LR, Shanahan EM, de Silva I, Hodgson JM, Mangoni AA. Diets high in n-3 fatty acids are associated with lower arterial stiffness in patients with rheumatoid arthritis: a latent profile analysis. Br J Nutr. 2019;121(2):182–94.

60. Arulkumaran K, Deisenroth MP, Brundage M, Bharath AA. Deep reinforcement learning: a brief survey. EEE Signal Process Mag. 2017;34(Nov):26–38.

61. Jonsson A. Deep reinforcement learning in medicine. Kidney Dis (Basel). 2019;5(1):18–22.

62. Zhang Z. When doctors meet with AlphaGo: potential application of machine learning to clinical medicine. Ann Transl Med. 2016;4(6):125.

63. Silver D, Huang A, Maddison CJ, Guez A, Sifre L, van den Driessche G, et al. Mastering the game of go with deep neural networks and tree search. Nature. 2016;529(7587):484–9.

64. Source GI. Google buys Deepmind for $500 million; 2022. Available from: https://guruit-source.com/google-buys-deepmind-for-500-million/.

65. Colleran K, DeepMind AI. Lab predicts structure of most proteins; 2022. Available from: https://techilive.in/deepmind-ai-lab-predicts-structure-of-most-proteins/.

66. Liu S, See KC, Ngiam KY, Celi LA, Sun X, Feng M. Reinforcement learning for clinical decision support in critical care: comprehensive review. J Med Internet Res. 2020;22(7):e18477.

67. Nowakowski K, El Kirat K, Dao TT. Deep reinforcement learning coupled with musculoskeletal modelling for a better understanding of elderly falls. Med Biol Eng Comput. 2022;60(6):1745–61.
68. Shah H. The DeepMind debacle demands dialogue on data. Nature. 2017;547(7663):259.
69. Powles J, Hodson H. Google DeepMind and healthcare in an age of algorithms. Health Technol (Berl). 2017;7(4):351–67.
70. Morley J, Taddeo M, Floridi L. Google health and the NHS: overcoming the trust deficit. Lancet Digit Health. 2019;1(8):e389.
71. McGraw D, Mandl KD. Privacy protections to encourage use of health-relevant digital data in a learning health system. NPJ Digit Med. 2021;4(1):2.
72. Grote T, Berens P. On the ethics of algorithmic decision-making in healthcare. J Med Ethics. 2020;46(3):205–11.
73. Baird A, Schuller B. Considerations for a more ethical approach to data in AI: on data representation and infrastructure. Front Big Data. 2020;3:25.
74. Harwich E, Laycock K. Thinking on its own: AI in the NHS. Reform Res Trust. 2018;
75. Scheetz J, Rothschild P, McGuinness M, Hadoux X, Soyer HP, Janda M, et al. A survey of clinicians on the use of artificial intelligence in ophthalmology, dermatology, radiology and radiation oncology. Sci Rep. 2021;11(1):5193.
76. Cristiano A, Musteata S, De Silvestri S, Bellandi V, Ceravolo P, Cesari M, et al. Older Adults' and Clinicians' perspectives on a smart health platform for the aging population: design and evaluation study. JMIR Aging. 2022;5(1):e29623.
77. Bzdok D, Altman N, Krzywinski M. Statistics versus machine learning. Nat Methods. 2018;15(4):233–4.
78. Lipton Z. The mythos of model interprtability. ACM Queue. 2018;16:31–57.
79. Mohar C. Interpretable machine learning: a guide for making black box models explainable. [GitHub Repository] 2019. Available from: https://christophm.github.io/interpretable-ml-book/example-based.html.
80. Amann J, Blasimme A, Vayena E, Frey D, Madai VI, Qc P. Explainability for artificial intelligence in healthcare: a multidisciplinary perspective. BMC Med Inform Decis Mak. 2020;20(1):310.
81. Vokinger KN, Feuerriegel S, Kesselheim AS. Mitigating bias in machine learning for medicine. Commun Med (London). 2021;1:25.
82. Informatics OHDSa. OHDSI; 2022. Available from: https://www.ohdsi.org/ohdsi-workgroups/.
83. (MACH) MACfH. Transformational data collaboration; 2020. Available from: https://mach-australia.org/projects/transformational-data-collaboration/.
84. Arute F, Arya K, Babbush R, Bacon D, Bardin JC, Barends R, et al. Quantum supremacy using a programmable superconducting processor. Nature. 2019;574(7779):505–10.
85. Solenov D, Brieler J, Scherrer JF. The potential of quantum computing and machine learning to advance clinical research and change the practice of medicine. Mo Med. 2018;115(5):463–7.
86. Rieke N, Hancox J, Li W, Milletari F, Roth HR, Albarqouni S, et al. The future of digital health with federated learning. NPJ Digit Med. 2020;3:119.
87. Waring J, Lindvall C, Umeton R. Automated machine learning: review of the state-of-the-art and opportunities for healthcare. Artif Intell Med. 2020;104:101822.
88. Cloud G. AutoML; 2022. Available from: https://cloud.google.com/automl.
89. He X, Zhao K, Chu X. AutoML: A survey of the state-of-the-art. Knowl-Based Syst. 2021;212:106662.
90. Kong HJ. Managing unstructured big data in healthcare system. Healthc Inform Res. 2019;25(1):1–2.
91. Wouters OJ, McKee M, Luyten J. Estimated research and development investment needed to bring a new medicine to market, 2009–2018. JAMA. 2020;323(9):844–53.
92. Vatansever S, Schlessinger A, Wacker D, Kaniskan HU, Jin J, Zhou MM, et al. Artificial intelligence and machine learning-aided drug discovery in central nervous system diseases: state-of-the-arts and future directions. Med Res Rev. 2021;41(3):1427–73.

93. Ahmed F, Soomro AM, Chethikkattuveli Salih AR, Samantasinghar A, Asif A, Kang IS, et al. A comprehensive review of artificial intelligence and network based approaches to drug repurposing in Covid-19. Biomed Pharmacother. 2022;153:113350.

94. Sharma PP, Bansal M, Sethi A, Poonam PL, Goel VK, et al. Computational methods directed towards drug repurposing for COVID-19: advantages and limitations. RSC Advances. 2021;11(57):36181–98.

95. Lv H, Shi L, Berkenpas JW, Dao F-Y, Zulfiqar H, Ding H, et al. Application of artificial intelligence and machine learning for COVID-19 drug discovery and vaccine design. Brief Bioinform. 2021;22(6)

96. Konig IR, Fuchs O, Hansen G, von Mutius E, Kopp MV. What is precision medicine? Eur Respir J. 2017;50(4):1700391.

97. McGrath S, Ghersi D. Building towards precision medicine: empowering medical professionals for the next revolution. BMC Med Genet. 2016;9(1):23.

98. Hingorani AD, Windt DA, Riley RD, Abrams K, Moons KG, Steyerberg EW, et al. Prognosis research strategy (PROGRESS) 4: stratified medicine research. BMJ. 2013;346:e5793.

99. Gutierrez-Valencia M, Izquierdo M, Cesari M, Casas-Herrero A, Inzitari M, Martinez-Velilla N. The relationship between frailty and polypharmacy in older people: a systematic review. Br J Clin Pharmacol. 2018;84(7):1432–44.

100. Coronato A, Naeem M, De Pietro G, Paragliola G. Reinforcement learning for intelligent healthcare applications: a survey. Artif Intell Med. 2020;109:101964.

101. Zheng H, Zhu J, Xie W, Zhong J. Reinforcement learning assisted oxygen therapy for COVID-19 patients under intensive care. BMC Med Inform Decis Mak. 2021;21(1):350.

Bio-Technologies to Understand Aging, Frailty, and Resilience

Carlo Custodero, Alberto Pilotto, and Luigi Ferrucci

13.1 The Dawn of New Era in Aging Research

The demographic transition that occurred in the last century led to a massive increase in the percentage of older persons in the population. Among the many effects, this transformation caused a progressively rising incidence and prevalence of chronic conditions that profoundly challenged the healthcare systems of both developed and developing countries still mostly organized around a model of single diseases [1]. Most healthcare systems handle health crises through hospital-centered emergency rooms. More and more such health crises occur in older persons and are reactivation and decompensation of medical conditions that are already present and are left unchecked until they precipitate, with inevitable consequences on quality of care for those affected and their direct environment, and cost for the societies. Indeed, while there have been substantial progresses in medicine for the prevention and cure of single diseases, such as cardiovascular diseases and even cancer, we have seen little progress in the cure and management of older persons with complex multimorbidity and disability. Actually, the care of such vulnerable older adults consists mainly of the mere provision of welfare services. This approach even causes social disparities, e.g., due to differences in offered services across and within same countries, and

C. Custodero (✉)
Department of Interdisciplinary Medicine, University of Bari Aldo Moro, Bari, Italy
e-mail: carlo.custodero@uniba.it

A. Pilotto
Department of Interdisciplinary Medicine, University of Bari Aldo Moro, Bari, Italy

Geriatrics Unit, Department of Geriatric Care, Orthogeriatrics and Rehabilitation, Galliera Hospital, Genoa, Italy

L. Ferrucci
Longitudinal Studies Section, Translational Gerontology Branch, National Institute on Aging, Baltimore, MD, USA

© The Author(s), under exclusive license to Springer Nature Switzerland AG 2023
A. Pilotto, W. Maetzler (eds.), *Gerontechnology. A Clinical Perspective*, Practical Issues in Geriatrics, https://doi.org/10.1007/978-3-031-32246-4_13

prefers wealthier patients. In addition, programs of care often have little ability to address the individual needs and requirements of those affected and pay little attention to quality of life.

The novel paradigm of *geroscience* tries to bolster a preventive medicine approach instead of the traditional mainly curative/supportive one [1]. According to the geroscience perspective, aging and diseases are two faces of the same coin. Mechanisms underlying the aging process might be strictly interconnected with morbidity. Aging is conceptualized as the ratio between damage accumulation under the effect of stochastic, internal, and environmental stressors on the one side, and resilience strategies of maintenance and repair on the other side, with progressive unbalance toward the first mechanisms that causes progressive accumulation of unrepaired and unrepairable damage [2]. The accumulation of molecular damage with aging creates the susceptibility for the emergence of chronic diseases, which take different forms based on heterogeneous genetic background, behaviors, and environmental exposures. Finding strategies to slowing down biological aging could potentially delay the onset and progression of multiple chronic diseases and functional decline and reduce the burden of multimorbidity.

This implies also that the point of view based on "one size fits all" for the management of older adults is no more reasonable and affordable. A better understanding of the specific aspects of the biology of aging that are dysfunctional in specific individuals should warrant the identification of effective targets and refinement of personalized preventive and therapeutic approaches.

13.2　The Search of Longevity: The Biogerontology

Since the dawn of human history, people, as the alchemists, struggled to find the elixir of eternal youth. The birth of a real scientific approach in the search for longevity could be traced back only to the beginning of the last century. The seminal experiments on the effects of caloric restriction in rodents showed that animals undergoing diet with reduced total calories intake (roughly 60% lower than normal) lived up to 40% longer than controls with no restriction to food [3]. Interestingly, this kind of intervention not only extended lifespan but also in parallel delayed all the age-related diseases. This finding has been successfully replicated in several species, although the effect of dietary restriction in non-human primates as well as in humans is questionable [4, 5]. A growing impulse on this research branch has been provided by deeper knowledge of cellular structures, the characterization of coding systems of biological information with the discoveries of DNA and RNA, the development of omics sciences, and the recognition of signaling and regulatory pathways.

By understanding the mechanisms of biological aging, including frailty and resilience, clinicians will be able to best orient diagnosis and prescribe therapeutic choices [6, 7]. Biologically, aging may be defined as the transition process from young to older age, usually parallel to the lifelong accumulation, at subclinical level, of consequences of acute (e.g., infections, trauma, cardiovascular accidents) and chronic diseases and conditions (e.g., diabetes, cancers, lung disease, liver disease, osteoarthritis, and osteoporosis, Alzheimer's disease), exposure to environmental risk factors (e.g., pollution, UV radiations, toxins), and lifestyle (e.g., diet, smoking, alcohol consumption, physical activity levels). During the life several mechanisms try to counteract the effects of these stressors, leading to progressive decline of the individual homeostatic capacities [2]. When these finally become exhausted, this moment could be identified as the turning point for biological aging. Overall the progressive burden of multiple stress factors, no more efficiently balanced by defensive barriers, may predispose to occurrence and progression of functional limitations which may finally lead to morbidity and mortality.

Based on these considerations, we predict that the geriatricians of the future will need a profound expertise in biogerontology, the science that studies the biological basis of aging and its relationship to disease, to capture also mechanisms underlying frailty and resilience. Indeed, several lines of evidence suggest that aging, despite its complexity and evolutionary conservation, can be slowed down and perhaps even reversed.

13.3 The Hallmarks of Aging

In 2013, the National Institute of Health (NIH) held a landmark conference with the aim to identify a core of few fundamental aging mechanisms that can serve as potentially eligible targets of therapeutic or preventative interventions for age-associated diseases [1]. Based on accumulating evidence from preclinical models [8], it was concluded that the cellular processes that drive the biology of aging can be summarized in seven "pillars" or "hallmarks" of aging: (1) epigenetics, (2) macromolecular damage, (3) proteostasis, (4) stem cells exhaustion, (5) metabolism, (6) adaptation to stress, and (7) inflammation.

Epigenetic modifications that occur with aging include stereotypic changes in the DNA methylation and acetylation of histones, the proteins around which DNA is packaged, but also nucleosome positioning and expression of non-coding RNAs, including long non-coding RNAs, microRNAs, and circular RNAs. Many lines of evidence suggest that a substantial portion of epigenetic changes are not stochastic or due to a "drift" but rather are meaningful mechanisms of aging, although their nature has not been yet elucidated [9]. Several experiments have demonstrated that the levels of DNA methylation is a very reliable marker of biological aging and can be assessed by "epigenetic clocks" [10]. Overall, changes in epigenetic are thought to regulate gene expression and may even affect genomic instability.

Another characteristic of aging is the accumulation of macromolecular damage to DNA, proteins, and lipids [11]. For example, above a certain level of severity, somatic mutations in nuclear and mitochondrial DNA or shortening of telomere length, short caps or repeated short sequences at the ends DNA strands that prevent the DNA from unraveling, and are shortened at each cell division, may activate apoptotic signals leading to a programmed cell death or, alternatively, trigger cellular senescence. Closely linked with this mechanism is the alteration of proteostasis (i.e., biogenesis, folding, trafficking, and degradation of proteins) with an impairment of chaperon-mediated autophagy and macro autophagy, which are critical mechanisms for the removal of damaged macromolecules and organelles [12].

During aging it occurs a progressive reduction of the stem cell pool that reduces the regenerative capacities of organs and tissues [13]. Aged stem cells have reduced ability to proliferate, poor differentiative capacity, and increased propensity for apoptosis and senescence. In addition, aging appears to affect the capacity to maintain stemness.

Metabolic dysregulation, such as insulin resistance, increases with age and can, at least partly, be traced back to the presence of a dysfunction of the mitochondria, the intracellular organelles responsible for energy production through the process of oxidative phosphorylation [14]. Bioenergetic derangement, occurring during aging and often driven by mitochondrial dysfunction, might also impair the capacity to mount an effective and specific stress response [15]. Evidence from preclinical models showed that increased resistance to stress ensured an increase in survival. In particular, following the theory of hormesis while acute and severe stressor events would expose to an earlier depletion of homeostatic capacities and accumulation of molecular damages, a repeated stimulation in response to mild stressors would favor increased resistance to stress and a better resilience.

Another important hallmark of aging is inflammation or, more precisely, the pro-inflammatory state of aging ("inflammaging") that is witnessed by rising levels of pro-inflammatory markers and is not associated with overt autoimmunity or infection [16]. Inflammaging is associated with a rearrangement of the immune system called immunosenescence with a shift from an immune system mainly based on adaptive immunity (more refined and based on specific antibody responses) toward one based on the innate immunity (a more primordial system basically founded on the phagocytic abilities of the macrophages).

All these mechanisms are strictly inter-connected with each other and some authors hypothesized that they can converge on a single unifying mechanism represented by inflammation, which could be fueled by all the dysfunction of one or more of the other remaining mechanisms [17].

13.4 Metrics of Aging

Aging is characterized by some highly prevalent and fundamental phenotypic characteristics, which are preserved between different species. Examples are gray hairs, reduction of visual and auditory acuity, osteo-articular problems, loss of muscle mass and function, reduction of aerobic capacity, and memory problems. However, these are not unavoidable events occurring with advancing age. Rather this aging process is shaped by stochasticity. The global rate of aging can be imagined as a dynamic equilibrium between different entropic forces and conserved homeostatic mechanisms [2]. The latter, also known under the term of "resilience", allows humans to maintain health and function over many years, but their efficiency eventually fades and, when entropy level exceed, frailty and mortality may occur [7]. The extreme variability by which these mechanisms maintain an equilibrium explains the variance of aging phenotypes with the advancing age, despite the leveling force of mortality. In fact, subjects with the same chronological age will always present a wide heterogeneity of health and clinical manifestations, from octogenarians able to perform a marathon with almost no deficit, to those who are fully bedridden with a terminal disease.

The heterogeneity in health and functional trajectories of aging has stimulated research to develop specific metrics of aging that could be used in clinical practice to identify individuals with "accelerated aging" [18] (Fig. 13.1). The first level of interpretation is indeed the "functional" level characterized by some of the features mentioned above and therefore the visible manifestations of aging including functional deficits, loss of independence, reduced mobility, cognitive impairment, depression, sleep disorders, multimorbidity, polypharmacy, and geriatric syndromes. The second level is that of pathophysiological mechanisms leading to clinical manifestations, the so-called "phenotypical" level which encompasses changes in body composition, energetics, homeostatic mechanisms, and neuronal function. The third level is "biological" aging, which is still largely hypothetical and may include the above-mentioned hallmarks of aging (e.g., mitochondrial dysfunction, DNA damages and methylation, telomere shortening, defecting autophagy, loss of stemness, immunosenescence).

This hierarchical system of measurement of aging with increasing levels of complexity, from the lowest stage represented by biology to the highest represented by

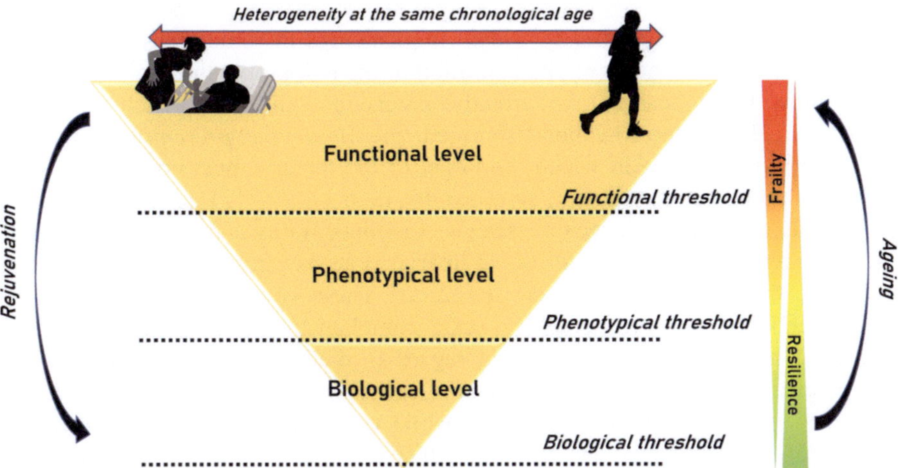

Fig. 13.1 The metrics of aging to understand discrepancies between chronological and biological age. The global rate of aging can be imagined as a dynamic equilibrium between different entropic forces (fueling frailty condition) and conserved homeostatic mechanisms (resilience). When the homeostatic mechanisms are fully saturated the damage becomes progressively evident at the biological, phenotypic, and finally to functional level. Rejuvenation therapies might be able to slow-down or revert aging process also in humans

the clinic, offers a better explanation of the observed discrepancies between chronological age and biological age (Fig. 13.1). In humans, and similarly also in other organisms, there is substantial physiological resilience that buffers damage accumulation (i.e., at biological and phenotypical levels) until the homeostatic mechanisms are fully saturated and the damage becomes progressively evident at the biological, phenotypic, and finally to functional level. In humans, this process takes several years, and the possibility of assessing it at an early stage could offer the opportunity to promote preventive interventions.

The main objectives of medical interventions for older adults should focus on: (1) maximizing the ability of an individual to function in his/her environment improving their resilience capacity and (2) maintaining autonomy and improving quality of life by reduction of frailty incidence and progression.

13.5   Biotechnologies in Aging Research

The multiomics revolution (i.e., genomics, proteomics, lipidomics, transcriptomics) through techniques such as next-generation sequencing (NGS) for genome analysis and the single molecule array (SiMoA) technology for detection of proteins and nucleic acids, provided ample, new opportunities for the discovery of biomarkers of aging and chronic diseases [19, 20]. The identification and dosage of biomarkers would not only be useful from diagnostic and prognostic points of view, but also, and above all, from a therapeutic one (Table 13.1). In fact, in this sense, a biomarker could represent a therapeutic target, and, following its trend over time, an indicator of response to therapy.

Borrowing a strategy already widely implemented in some areas of medicine (e.g., oncology, immunology), the definition of the risk profile through biomarkers could allow the application of an effective precision medicine approach also in the geriatric field. It is the so-called "4P" medicine: *predictive, preventive, personalized,* and *participatory*, in which the target of the therapy must no longer be the single pathology but the subject, even healthy, in its entirety [21].

To date, the main evidence on strategies to reduce frailty and increase resilience in human aging is based on nutritional interventions as caloric restriction or intermittent fasting, or on physical exercise [22, 23]. These strategies, although strongly recommendable, are hampered by poor compliance over prolonged periods. Changing behaviors of individuals in regard to dietary and exercise habits has proven difficult, in part because the overall cultural view is that research on aging should address only older persons. Thus, while a cultural transformation remains at the core of the geroscience revolution, it will be important to find new treatment that oppose the deleterious effect of aging. From this point of view, the advances in biotechnology are offering opportunities unimaginable until a few years ago [24]. Biotechnology pursues the integration between the natural sciences and the engineering sciences and is aimed at transforming knowledge about organisms, parts of them or molecular analogs for the developments of new solutions for diagnostics and therapeutics. Biotechnology is already behind blockbuster drugs for treating

Table 13.1 Biomarkers of the hallmarks of aging and related potential rejuvenating strategies

Hallmark	Biomarker	Rejuvenation strategy
Epigenetics	DNA methylation	Cellular reprogramming
	Histone acetylation	Metabolic manipulation
	Nucleosome positioning	Senescent cells ablation
	Non-coding RNAs	
Macromolecular damage	Single-cell/NGS, SNP analyses	Cellular reprogramming
	DNA repair	
	Measures of DNA modifications	
	Long interspersed nuclear elements (LINEs)	Metabolic manipulation
	Reverse transcriptase	
	Telomere length	
	Markers of DNA damage response	Systemic factors
	Telomerase activity	
	Telomere-associated foci	
Proteostasis	Autophagy markers and flux	Metabolic manipulation
	Chaperone proteins	
	Advanced glycation end products (AGEs)	Systemic factors
	Protein aggregates	Cellular reprogramming
Stem cell exhaustion	Replication/differentiation potential	Systemic factors
	Tissue regeneration	Senescent cells ablation
		Metabolic manipulation
		Cellular reprogramming
Metabolism	IGF-1 pathway	Metabolic manipulation
	mTOR signaling	
	Mitochondrial function	
	Mitochondrial volume, number, shape	
	Markers of biogenesis	Cellular reprogramming
	mtDNA copy number, mutations, haplotypes	
	NAD+ metabolites	
	Sirtuins	
Adaptation to stress	o-tyrosine	Systemic factors
	3-chlorotyrosine	
	3-nitrotyrosine	Senescent cells ablation
	8-iso prostaglandin F2α	
	8-hydroxy-2′-deoxyguanosine	Metabolic manipulation
	8-hydroxyguanosine	Cellular reprogramming
Inflammation	Senescence-associated secretory phenotype	Systemic factors
		Metabolic manipulation
		Senescent cells ablation
		Cellular reprogramming

several non-communicable diseases (NCDs) and the development of largely recommended vaccines for influenza, herpes zoster, pneumococcal disease, and more recently against Sars-CoV-2 infection. A very ambitious future goal of biotechnologies could be to transfer the preclinical results of rejuvenation therapies to humans.

## 13.6	Biotechnologies to Prevent Frailty and Increase Resilience

Several rejuvenation strategies have been proposed to increase resilience and slow down the aging process [25]. These fall into four broad categories: systemic factors, metabolic manipulations, senescent cell ablation, and cellular reprogramming (Table 13.1).

The role of biotechnologies in metabolic manipulation strategies involves the use of compounds acting on nutrient-sensing pathways. The inhibition of high-nutrient sensing targets as the mechanistic target of rapamycin (mTOR) and the insulin–insulin-like growth factor (IGF) signaling cascade, or the activation of low-nutrient sensing targets as the 5′ AMP-activated protein kinase (AMPK) and sirtuins could produce life extension [26]. Among the compounds acting on these pathways are worth of mention the rapamycin, an mTOR inhibitor and potent immunosuppressant, which has been proven to extend lifespan in mice through the improvement of stemness and increasing autophagy [27]; and the metformin, a drug commonly used in type 2 diabetes, which increases AMPK activity, preserving mitochondrial function and reducing inflammation [28]. Moreover, the sirtuins activators, resveratrol (a natural antioxidant compound) and nicotinamide riboside (a nicotinamide adenine dinucleotide (NAD+) precursor) have been shown to promote survival through anti-inflammatory activity [29, 30].

Another category of rejuvenating interventions is represented by circulating systemic factors [25]. Experiments on heterochronic parabiosis in which the coupling of circulations of a young and an aged mouse reversed the age-dependent decline improving staminality and genomic instability, sustain the hypothesis that some blood factor might be involved in lifespan extension [31]. Administration of compounds like oxytocin, growth differentiation factor 11 (GDF11) or tissue inhibitor of metalloproteinases-2 (TIMP2), all normally reduced in aged mice, showed promising findings to enhance the function of stem cells in different organs and tissues (e.g., heart, muscle, nervous system) [25].

Cellular senescence is an intrinsic mechanism of protection against damaged cells and thus against carcinogenesis, implying the irreversible replicative arrest, but with resistance to apoptosis [32]. Senescent cells accumulate with aging and in several chronic diseases. Markers of cellular senescence include senescence-associated β-galactosidase activity, the cell-cycle inhibitors p16INK4a and p21CIP1, and other inflammatory factors collectively referred as the senescence-associated secretory phenotype (SASP) [33]. A novel class of drugs called "senolytics", including dasatinib, quercetin, fisetin, and navitoclax, have the selective ability to clear senescent cells and demonstrated in preclinical models to mitigate or prevent frailty and several NCDs [34].

Finally, the discovery of cellular reprogramming, a way of conversion of terminally differentiated somatic cells back into induced pluripotent stem cells, has been received with great interest [35]. The cyclic administration, to avoid teratogenesis, of a complex of four transcription factors (OCT4, SOX2, KLF4, and MYC) collectively termed OSKM or "Yamanaka factors" via adenovirus vectors erased features of aging (e.g., DNA damage, dysregulation of histone marks, expression of senescence-associated genes) probably through epigenetic remodeling and in particular histone modifications [36].

13.7 Future Perspective

Further development of biotechnologies will warrant a more efficient and precise measure of the biological mechanisms of aging in humans and will be informative on trajectories of accelerated aging early in the process. Screening individuals for subclinical diseases will provide targets for future interventions that globally affect aging, improving resilience and delaying frailty. Ultimately, interventions that effectively slow, delay, or even revert the mechanisms of aging in subjects diagnosed with "accelerated aging" will need to be identified and properly tested. Current research agendas encompass studies on more than 200 *geroprotective* compounds which need to be tested and implemented in humans [37].

Nevertheless, it should be always kept in mind that the final goal of "anti-aging" strategies cannot be a mere extension of life span, but rather provide a longer healthspan and improve quality of life during the diseased phase.

References

1. Kennedy BK, et al. Geroscience: linking aging to chronic disease. Cell. 2014;159(4):709–13.
2. Ferrucci L, et al. Measuring biological aging in humans: a quest. Aging Cell. 2020;19(2):e13080.
3. McCay CM, Crowell MF, Maynard LA. The effect of retarded growth upon the length of life span and upon the ultimate body size: one figure. J Nutr. 1935;10(1):63–79.
4. Mattison JA, et al. Impact of caloric restriction on health and survival in rhesus monkeys from the NIA study. Nature. 2012;489(7415):318–21.
5. Dirks AJ, Leeuwenburgh C. Caloric restriction in humans: potential pitfalls and health concerns. Mech Ageing Dev. 2006;127(1):1–7.
6. Walston J, et al. Moving frailty toward clinical practice: NIA intramural frailty science symposium summary. J Am Geriatr Soc. 2019;67(8):1559–64.
7. Hadley EC, et al. Report: NIA workshop on measures of physiologic resiliencies in human aging. J Gerontol A Biol Sci Med Sci. 2017;72(7):980–90.
8. Lopez-Otin C, et al. The hallmarks of aging. Cell. 2013;153(6):1194–217.
9. Levine ME, et al. An epigenetic biomarker of aging for lifespan and healthspan. Aging (Albany NY). 2018;10(4):573–91.
10. Horvath S, Raj K. DNA methylation-based biomarkers and the epigenetic clock theory of ageing. Nat Rev Genet. 2018;19(6):371–84.

11. Richardson AG, Schadt EE. The role of macromolecular damage in aging and age-related disease. J Gerontol A Biol Sci Med Sci. 2014;69(Suppl 1):S28–32.
12. Morimoto RI, Cuervo AM. Proteostasis and the aging proteome in health and disease. J Gerontol A Biol Sci Med Sci. 2014;69(Suppl 1):S33–8.
13. Wang MJ, et al. Rejuvenating strategies of tissue-specific stem cells for healthy aging. Aging Dis. 2019;10(4):871–82.
14. Gonzalez-Freire M, et al. Reconsidering the role of mitochondria in aging. J Gerontol A Biol Sci Med Sci. 2015;70(11):1334–42.
15. Epel ES, Lithgow GJ. Stress biology and aging mechanisms: toward understanding the deep connection between adaptation to stress and longevity. J Gerontol A Biol Sci Med Sci. 2014;69(Suppl 1):S10–6.
16. Franceschi C, et al. Inflamm-aging. An evolutionary perspective on immunosenescence. Ann N Y Acad Sci. 2000;908:244–54.
17. Franceschi C, et al. Inflammaging: a new immune-metabolic viewpoint for age-related diseases. Nat Rev Endocrinol. 2018;14(10):576–90.
18. Ferrucci L, et al. Time and the metrics of aging. Circ Res. 2018;123(7):740–4.
19. LeBrasseur NK, et al. Identifying biomarkers for biological age: Geroscience and the ICFSR task force. J Frailty Aging. 2021;10(3):196–201.
20. Xia X, et al. Molecular and phenotypic biomarkers of aging. F1000Res. 2017;6:860.
21. Flores M, et al. P4 medicine: how systems medicine will transform the healthcare sector and society. Per Med. 2013;10(6):565–76.
22. Lee C, Longo V. Dietary restriction with and without caloric restriction for healthy aging. F1000Research. 2016;5:F1000. Faculty Rev-117
23. Goh J, et al. Targeting the molecular & cellular pillars of human aging with exercise. FEBS J. 2021;
24. Ho D, et al. Enabling technologies for personalized and precision medicine. Trends Biotechnol. 2020;38(5):497–518.
25. Mahmoudi S, Xu L, Brunet A. Turning back time with emerging rejuvenation strategies. Nat Cell Biol. 2019;21(1):32–43.
26. Longo VD, et al. Interventions to slow aging in humans: are we ready? Aging Cell. 2015;14(4):497–510.
27. Harrison DE, et al. Rapamycin fed late in life extends lifespan in genetically heterogeneous mice. Nature. 2009;460(7253):392–5.
28. Martin-Montalvo A, et al. Metformin improves healthspan and lifespan in mice. Nat Commun. 2013;4:2192.
29. Hubbard BP, Sinclair DA. Small molecule SIRT1 activators for the treatment of aging and age-related diseases. Trends Pharmacol Sci. 2014;35(3):146–54.
30. Custodero C, et al. Nicotinamide riboside-a missing piece in the puzzle of exercise therapy for older adults? Exp Gerontol. 2020;137:110972.
31. Conboy IM, et al. Rejuvenation of aged progenitor cells by exposure to a young systemic environment. Nature. 2005;433(7027):760–4.
32. Campisi J. Aging, cellular senescence, and cancer. Annu Rev Physiol. 2013;75:685–705.
33. Coppe JP, et al. The senescence-associated secretory phenotype: the dark side of tumor suppression. Annu Rev Pathol. 2010;5:99–118.
34. Kirkland JL, Tchkonia T. Senolytic drugs: from discovery to translation. J Intern Med. 2020;288(5):518–36.
35. Denoth-Lippuner A, Jessberger S. Mechanisms of cellular rejuvenation. FEBS Lett. 2019;593(23):3381–92.
36. Mendelsohn AR, Larrick JW. Epigenetic age reversal by cell-extrinsic and cell-intrinsic means. Rejuvenation Res. 2019;22(5):439–46.
37. Trendelenburg AU, et al. Geroprotectors: a role in the treatment of frailty. Mech Ageing Dev. 2019;180:11–20.

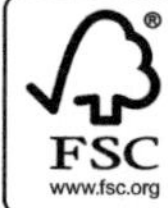

MIX
Papier aus verantwortungsvollen Quellen
Paper from responsible sources
FSC® C105338

If you have any concerns about our products,
you can contact us on
ProductSafety@springernature.com

In case Publisher is established outside the EU,
the EU authorized representative is:
Springer Nature Customer Service Center GmbH
Europaplatz 3, 69115 Heidelberg, Germany

Printed by Libri Plureos GmbH
in Hamburg, Germany